PEOPLE IN CRISIS

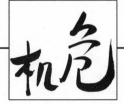

PEOPLE IN CRISIS

Understanding and Helping

FOURTH EDITION

Lee Ann Hoff

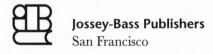

Jossey-Bass Publishers
San Francisco

Substantial discounts on bulk quantities of Jossey-Bass books are available to corporations, professional associations, and other organizations. For details and discount information, contact the special sales department at Jossey-Bass Inc., Publishers. (415) 433–1740; Fax (800) 605–2665.

For sales outside the United States, please contact your local Paramount Publishing International Office.

Library of Congress Cataloging-in-Publication Data

Hoff, Lee Ann.
    People in crisis: understanding and helping / Lee Ann Hoff. —
1st ed.
        p. cm. — (The Jossey-Bass social and behavioral science
series)
    Includes bibliographical references and index.
    ISBN 0–7879–0084–2 (acid-free paper)
    1. Crisis intervention (Psychiatry)   I. Title.   II. Series.
RC480.6.H64 1995
616.89′025—dc20   94-46309
                                                                              CIP

FOURTH EDITION
PB Printing   10 9 8 7 6 5 4 3 2 1

CONTENTS

4.   HELPING PEOPLE IN CRISIS   105

5.   FAMILY AND SOCIAL NETWORK STRATEGIES DURING CRISIS   133

LIST OF TABLES, FIGURES, AND EXHIBITS

Tables

Figures

Exhibits

PREFACE

This book is about people in crisis and those who help them. As social beings, most of us need help to weather the storm of events such as sickness, divorce, violent attack, or the death of a loved one. This book offers those who provide that help—health and social service professionals and others—a comprehensive yet concise view of how people feel, think, and act when navigating the emotional storm of a crisis. Understanding the crisis experience lays the foundation for learning the strategies and resources we can use to help distressed people. While mental health and other professionals have traditionally helped upset and highly anxious people, this book situates emotional crisis within the *normal* range of human experience. At the same time, it shows how crisis intersects with serious health and mental health problems when necessary help is not available to people threatening suicide, violence, or otherwise making desperate responses to crisis.

Personal crises do not occur in a social or cultural vacuum. *People in Crisis: Understanding and Helping* is unique among contemporary texts in the extent to which it recognizes this fact. The inclusion of cultural and social content; the clearly drawn relationship between crisis theory and practice; the emphasis on human development; the blending of individual, family, and group approaches to intervention; and the humanistic thrust of the book all reflect a view of crisis in sociocultural context and with sensitivity to the unique experience of each person.

Audience

The comprehensiveness and interdisciplinary facets of this book also reflect the fact that *helping people in crisis is everybody's business* and not just the specialty of any one helping profession. All of us can grow in the knowledge and art of helping ourselves and others in crisis. *People in Crisis* was written to help readers in that learning process, in particular:

- Frontline crisis workers: nurses, social workers, physicians, police, clergy, teachers, and rescue workers
- Therapists and specialized crisis workers, both volunteers and others
- Health and mental health educators who train physicians, nurses, social workers, psychologists, and counselors
- Human service administrators and program coordinators who must plan, develop, and supervise crisis services
- Social science teachers and researchers interested in the application of sociocultural theory in health and other human service practice
- The general reader who seeks a better understanding of personal crises

New in Fourth Edition

Since the earlier editions of *People in Crisis*, published in 1978, 1984, and 1989, new world developments have underscored two facts featured in this book: (1) crisis intervention is an integral aspect of human service delivery systems, and (2) crisis work should be sensitive to the relationship between personal, family, and sociocultural issues. Some of these issues include: national and international initiatives to stem the tide of violence in public and domestic arenas; continuing escalation of health care costs; the lack of health insurance for millions and the increasing emphasis on primary health care; the growing epidemics of alienation, suicide, and violence among youth; the persistence of homelessness for millions who are poor, lack community-based health care, or are refugees of political persecution and civil wars; environmental, farm, and fisheries crises; continuing controversy over reproductive technologies; the widening gap between rich and poor; health and safety hazards in the natural and work environment; the continuing AIDS pandemic and apparent failure of individualistic preventive approaches.

To meet the challenges posed by these developments, this fourth edition presents updated information along with an expanded theory and research foundation for the book, as reflected in current references. The research-based Crisis Paradigm featured in the second and third editions continues as this book's conceptual framework, with further clarification of the relationship between violence, victimization, and suicide. Reflecting current concerns about violence and the integration of crisis concepts in general health practice, two new Chapters (Nine and Eleven) were developed for this edition from the former Chapters Eight and Ten, respectively. Content has been revised or expanded in the following areas:

- Primary care and the interrelationship between violence, victim-blaming, depression, and negative sequelae of victimization (Chapters One and Two)
- Cohousing and its implications for social support and crisis prevention (Chapter Five)
- Ethics of assisted suicide; self-mutilation as distinguished from suicidal behavior; issues regarding "no suicide contracts" (Chapters Six and Seven)
- Suggested screening questions for assessment in life-threatening situations: victimization; suicide risk; assault or homicide risk (Chapters Eight and Nine)
- Illustration of a service contract and crisis counseling with a battered woman; lesbian battering (Chapter Eight)
- Youth violence and its intersection with abuse and alienation; dynamics of and treatment programs for violent men; primary prevention and social change strategies concerning violence and antisocial behavior (Chapter Nine)
- Environmental crises and the special vulnerability of disadvantaged groups during disaster (Chapter Ten)
- Crisis vulnerability of people with disabilities and without health insurance (Chapter Eleven)
- Sexual identity crisis and application of the Crisis Paradigm to gay, lesbian, and bisexual youth at particular risk of suicide (Chapter Thirteen)
- Presentation of a possible paradigm shift toward primary prevention in response to the global AIDS crisis (Chapter Fourteen)

As in previous editions, the examples were drawn from all major racial, ethnic, and socioeconomic groups in the United States and Canada so that the variety of people seeking help in crisis would be accurately conveyed. In writing case examples, I have also used my experience and study in urban and rural settings both in the United States and abroad, including volunteer work with battered women and people with AIDS. The cases are real but have been disguised to protect the identity of the people concerned.

While drawing on insights from several health and social sciences—among them nursing, psychology, social work, medicine, anthropology, and sociology—I have tried to avoid technical jargon. The book should thus be understandable to students, professional people, and lay readers alike, with additional references provided for those who wish to continue their study of a particular topic.

Organization

The book consists of three parts: Part One presents the basic concepts and strategies necessary to understand, identify, and help people in crisis. It lays the foundation for considering major crisis experiences in greater depth in the book's later chapters. Part Two deals with violence, both as an *origin* of crisis (e.g., victimization) and as a *response* to crisis (e.g., suicide or violence). Rather than the usual public/private categorization of violence, Chapters Eight and Nine focus respectively on the victim-as-survivor and the assailant regarding prevention, crisis intervention, and follow-up care. The growing and fearsome presence of violence, not only in U.S. society but throughout the world, necessitated the expanded treatment of topics such as routine assessment for victimization and assault/homicide danger, disasters originating from technological and human factors, and economic disparities between nations. Part Three discusses those crisis states traditionally defined as situational and transitional, with an emphasis on the theme of passage, cultural context, and the need for "contemporary rites of passage" to assist individuals through these normal life events. The concluding chapter on AIDS illustrates the danger and opportunity presented by this unprecedented pandemic and its typification of interrelated situational, transitional, and sociocultural facets of life crises. It also presents evidence of a possible paradigm shift in addressing the global AIDS crisis and its linkage to other critical issues faced by vulnerable groups.

Final Word

Crisis is intrinsic to life, but crisis intervention is not a panacea for all of life's problems. The Chinese symbol for *crisis* appears throughout this book. The symbol depicts crisis as a two-part character—danger and opportunity. We can determine for ourselves whether we come through a crisis enriched and stronger or stagnating and hopeless; whether we gain new awareness and coping ability or lose our emotional and physical health and the opportunity to die a peaceful death. It is my hope that this book will make a difference for all those who read it.

March 1995   Lee Ann Hoff
Boston, Massachusetts

ACKNOWLEDGMENTS

For more than twenty-five years I have worked with people in crisis, studied the dynamics and outcomes of this pivotal life experience, and shared what I have learned with numerous students, colleagues, and others. This book is the result of that special opportunity to grow and learn from the pain and joy of people who live through life's crises. As this fourth edition goes to press, I remember with gratitude all those who read and provided feedback to earlier editions of *People in Crisis*. These readers include thousands of students, colleagues, workshop participants, and others. You have affirmed the need to produce this edition and to keep people current with a comprehensive book on life crises.

Very special thanks go to the formal reviewers of this edition's first draft: Kazimiera Adamowski and Janet Douglas. Your careful reading, affirmation, and detailed recommendations for revision were particularly helpful.

Valerie McLennan's steadfast assistance with the literature review was fundamental to the book's current relevance based on research and clinical practice. And the new content on sexual identity crisis was developed with the special help of Trudy Cox. Without the technical assistance of Leonard and Suzanne Thomas Buckle and Mark Gottlieb through various computer crises, this book could never have gone to press. I thank you all.

At Jossey-Bass, I especially thank Becky McGovern for her hours of time and most constructive editorial suggestions in developing and launching this fourth edition. Mary White's patience and persistence assured the timely interface between author, reviewers, and production manager. I also thank Mary O'Briant for her precise and sensitive copyediting of the manuscript; Frank Welsch for his direction and supervision of the production process; Margaret Sebold for managing the marketing program; and Sarah Miller and Karen Warner for assistance with production and marketing. Your friendly support, encouragement, and patience were a major boon in completing the work. Last but not least, I thank my family and friends, who continued to understand and support me when manuscript preparation demanded time I would like to have spent with them.

THE AUTHOR

Lee Ann Hoff was born and raised in North Dakota, where she worked as a clinical specialist, teacher, and supervisor in psychiatric/mental health nursing. She started one of the first twenty-four–hour crisis services and pioneered in the community mental health movement of the 1960s. In 1969, she extended this work through a suicidology fellowship at Johns Hopkins University. During her years as a clinician, consultant, and administrator, her special achievements included development of the first crisis outreach program and initiation of a program for the national certification of crisis programs. She also spearheaded the program for national certification of individual crisis workers. In recognition of her work, she received the first Service Award from the American Association of Suicidology. Acting on her long-standing cross-cultural interests, in 1978 she obtained a master's degree in social anthropology from the London School of Economics, and in 1984, a Ph.D. degree from Boston University, specializing in women's health issues and a sociocultural analysis of violence.

Drawing on the holistic traditions of nursing and social anthropology, Hoff now focuses on building bridges, for example, between theory and practice regarding people at risk; academics and activists; feminist and mainstream analysis; cross-cultural distinctions and commonalities; and individual and social interventions.

Her teaching experience spans undergraduate, graduate, and continuing education programs in nursing, mental health disciplines, police departments, women's studies, and social sciences in U.S. and Canadian universities. She is also a frequent presenter at national and international conferences in women's health, nursing, anthropology, public health, psychiatry, suicidology, and victimology.

Hoff is founding director of the Life Crisis Institute, an international not-for-profit organization based in Boston and Ottawa and is Adjunct Professor at the University of Ottawa, Faculty of Health Sciences. Her current research is on the interface between violence, victimization, and suicide. Some of her other major publications include *Battered Women as Survivors* (1990); *Violence Issues: An Interdisciplinary Curriculum Guide for Health Professionals* (1995); and *Programs for People in Crisis* (with Nina Miller, 1987).

Balancing her antiviolence and bridge-building efforts, she swims, hikes, enjoys the wonders of New England, Ontario, Quebec, and the Maritimes, and maintains her avid belief in human resilience and generosity through crisis and beyond.

PEOPLE IN CRISIS

To the memory of my mother, Elizabeth, and my father, Lee, who first taught me about crisis, hope, and resilience

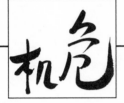

PART ONE

THE UNDERSTANDING AND PRACTICE OF CRISIS INTERVENTION

The concepts and strategies that form the nucleus of crisis theory and practice are fundamental to understanding and helping people in crisis. Chapter One sets the concepts in historical context, linking contemporary crisis intervention to the theories and practices that preceded it. A psychosociocultural perspective is highlighted in a Crisis Paradigm that is introduced in Chapter One, is discussed in detail in Chapter Two, and provides the theoretical framework for the entire book. In Chapter Three, the concepts are applied to the process of assessing individuals and families for crisis risk. Chapter Four focuses on planning and implementing helping strategies, while Chapter Five extends the helping process to family, group, and community crisis situations. The concepts and strategies discussed in Part One constitute the foundation for all remaining chapters.

CHAPTER ONE

CRISIS THEORY AND PRACTICE: INTRODUCTION AND OVERVIEW

Deborah, age fifty, is married and the mother of two teenage children. One day at work, she has a heart attack and is taken to the hospital by ambulance. This is clearly a medical emergency and a source of stress for Deborah and her family. However, a life-threatening event like this may also precipitate an emotional crisis for everyone involved. Chronic stress following Deborah's physical illness can lead to an emotionally troubled family or to the mental breakdown of individual family members, depending on the various psychological, social, and cultural factors involved in the crisis. Whether this crisis experience results in growth and enrichment for Deborah and her loved ones or in a lower level of functioning for one or all of them depends largely on their problem-solving abilities, cultural values regarding illness and health, and current levels of social and economic support (Brown, 1993; Robinson, 1971).

Deborah, it turns out, is a health care executive who has just received a promotion. She comes from a working-class family. One of her major life ambitions is to achieve professional success while also maintaining a stable family life. Deborah's husband and children are devoted to her, but she feels constant pressure to set an example of strength and to perform to an exacting standard. Being a responsible wife and mother and a successful professional are all-important to Deborah. These facts of Deborah's life and the lives of people like her suggest that the crisis experience is subjective. This subjectivity contributes to the difficulty of scientific research and theory-building about crisis (Antonovsky, 1987; Hoff, 1990; Smith, 1978; Taplin, 1971).

What Is Crisis and Crisis Intervention?

There are meaningful differences and relationships among the following key terms: *stress, predicament, emergency, crisis,* and *emotional or mental breakdown.* Stress is not crisis; stress is tension, strain, or pressure. Predicament is not crisis either; predicament is a condition or situation that is unpleasant, dangerous, or embarrassing. Emergency is not crisis; emergency is an unforeseen combination of circumstances calling for immediate action, often with life or death implications. Finally, crisis is not emotional or mental illness. Crisis may be defined as a serious occasion or turning point presenting both danger and opportunity.

If Deborah or members of her family become extremely upset as a result of her heart attack and feel emotionally unable to handle the event, they are said to be in crisis. In this book, *crisis,* in clinical context, refers to *an acute emotional upset arising from situational, developmental, or sociocultural sources and resulting in a temporary inability to cope by means of one's usual problem-solving devices.* A crisis does not last long and is self-limiting. *Crisis management* refers to the entire process of working through a crisis to its resolution, a process that usually includes activities not only of the individual in crisis but also of various members of the person's natural and/or institutional network. Whether the resolution of a crisis is positive or negative often depends on *crisis intervention,* that aspect of crisis management carried out by a crisis worker—nurse, social worker, police officer, physician, counselor, or minister. Crisis intervention is a short-term helping process. It focuses on resolution of the immediate problem through the use of personal, social, and environmental resources. Crisis intervention is related to but differs from psychotherapy. *Emergency psychiatry* is a branch of medicine that deals with acute behavioral disturbances related to severe mental or emotional instability. It may overlap with crisis intervention, but it also implies the need for distinct medical intervention such as medication or admission to an inpatient psychiatric service. The paradigm for this helping process during crisis and the theory supporting it constitute the *crisis model.*

Predicaments, conflicts, and emergencies such as Deborah's lead to stress that can sometimes evolve into a crisis state. But stress is a common denominator in everyone's passage from infancy through childhood to adolescence, adulthood, and old age, and its effects vary. For example, your son finds himself in turmoil during adolescence; your son's friend does not. You face midlife as a normal part of human development; your friend becomes depressed; a neighbor becomes suicidal. Part of the beauty of life, though, is the rebirth of peace following turmoil and pain; few escape the lows—and the subsequent highs—of living through stressful events, such as the death of a loved one, a serious illness, or victimization by violence.

Although stressful events, emotional upsets, and emergency situations are part of life—and they are potential crises—a crisis does not necessarily follow a traumatic event. Nor does crisis imply, or inevitably lead to, emotional or mental breakdown. Something that is a crisis for me may not be a crisis for you. As long as we are able to handle stressful life events, we will not experience a crisis. But if stress overwhelms us, and we are unable to find a way out of our predicament, a crisis may result. Crises must be resolved constructively, or emotional or mental illness, addictions, suicide, or violence against others can be the unfortunate outcome. And once emotional breakdown occurs, a person is more vulnerable to other stressful life events, thus beginning an interacting cycle between stress, crisis, and destructive crisis outcomes. Crisis does not occur in isolation but is usually experienced in dynamic interplay with stress and illness in particular cultural contexts.

Note that the events of our lives do not themselves activate crisis. Crisis occurs when our interpretation of these events, our coping ability, and the limitations of our social resources lead to stress so severe that we cannot find relief. Accordingly, understanding people in crisis and knowing how to help them involves attention not only to the emotional tension experienced but also to the social, cultural, and material factors that influence how people respond to stressful life events.

Key words of this book will be explicated in the remainder of this chapter and throughout the following chapters. The principles and strategies necessary to understand and effectively assist people in crisis form the core of this text. They can be summarized in the following aspects of crisis theory and practice:

1. The nature of the person in crisis (Chapter One)
2. The crisis experience (Chapter Two)
3. The environment and context of crisis management and resolution (Chapters One and Two)
4. The formal process of crisis assessment, intervention, and management (all remaining chapters)

Views and Myths About People in Crisis and How to Help Them

People have been experiencing stress, predicaments, and life crises from the beginning of time. They have also found a variety of ways to resolve predicaments and live through crises. People have always helped others cope with life events as well. Hansell (1976, pp. 15–19) cites the biblical Noah anticipating the great flood as an example of how our ancestors handled crises. Noah was warned of the serious predicament he and his family would be facing shortly; they prepared for the event and, through various clever maneuvers, avoided being overwhelmed by the flood waters.

Insights developed through the psychological and social sciences have helped people understand themselves and others in crisis. The advent of a more enlightened view of people in crisis has helped put to rest some old myths about people who are upset. It is not so easy anymore to write off as "crazy" and to institutionalize people who seem to be behaving strangely in the face of an upsetting event. Modern crisis theory has helped establish a new approach to people with problems.

Crisis theory, with its emphasis on the growth potential of the crisis experience, raises questions about several notions:

1. *Myth:* People in crisis are suffering from a form of mental illness. *Fact:* People who are acutely upset or in crisis may have had a chronic emotional or mental disturbance before the crisis. Or, a negative resolution of a crisis may have resulted in emotional or mental breakdown. Both of these statements are different from asserting that a crisis state is essentially the same as emotional or mental disturbance; this distinction is crucial. Although not everyone claims that people in crisis are ill, the common reference to crisis *therapy* implies such a belief (see Myth Five and "Interrelationships Between Crisis Origins and Development" in Chapter Two).

2. *Myth:* People in crisis cannot help themselves. *Fact:* Not only is this proposition untrue but action on such a belief can be very damaging to prospects for positive crisis resolution. This fact is based on recognition of our basic human need for self-mastery. It also speaks to the resentment (usually repressed, with depression often resulting) most of us feel when we are denied the opportunity for self-determination, even when we are in crisis. Conscious resistance to this myth is important in counteracting some human service workers' tendency to rescue or "save" distressed people. Such tactics often result in workers' own burnout. The persistence of this myth compromises the possibilities for a healthy crisis outcome, whereas active fostering of doing for oneself contributes to the sense of control needed for positive crisis resolution. This is true especially when a fear of losing control is a major part of the crisis experience.

3. *Myth:* Only psychiatrists or highly trained therapists can effectively help people in crisis. *Fact:* A great deal of crisis work has been done by lay volunteers, police officers, ministers, and other frontline workers. In some communities today, crisis intervention by these groups often occurs in the absence of psychiatric and mental health professionals. To date, many mental health professionals—in contrast to lay and professional staff of certified crisis centers—still do not receive the minimum forty hours of training in crisis theory and practice recommended by the American Association of Suicidology, a national standard-setting body for crisis services. This fact is related to the next myth.

4. *Myth:* Crisis intervention is a mere Band-Aid, a necessary preliminary action, but trivial in comparison to the real treatment carried out by professional

psychotherapists. *Fact:* This myth is fading fast as growing numbers of health and mental health professionals recognize the effectiveness and economy of the crisis approach to helping distressed people. It is also giving way to acceptance of crisis intervention as the third of three revolutionary phases that have occurred since the turn of the century in the mental and public health fields: (1) Freud's discovery of the unconscious; (2) the discovery of psychotropic drugs in the 1950s; and (3) crisis intervention in the 1960s and later. The Band-Aid myth is curiously related to the next misconception in the helping arena.

   5. *Myth:* Crisis intervention is a form of psychotherapy. *Fact:* Crisis intervention is not merely a Band-Aid, but neither is it psychotherapy. This myth follows from the myth of "crisis as illness" (Myth One). The fact that techniques such as listening intently and giving feedback are used by psychotherapists and crisis workers alike does not equate psychotherapy and crisis intervention any more than either can be equated with friendship or consultation, which also employ listening. The *Shorter Oxford English Dictionary* defines psychotherapy as "the treatment of disorders of emotion or personality by psychic or hypnotic influence." Psychotherapy is a helping process directed toward changing a person's feelings and patterns of thought and behavior. It involves uncovering unconscious conflict and relieving symptoms that cause distress to the person seeking treatment. In contrast, crisis intervention avoids probing into deep-seated psychological problems.

   Ironically, as long as traditionally trained mental health professionals did not generally do crisis intervention, it was popularly referred to as a Band-Aid approach. But now that crisis intervention is more commonly incorporated into human services as an essential element, it is often defined as a form of psychotherapy. This definition of crisis work and its relationship to "medicalization,"—the tendency to interpret life's problems in a medical framework—(Freidson, 1970; Illich, 1976; McNamee & Gergen, 1992) have important implications for crisis theory development and practice. For example, the fact that people in crisis need support from others for positive crisis resolution can be explained in terms of the social nature of human beings rather than in terms of illness. Thus, the person who helps someone in crisis need not be a psychotherapist, and the helping process need not be defined as crisis therapy. Even when therapy is defined more broadly to include the social, cultural, and environmental facets of life, the word itself implies illness, which in turn has historically implied individual rather than sociocultural considerations. Since those who define crisis intervention as psychotherapy (e.g., Ewing, 1978) stress the importance of approaches that psychotherapists generally avoid (such as active engagement with the client in solving identified problems), one might ask: Why call it psychotherapy?

   The ramifications of these myths and the differences and interrelationships between crisis and illness are explored in greater depth in later sections of this book, as are the foundation of these myths in social and cultural theory and in research.

Views about people in crisis and how to help them vary according to one's value system and the philosophical assumptions guiding practice. But whatever these values and assumptions are, they must be made explicit. People who are involved in crisis intervention—parents, spouses, social workers, nurses, physicians, counselors, teachers—can be most helpful if they recognize that everyone has vast potential for growth and that crisis is a point of *opportunity* as well as *danger.* For most of us, our healthiest human growth and greatest achievements can often be traced to the trust and hopeful expectations of significant others. Successful crisis intervention involves helping people take advantage of the opportunity and avoid the danger inherent in crisis. Our success in this task may depend on our values and beliefs about the nature of the person experiencing crisis. In this book, the following values are assumed:

- People in crisis are basically normal from the standpoint of diagnosable illness, even though they are in a state of high tension and anxiety. However, the precrisis state for some persons in crisis may be one of emotional or mental disturbance. In these instances, the person can be viewed as ill while simultaneously experiencing a crisis.
- People in crisis are social by nature and live in specific cultural communities by necessity. Therefore, their psychological responses to hazardous events cannot be properly understood apart from a sociocultural context.
- People in crisis generally want to, and are capable of, helping themselves, although this capacity may be impaired to varying degrees. Their capacity for growth from the crisis experience is usually enhanced with timely help from friends, family, neighbors, and, sometimes, trained crisis workers. Conversely, failure to receive such help when needed can result in diminished growth and disastrous crisis resolution in the form of addictions, suicide, or assault on others. The strength of a person's desire for self-determination and growth, along with available help from others, will usually influence the outcome of crisis in a favorable direction.

Growing numbers of counselors, family members, and others regard the stress and crises of life as normal, as opportunities to advance from one level of maturity to another. Such was the case for the self-actualized individuals studied by Maslow (1970). His study, unique in its time for its focus on normal rather than disturbed people, revealed that people are capable of virtually limitless growth and development. Growth rather than stagnation and emotional breakdown occurred for these people in the midst of the pain and turmoil of events such as divorce and physical illness. This optimistic view of people and their problems is becoming a viable alternative to the popular view of life and human suffering in an illness paradigm. Interpreting crisis as illness implies treatment or tranquilization, whereas viewing it as opportunity invites a human, growth-promoting response to people in crisis.

The Evolution of Crisis Theory and Intervention Contexts

In the broadest sense, crisis and crisis intervention are as old as humankind. Helping other people in crisis is intrinsic to the nurturing side of human character. The capacity for creating a culture of caring and concern for others in distress is implicit in the social nature of humans. In a sense, then, crisis intervention is human action embedded in culture and in the process of learning how to live successfully through stressful life events among one's fellow human beings.

When considered in the context of professional human services, however, crisis intervention is very new—only a few decades old. As an organized body of knowledge and practice, crisis intervention is based on humanistic foundations. However, knowledge and experience from the social and health sciences can often enhance our ability to help others.

Crisis intervention has interdisciplinary roots that are revealed by the growing attention it is receiving from many health and human service practitioners. In discussing the multifaceted foundation of contemporary crisis theory and practice, the focus will be on the distinctive contributions of each area or pioneer in the field, along with critiques of current issues and differences.

Freud and Psychoanalytic Theory

Decades ago, Freud made pioneering contributions to the study of human behavior and the treatment of emotional conflict. He laid the foundation for a view of people as complex beings capable of self-discovery and change. Through extensive case studies, he demonstrated the profound effect that early life experiences can have on later development and happiness. He also found that people can resolve conflicts stemming from traumatic events of childhood and thereby live fuller, happier lives. His conclusions, however, are based largely on the study of disturbed rather than normal individuals. Psychoanalysis, the treatment method he developed from his theory, is costly, lengthy, available to few, and generally not applicable to the person in crisis.

Another limitation of Freudian theory is its foundation in biology, resulting in a mechanistic model of personality. Freud's model states that the three-part system of personality—id, ego, and superego—must be kept in balance (equilibrium) to avoid unhealthy defense mechanisms and psychopathology. There are widespread objections to the determinism found in classical psychoanalytic theory (Greenspan, 1983; Rieker & Carmen, 1984; Walsh, 1987). Determinism is based on the idea that our personalities and later life problems are determined by early childhood experiences. However, the concept of equilibrium is commonplace in the literature on crisis (e.g., Aguilera, 1989; Janosik, 1984). Besides appearing in the works of Freud, the concept of equilibrium can also be traced to the use of the scientific method in the helping professions and the search for laws (as in the natural sciences) to explain human behavior.

In spite of the limitations of Freudian theory, certain psychoanalytic techniques such as listening and evoking catharsis (the expression of feelings about a traumatic event) are useful in human helping processes, including crisis intervention and brief psychotherapy (Cade & O'Hanlon, 1993; Friedman & Fanger, 1991).

Ego Psychology

Awareness of the static nature of Freudian theory led to the development of new, less deterministic views of human beings. In the last fifty years, ego psychologists such as Fromm (1941), Maslow (1970), and Erikson (1963) did much to lay the philosophical base for crisis theory. They stressed the person's ability to learn and grow all through life—a developmental concept used throughout this book. Their views about people and human problems are based on the study of normal rather than disturbed individuals. Recently, however, Erikson has come under critical scrutiny because his theory supports patriarchal family structures (Buss, 1979, pp. 326–329; Panchuck, 1994). These traditional family structures produce more stress for women, partly because they require women to bear disproportionately the burden of a caretaking role throughout their lives (Kessler & McLeod, 1984; Turner & Avison, 1987).

Military Psychiatry

During World War II and the Korean War, members of the military who felt distressed were treated at the front lines whenever possible rather than being sent back home to psychiatric hospitals. Studies reveal that the majority of these men were able to return to combat duty rapidly as a result of receiving immediate help, that is, crisis intervention, either individually or in a group (Glass, 1957; Hansell, 1976).

This approach to psychiatric practice in the military assumed that active combat was the normal place for a soldier and that the soldier would return to duty in spite of temporary problems. Thus, while military psychiatrists used crisis intervention primarily to expedite institutional goals, they made a useful discovery for the crisis field as a whole.

Preventive Psychiatry

In 1942, a terrible fire raged through the Cocoanut Grove Melody Lounge in Boston, killing 492 people. Lindemann's (1944) classical study of bereavement following this disaster defined the grieving process people went through after the sudden death of a relative. Lindemann found that survivors of this disaster who developed serious psychopathologies had failed to go through the normal process of grieving. His findings can be applied when working with anyone suffering a serious, sudden loss. Since loss is a common theme in the crisis experience, Lindemann's work constitutes one of the most important foundations of contemporary crisis theory. Unfortunately, several decades later, even as some recount the tragedy (Thomas, 1992), many others still lack the assistance and social approval necessary for grief work following loss and instead are offered medication (see Chapter Four, "Tranquilizers: What Place in Crisis Intervention?" and "Loss, Change, and Grief Work"). Grief work consists of the process of mourning one's loss, experiencing the pain of such loss, and eventually accepting the loss and adjusting to life without the loved person or object. Encouraging people to allow themselves to go through the normal process of grieving can prevent negative outcomes of crises due to loss.

Tyhurst (1957), another pioneer in preventive psychiatry, has helped us understand a person's response to community crises such as natural disasters. During the 1940s and 1950s, Tyhurst studied transition states such as migration, parenthood, and retirement. His work examined many crisis states that occur as a result of social mobility or cultural change.

Among all the pioneers in the preventive psychiatry field, perhaps none is more outstanding or more frequently quoted than Gerald Caplan. In 1964, he developed a conceptual framework for understanding crisis, including the process of crisis development, discussed in detail in Chapter Two. Caplan also emphasized a community-wide approach to crisis intervention. Public education programs and consultation with various caretakers such as teachers, police officers, and public health nurses were cited as important ways to prevent destructive outcomes of crises. Caplan's (1964, 1974, 1981) focus on crisis prevention, mastery, and the importance of social, cultural, and material "supplies" necessary to avoid crisis seems highly suitable to explaining the development and resolution of crises. All community mental health professionals should be familiar with his classic work, *Principles of Preventive Psychiatry* (1964).

Caplan's contribution to the development of crisis theory and practice is so basic that virtually all writers in the field rely on or adapt his major concepts (see Aguilera, 1989; Golan, 1978; Hansell, 1976; Janosik, 1984; Smith, 1978). However, because of the centrality of Caplan's work in the entire crisis field and the controversy surrounding his work and the medical model (e.g., Danish, Smyer, & Nowak, 1980; Hoff, 1990; Taplin, 1971), a brief examination of his work is in order.

Caplan's conceptual framework can be questioned for its reliance on disease rather than health concepts. This limitation is offset, however, by his emphasis on prevention rather than treatment of disease. In developing crisis theory from the foundations laid by Caplan, the useful concepts of his theory should not be re-

jected along with those that are controversial. Let us consider what should probably be preserved and what should be questioned. This critique lays the foundation for the next chapter, which relies heavily on Caplan in explaining the phases
of crisis development and will be supported by analysis and case examples
throughout the text.

Caplan grounds his work in the mechanistic concepts set forth by Freud and
in one of the most popular theories in the social and health sciences: general
systems theory.[1] The concepts of *homeostasis* and *equilibrium* are central to general
systems theory. They are more suited to explaining physical disease processes than
emotional crisis, yet they are pivotal in much of crisis theory. Systems authority
Ludwig von Bertalanffy (1968), a biologist, cites several limitations to the systems concept of homeostasis as applied in psychology and psychiatry. For example, homeostasis does not apply to processes of growth, development, creation,
and the like (p. 210). Bertalanffy also describes general systems theory as a "pre-
eminently mathematical field" (p. vii). This mathematical base of systems theory
as applied to the crisis field is illustrated by the modified square root symbol
(√ ⌐ ⌐ ⌐): the downward stroke represents the loss of functioning during crisis, while the varying positions of the horizontal line symbolize the return to higher,
the same, or lower levels of equilibrium following a crisis (Jacobson, 1980, p. 8;
Smith, 1978, p. 399).

This interpretation of the crisis experience implies that people in crisis are
unable to take charge of their lives. People who accept this view of themselves
when in crisis will be less likely to participate actively in the crisis resolution process
and thereby diminish their potential for growth. General systems theory also highlights the concept of equilibrium as a static notion. This idea comes from consensus theory in the social sciences, which states that people in disequilibrium are
out of kilter with respect to both their personality and the social system; they are
unbalanced rather than in the ideal state of equilibrium. In a system in equilibrium, people and behavior fit according to established norms (consensus). Parsons'
(1951) definition of the "sick role" as a "state of deviance" is one of the most classic and controversial examples of consensus theory (Levine & Kozloff, 1978). Systems theory appeals to our desire and need for precision and a sense of order in
our lives. However, the reality of our lives and the world at large suggests that dynamic, interactional theories correspond more closely to the way people actually
feel, think, behave, and make sense of the crises they experience.

[1]Some advocates of general systems theory have declared it a "new humanistic philosophy of
man" and a "new skeleton of science," while critics accuse it of being more "general" than
"theory" (Broderick & Smith, 1979, p. 112). Urban (1978, p. 62) cites this asset of systems
theory: "The language of the systems view permits one to operate disencumbered by the het-
erogeneous meanings attached to our concepts arising from our everyday language, our prior
technical attempts, and our personal, private, and idiosyncratic experience." In my opinion,
nothing could be more contrary to the subjective nature of the crisis experience and to the
importance of communication and personal meaning in understanding and helping people in
crisis.

Another major criticism of the concept of equilibrium in crisis theory is that it is reductionist. It attempts to explain a complex human phenomenon in the framework of a single discipline, psychology, whereas the explanation of human behavior demands more than psychological concepts. Furthermore, existential philosophy, learning, and other humanistic frameworks are ignored by this deterministic notion borrowed from mathematics, engineering, and the natural sciences (Taplin, 1971). For example, how can the concept of equilibrium explain the different responses of people to the crises encountered in concentration camps and atomic bomb blasts? Or, after the death of a child, a parent's equilibrium may still waver at the thought of the tragic loss, yet she or he may have resolved this crisis within a religious framework.

Still another problem with the concept of equilibrium in crisis theory is its implication for practice. For example, Bograd (1984) discusses the negative impact of a family systems approach in attempts to help battered women in crisis. A systems approach here implies the importance of keeping the family intact in spite of abuse and often with heavy reliance on tranquilizers. Chemical restoration of homeostasis with psychoactive drugs is common. It might be argued that other rationales explain the pervasive use of tranquilizers in crisis situations, yet attention to the theory underlying this practice might reduce this prevalent but misguided approach to people in crisis. It is possible that chemical stabilization practiced without humanistic crisis intervention is related to iatrogenesis, that is, illness induced by physicians and other helpers (Ehrenreich, 1978; Fuchs, 1974; Johnson, 1990; McKinlay, 1990). Indeed, general systems theory supports the notion that within the complementary health delivery and economic systems, budgets can be balanced and higher profits secured if a sufficient number of drugs (in addition to other technological devices) are sold, regardless of clinical contraindications for their use for people in crisis. Other frameworks, such as conflict and change theory, are needed to support the awareness and social action necessary to address some of these damaging practices in the crisis field.

In summary, since human beings are more than their bodies, one might ask: Why rely so heavily on natural science models when philosophy, the humanities, and political science are also available to help explain human behavior?

Community Mental Health

Caplan's concepts about crisis emerged during the same period in which the community mental health movement was born. An important influence on crisis intervention during this era was the 1961 Report of the Joint Commission on Mental Illness and Health in the United States. This book, *Action for Mental Health* (1961), laid the foundation for the community mental health movement in the United States. It documented through five years of study the crucial fact that people were not getting the help they needed, when they needed it, and where they needed it—close to their natural social setting. The report revealed that (1) people in crisis were tired of waiting lists; (2) professionals were tired of lengthy and expensive therapy that often did not help; (3) large numbers of people (42 percent) went initially to a physician or to clergy for any problem; (4) long years of training were not necessary to learn how to help distressed people; and (5) volunteers and community caretakers (e.g., police officers, teachers, ministers) were a large, untapped source for helping people in distress.

One of the many recommendations in this report was that every community should have a local emergency mental health program. In 1963 and 1965, legislation made federal funds available to provide comprehensive mental health services through community mental health centers. Hansell (1976) refined many of the findings of Caplan, Tyhurst, military psychiatry, and community mental health studies into an entire system of response to the person in distress. His work is especially important to crisis workers in community mental health agencies because many people in high-risk groups go there for help. However, some communities still do not have such programs. And even among those that do, emergency and other services are often far from ideal. Political and fiscal policies in the 1980s resulted in further departures from community mental health ideals worldwide (Hoff, 1993; Marks & Scott, 1990). Reform movements in Canada, Italy, and the United States have attempted to reverse this trend (Mosher & Burti, 1989; *Putting People First*, 1993; Scheper-Hughes & Lovell, 1986).

Primary Health Care

Since the Alma Ata Declaration by the World Health Organization (WHO) in 1978, international and national agencies, both public and private, have committed themselves to the concept of primary health care as fundamental to the health status of citizens (Kaseje & Sempebwa, 1989). WHO's original declaration focuses on immunization, sanitation, nutrition, and maternal and child health, as well as the economic, occupational, and educational underpinnings of health status. But health planners and policy makers increasingly recognize that mental health status is tied to socioeconomic, political, and cultural factors affecting individuals. One of the most important implications of this interrelationship is the significance of the socioeconomic and cultural *context* within which violence is used as a response to individual and interpersonal stressors. Fiscal constraints worldwide have forced even greater attention to the centrality of primary health care in various health reform efforts (Fiedler & Wight, 1990; Hoff, 1993). However, despite savings in cost and human pain, crisis intervention as part of primary care is still not fully recognized for its contribution to preventing illness and maintaining health (Paykel, 1990).

Crisis Care and Psychiatric Stabilization

Similar to the growing emphasis on primary health care is the integration of crisis approaches on behalf of those suffering from acute psychotic episodes. Typically, such persons are seen in the crisis unit of community mental health centers or in the emergency service of general hospitals where the emphasis is on triage and rapid disposition; psychopharmacological agents are often used to stabilize distressed people. The strong medical orientation in such units warrants greater caution than usual by providers to assure that crisis intervention techniques are not supplanted rather than supplemented by tranquilization of acutely upset persons. When these units are not tightly integrated with other services, staff burnout and rapid turnover is one of the costly results. Ideally, all mental health staff members should be trained in crisis intervention. In that way, coverage of the crisis service could be rotated and greater continuity of care assured.

Crisis Care and Chronic Problems

While people with chronic problems are generally more vulnerable to crisis episodes, their vulnerability is exacerbated by the fiscal and other policies that have left thousands of seriously disturbed people without the mental health services they need after years of institutionalization (Chandler, 1990; Hoff, 1993; Johnson, 1990). One result of these actions is that community-based crisis hotlines serve by default as the routine support service to seriously disturbed people whose care is not always well coordinated among an array of agencies and providers. Routine training in crisis care for those serving this vulnerable population would prevent a misuse of hotlines as well as frequent readmissions to costly psychiatric services (Marks, 1985).

Suicide Prevention and Other Specialized Crisis Services

Another important influence is the suicide prevention movement. McGee (1974) has documented in detail the work of the Los Angeles Suicide Prevention Center and other groups in launching the suicide prevention and crisis intervention movement in the United States. The Los Angeles Suicide Prevention Center was born out of the efforts of Norman Farberow and Edwin Shneidman. In the late 1950s, these two psychologists led the movement by studying suicide notes. Through their many projects and those of numerous colleagues, suicide prevention and crisis centers were established throughout North America and Western Europe. The Samaritans, founded in 1953 in London by Chad Varah, is the most widespread and visible suicide prevention group, with 182 branches in the United Kingdom; 117 branches of Befrienders International are now established in twenty-six countries. Another international group, Lifeline Contact Teleministry (now Contact USA), was founded in 1963 in Sydney, Australia.

The suicide prevention and crisis movement emerged in the United States during the decade when professional mental health workers had a mandate (*Action for Mental Health*, 1961) and massive federal funding to provide emergency services along with other mental health care. Remarkably, however, most crisis centers were staffed by volunteers and often were started by volunteer citizen groups such as mental health or ministerial associations. It would seem that volunteers were often willing and able to respond to an unmet community need, whereas professionals in mental health either could not or would not respond. This situation is currently changing, but it is still noteworthy in light of some of the myths discussed earlier (Kalafat, 1984; Levine, 1981).

In recent years, a number of these crisis centers in the United States have closed because of insufficient funds or inadequate leadership. Others have merged with community mental health programs. Still others have adapted and expanded their services or have begun new programs to meet the special needs of rape victims, abused children, runaway youths, battered women, or people with AIDS.

Currently, suicide prevention and crisis services exist in a variety of organizational frameworks. For example, many shelters for battered women offering around-the-clock telephone response and physical refuge avoid traditional hierarchies in favor of a collective structure. Regardless of the models used, however, every community should have a comprehensive crisis program, including services for suicide emergencies, discharged mental patients, and victims of violence (Hoff & Miller, 1987).

The increasing recognition of the need for comprehensive crisis services has resulted in some relief from the dichotomy in practice between traditional psychiatric emergency care and grassroots suicide prevention, along with other specialized crisis services. The separation and territorial conflicts between these two aspects of crisis service are at best artificial and at worst a disservice to people experiencing life crises or psychiatric emergencies, the boundaries of which often overlap.

Unfortunately, some staff members of these specialized services are initially suspicious and disdainful of anything associated with traditional psychiatric care, only to find that some professional skills and services are needed in spite of objections to how these services are sometimes delivered. Conversely, traditional mental health professionals often assume that they are the only real professionals. They may regard alternative crisis service providers as naive do-gooders, usually without having observed firsthand the quality of their work or assisted with the funding and other types of problems faced in responding to community needs. For example, if a battered woman in a shelter run by volunteers becomes suicidal or psychotic, staff members without crisis intervention training usually must call on psychiatric professionals for assistance. On the other hand, a health or mental health professional treating a battered woman in a hospital emergency facility may compound the problem by a victim-blaming attitude that is revealed in words and in practice.

Greater collaboration between psychiatric and indigenous specialized crisis services is needed as survivors of abuse and increasing numbers of crisis-prone patients discharged from mental institutions seek assistance from twenty-four–hour community crisis programs.

Sociological Influences

Discussion of the evolution of crisis theory and practice thus far suggests that the momentum has come largely from psychological, psychiatric, or community sources. It is true that the strongest influences on crisis theory and practice have stressed the individual rather than the social aspects of crisis. Nevertheless, the relative neglect of social factors in crisis theory does not reflect their unimportance but rather represents a serious omission. Caplan (1964, pp. 31–34) refers to the psychological, social, cultural, and material supplies necessary to maintain equilibrium and avoid crisis. Yet in practice, while acknowledging the place of social support in the crisis development and resolution process, most writers focus on reducing psychological tension and returning to precrisis equilibrium without emphasizing how social factors influence these processes (see Chapter Five). Among all writers in the field, Hansell (1976) has done the most to stress social influences on the development and management of crisis. His social psychological approach to crisis theory and practice will be explained further in Chapters Two and Three, in concert with cross-cultural influences in the field.

Cross-Cultural and Diversity Influences

Political, social, and technological developments have contributed to more permeable national boundaries and at the same time have sharpened cultural awareness, ethnic identities, and sensitivity to diversity issues. For instance, international relations are becoming more critical; cross-continental travel and communication are more accessible; gay, lesbian, and bisexual activists have made visible the toll of discrimination on suicide rates among youth in this group. These observations have implications for cross-cultural and diversity issues in the experience of crisis as well as the variance in response to people in crisis. The rich data on rites of passage marking human transition states in traditional societies are another significant contribution of cultural and social anthropology to the understanding of life crises. These insights from other cultures are particularly relevant to crises around transition states, as discussed in Chapter Thirteen. In North American society, contributions to crisis theory from First Nations people, from immigrant ethnic groups, and from women have illuminated their responses to crises arising out of the social structure, associated values, and various discriminatory practices (see Chapter Two).

Feminist and Victimology Influences

Women increasingly reject theories and practices that damage them outright or prevent their human growth and development (Boston Women's Health Book Collective, 1992; Mirkin, 1994). The influence of feminism on crisis theory has increased considerably along with the growing literature on violence, as women and children are seen as primary objects of abuse worldwide (Hoff, 1990; Mawby & Walklate, 1994; Pan American Health Organization, 1994; Stanko, 1990). In particular, feminist and complementary critical analysis reveals dramatically the intersection between violence, victimization, crisis, and suicide. Thus, while cross-cultural, ethnic, and feminist experiences are the newest in the historical development of contemporary crisis theory and practice, in a real sense they are the oldest influences, as suggested earlier by the origins of crisis intervention. Thus we come full circle in this historical review.

Life Crises: A Psychosociocultural Perspective

Our review of the diverse sources of crisis theory and practice suggests that understanding and helping people in crisis is a complex, interdisciplinary endeavor. Since human beings encompass physical, emotional, social, and spiritual functions, no one theory is adequate to explain the crisis experience, its origins, or the most effective approach to helping people in crisis.

Accordingly, this book draws on insights, concepts, and strategies from psychology, nursing, sociology, psychiatry, anthropology, philosophy, political science, and critical analysis to propose a dynamic theory and practice with these emphases:[2]

• Individual, social, cultural, and material origins of crisis
• Development of the psychological crisis state
• Emotional, behavioral, and cognitive manifestations of crisis
• Interactive relationships between stress, crisis, and illness
• Issues involved and skills needed to deal with suicidal crises, violence against others, disaster, and transition states
• Resolution of crises by use of psychological, social, material, and cultural resources
• Collaboration between the person or family in crisis and various significant others in the effective management of crisis
• The social/political task of reducing the crisis vulnerability of a society's various disadvantaged groups through social change strategies

These elements of crisis theory and practice are illustrated relationally in the Crisis Paradigm as a preview of Chapter Two (see Figure 1.1). The Crisis Paradigm depicts (1) the *crisis process* experienced by the distressed person from origin through resolution, and (2) the sensitive application of natural and formal crisis

[2]Sol Levine, a medical sociologist, refers to this approach as "creative integrationism," not to be confused with superficial eclecticism (1983, personal communication).

FIGURE 1.1. CRISIS PARADIGM.

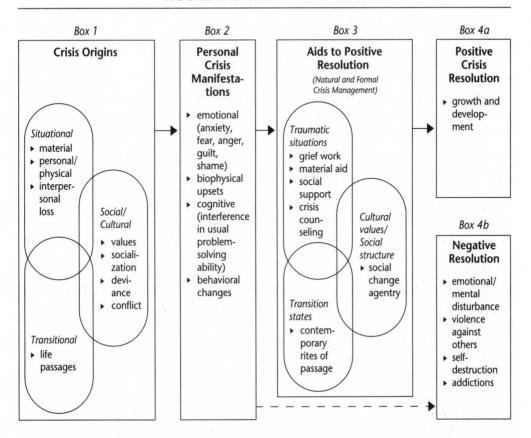

Crisis origins, manifestations, and outcomes, and the respective functions of crisis management have an interactional relationship. The intertwined circles represent the distinct yet interrelated origins of crisis and aids to positive resolution, even though personal manifestations are often similar. The arrows pointing from origins to positive resolution illustrate the *opportunity for growth and development* through crisis; the broken line at bottom depicts the potential *danger of crisis* in the absence of appropriate aids.

management strategies in promoting growth and avoiding negative crisis outcomes. This paradigm draws on research and clinical experience with victims of violence (Hoff, 1990), other life-event literature (e.g., Antonovsky, 1980; Cloward & Piven, 1979; Gerhardt, 1979), and work with survivors of man-made disasters. The inclusion of sociocultural origins of crisis extends the traditional focus of crisis intervention on situational and developmental life events—a framework found inadequate to guide practice with people intentionally injured through violence, prejudice, or neglect. The paradigm suggests a tandem approach to the crisis management process, that is, attending to the immediate problem while not losing sight of the social change strategies needed to address the complex origins of certain crisis situations. This psychosociocultural perspective on life crises is examined in detail throughout the book.

Approaches to Helping People in Crisis

The approaches to crisis intervention used by helpers will vary according to their exposure to historical influences, their values, and their professional preparation in various disciplines.

Differentiating Approaches to Helping People in Distress

There are several approaches to helping people in crisis. The following discussion illustrates the differences, overlap, and similarities among these approaches and suggests the relationship between crisis intervention and other ways of helping distressed people.

Certainly crisis intervention should not be regarded as a panacea for all social, emotional, and mental problems. It is not synonymous with psychotherapy, even though some techniques, such as listening and catharsis, are used in both. Nor is crisis intervention a mode of helping only poor people while reserving psychotherapy for the financially secure (Hallowitz, 1975). The occurrence of crisis does not depend on a person's socioeconomic status, and crisis intervention can be helpful regardless of that status.

It may be just as damaging to use a crisis intervention approach when it is inapplicable as *not* to use it when it is. For example, when suicide and crisis hotlines are ineffectively supervised and are not linked with other mental health services, there can be negative side effects, sometimes called "systems problems" (Hoff, 1983). Callers seeking help from crisis centers know they must at least act as though they are in crisis in order to get attention and help. Thus, some callers may appear to be in crisis when they are not. For example, a person who is crying may or may not be in crisis. Judgment of crisis should be based on an assessment of the caller's total situation.

If workers are unskilled in crisis assessment, they may unwittingly encourage crisis-like behavior by discounting what people in crisis say—much as the little boy crying "wolf" in the fable was discounted because he had cried wolf so many times when there was none that no one believed him when there was. In other words, if workers assume that a person is exaggerating or pretending—crying wolf—and thus fail to accurately assess the situation through questioning, they could miss the real and urgent message the person is trying to convey. Suicide or other-directed violence may be the eventual outcome.

Table 1.1 illustrates the range of services and differences among various services available to people with psychosocial problems. Crisis intervention is just one of the many services people need. Effective crisis intervention can be an important link to a mode of treatment such as psychotherapy (Perlmutter & Jones, 1985). This is because during crisis, people are more likely than at other times to consider getting help for chronic problems that made them crisis prone in the first place. Crisis intervention is also a significant means of avoiding last-resort measures such as institutional care. Evaluation of a regional mental health center's clinical services revealed that short-term community-oriented crisis approaches were not enough for people with serious mental and social disabilities (Smith, 1975). Such individuals need long-term rehabilitation programs as well, including, for example, training for jobs and instruction in home management (Johnson, 1990; Leff, 1990).

The limitations of crisis intervention and the need to see it in a larger sociocultural and political perspective are dramatically illustrated in the following vignette. McKinlay (1990, p. 502) discusses this need in terms of the "manufacture of illness" and the futility of tinkering with "downstream" versus "upstream" endeavors:

> My friend, Irving Zola, relates the story of a physician trying to explain the dilemmas of the modern practice of medicine: "You know," he said, "sometimes it feels like this. There I am standing by the shore of a swiftly flowing river and I hear the cry of a drowning man. So, I jump into the river, put my arms around him, pull him to shore and apply artificial respiration. Just when he begins to breathe, another cry for help. So back in the river again, reaching, pulling, applying, breathing and then another yell. Again and again, without end, goes the sequence. You know, I am so busy jumping in, pulling them to shore, applying artificial respiration, that I have no time to see who the hell is upstream pushing them all in."

This story underscores the need for crisis practitioners to take time to see their work in a broader perspective not only for the sake of people in crisis but in order to prevent burnout and the accompanying loss of meaning in their work. Within the array of services available to people in crisis, the different helping modes obviously overlap (see Table 1.1). But charts and models are intended to clarify points and issues in theoretical discussion rather than represent an exact picture of reality. Also, while the Crisis Paradigm presented in this book is strongly linked to public and community services, the intervention strategies outlined can be applied using telephone, face-to-face, and outreach modes in various settings: homes in different cultural milieux, clinics, hospitals, and social agencies. In spite of hazy boundaries between crisis and other service models, there are fundamental differences between their purposes and assumptions about people needing help. For example, in the medical model, intervention consists of treatment or therapy directed toward cure or the alleviation of symptoms of a person presumed ill or

TABLE 1.1. COMPARISON OF THERAPIES AND THE CRISIS INTERVENTION MODEL.

Psychotherapy	Medical-Institutional Therapy	Social-Service-Rehabilitation Therapy	Crisis Intervention
Type of People Served			
Those who wish to correct neurotic personality or behavior patterns	People with serious mental or emotional breakdowns	Those who are chronically disabled	Individuals and families in crisis or precrisis states
Service Goals			
Work through unconscious conflicts	Control, adjust, stabilize	Rehabilitation; return to normal functioning in society insofar as possible	Growth-promoting
Reconstruct behavior and personality patterns	Recover from acute disturbance		Personal and social integration
Grow personally and socially			
Service Methods			
Introspection	Medication	Work training	Social and environmental manipulation
Catharsis	Behavior modification	Resocialization	Focus on feelings and problem solving
Interpretation	Electric shock	Training in activities of daily living	May use medication to promote goals
Free association	Group activities	Peer and counselor support and advocacy	Decision counseling
(Use of additional techniques depends on philosophy and training of therapist)	(Use of additional techniques depends on philosophy of institution)		
Activity of Workers			
Exploratory	Direct, non-involved or indirect	Structured but less so than in crisis intervention	Active/direct (depends on functional level of client)
Nondirective			
Interpretive			

Psychotherapy	Medical-Institutional Therapy	Social-Service Rehabilitation Therapy	Crisis Intervention
Length of Service			
Usually long-term	Short or long (depends on degree of disability and approach of psychiatrist) High repeat rate	Long-term—a few months to 2–3 years	Short—usually 6 sessions or less
Beliefs About People			
Individualistic or social (depends on philosophy of therapist)	Individualistic—social aspect secondary Institution and order often more important than people	People can change Mental disability or a diagnosis should not spell hopelessness	Social—people are capable of growth and self-control
Attitudes Toward Service			
Emphasis on wisdom of therapist and 50-minute hour Flexibility varies with individual therapist	Scheduled Staff attitudes may become rigid and institutionalized	Willingness to stick with it and observe only slow change Hopefulness and expectation of goal achievement	Flexible, any hour

diseased. The focus is on the *individual*, who is generally assumed to harbor the source of difficulty within himself or herself (Barney, 1994). In contrast, the crisis model proposed in this book stresses the following:

- Social, cultural, and environmental factors in addition to personal origins of crisis
- Prevention of destructive crisis outcomes such as suicide or mental breakdown (or, if psychopathology was present prior to the crisis, the prevention of further breakdown and chronic pathology)
- Psychosocial growth and development as the ideal outcome of crisis—a possibility greatly enhanced through social support and other crisis management strategies

Prevention strategies are usually associated conceptually with public health and medical (disease) models. In growth and development theory, the term *enhancement* is used to describe health and development-promoting activities (Danish, Smyer, & Nowak, 1980, pp. 348–359). The theoretical distinction between prevention and enhancement has not been well documented in practice. Therefore, these concepts are considered together in the next section, on the assumption that crisis intervention is relevant for preventing disease (and other negative outcomes) as well as for enhancing growth and development.

Preventing Crisis and Promoting Growth

Viewing crisis as both an opportunity and a danger means that knowing about some upcoming events can allow us to prepare for normal life events and usually prevent the development of crises. For many people, however, these normal events do lead to hazard rather than opportunity.

While we cannot predict events such as sudden death of a loved one, the birth of a premature child, or natural disaster, we can anticipate how people will react to them. In his study of survivors of the Cocoanut Grove fire, Lindemann (1944) demonstrated the importance of recognizing crisis responses and preventing negative outcomes of crisis. Once a population or individual is identified as being at risk of crisis, we can use a number of time-honored approaches to prevent crisis and enhance growth. Caplan and others (Schulberg & Sheldon, 1968) speak of primary, secondary, and tertiary prevention in the fields of public health and mental health.

Primary Prevention and Enhancement. *Primary prevention,* in the form of education, consultation, and crisis intervention, is designed to reduce the occurrence of mental disability and to promote growth, development, and crisis resistance in a community. There are several means of doing this:

1. *Eliminate or modify the hazardous situation.* The practice of immunizing children against smallpox and diphtheria, for example, is based on the fact that failure to immunize can expose large numbers of people to the hazards of disease. Knowledge of sociopsychological hazards should inspire similar efforts to eliminate or modify these hazards.

For example, we can alter hospital structures and practices to reduce the risk of crisis for hospitalized children and adult surgical patients; eliminate substandard housing for crisis-prone older people and others disadvantaged by poverty; and educate people about the nature and effects of these hazards.

2. *Reduce exposure to hazardous situations.* For example, a flood warning allows people to escape disaster. In the psychosocial sphere, crisis can be prevented by advising and screening people entering potentially stressful situations such as college, or unusual occupations such as working in a foreign country, or demand-

ing occupations such as crisis counseling or firefighting. With respect to the AIDS pandemic, physical and psychosocial preventive practices must be combined. The current lack of a vaccine for immunization against AIDS underscores the importance of reducing people's exposure to HIV through education and the modification of sexual behavior.

3. *Reduce vulnerability by increasing coping ability.* In the physical health sector, people with certain diseases are directed to obtain extra rest, eat certain foods, and take prescribed medicines. In the psychosocial sphere, older people and the poor are most often exposed to the risk of urban dislocation. They can be provided with extra physical resources, social services, and social action skills to counter the negative social and emotional effects of a hazardous event. New parents will feel less vulnerable if they are prepared for the challenge of rearing their first child. Marriage and retirement are other important life events that we can prepare for so that they become occasions for continued growth rather than deterioration.

The success of anticipatory preventive measures depends largely on a person's openness to learning, cultural values, previous problem-solving success, and general social supports. Jacobson, Strickler, and Morley (1968) refer to anticipatory prevention as generic; that is, it is applicable to general target groups known to be at risk. Anticipatory prevention is similar to the developmental notion of using education to help people who are at risk handle stressful life events (Danish, Smyer, & Nowak, 1980, pp. 349–350).

When hazardous events or a person's vulnerability to events cannot be accurately predicted, or people are unable to respond to generic, anticipatory prevention, participatory techniques are indicated for the person or family in crisis (Caplan 1964, 1974; Caplan & Grunebaum, 1967). These involve a thorough psychosocial assessment and counseling of individuals or families by skilled crisis workers. Participatory techniques correspond to Morley's concept of individually tailored intervention (1980, p. 16) and are discussed in detail in later chapters. In developmental frameworks, the individual and the family participate actively in resolving the crisis. If such participation is not sought, the style of service might more appropriately be identified with the medical model, in which there is often an assumption of illness and loss of normal functioning (Danish, Smyer, & Nowak, 1980). For a further discussion of primary prevention in relation to crisis, see Hoff and Miller, 1987, Chapter Eight.

Secondary Prevention. The term *secondary prevention* implies that some form of mental disability has already occurred because of the absence of primary activities or because a person is unable to profit from those activities. The aim of secondary prevention is to shorten the duration of disability. A major means of doing this is to provide easily accessible crisis intervention services. If such services are offered, emotionally and mentally disturbed people can be kept out of psychiatric facilities. The disabling effects of institutional life and increased cost are thereby avoided, as are the destructive results of removal from one's natural community. Since mentally disturbed individuals are more crisis prone than others, they need more active help than might others in crisis. The thousands of homeless mentally ill persons illustrate this principle.

Tertiary Prevention. The goal of this level of prevention is to reduce long-term disabling effects for those who are recovering from a mental disorder. Social and rehabilitation programs are an important means of helping these people return to former social and occupational roles or learn new ones (Paykel, 1990). Crisis intervention is also important for the same reasons noted in the discussion of secondary prevention. The recovery process includes learning new ways of coping with stress through positive crisis resolution. Thus, even if the precrisis state is one of mental disability, it is never too late to learn new coping devices, as implied in a growth and development model.

Crisis Services in a Continuum Perspective

Anticipatory and participatory techniques can be viewed as a continuum of services for people with different kinds of psychosocial problems (see Figure 1.2). The continuum suggests that people with problems vary in their dependency on other people and agencies for help. It also illustrates the economic implications of cri-

FIGURE 1.2. CONTINUUM OF MENTAL HEALTH SERVICES: COST AND CLIENT INDEPENDENCE.

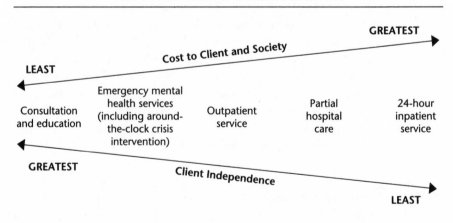

Assisting distressed people in their natural social roles (homemaker, paid worker, student) through consultation, education, and crisis services is the *least* costly means of service and allows the *greatest* client independence; institutional-based care is the *most* costly means and allows the *least* client independence.

sis intervention in addition to its clinical and humanistic benefits. However, in the United States, health and human service workers trying to implement community-based crisis approaches in their individual practices are often frustrated by insurance policies that reimburse only for hospital-based care. Current efforts to develop a national health plan suggest the possibility that this situation could change.

Services in the continuum include the basic elements of community mental health programs. These five essential services were originally mandated by the Community Mental Health Acts of 1963 and 1965. Recommendations by the U.S. Joint Commission on Mental Illness and Health formed the basis of these mental health acts (1961). Recent federal guidelines for basic services include rehabilitation, addiction services, victim services, services for the elderly and children, and evaluation programs, although policy decisions have curtailed many of these programs. Crisis intervention is considered a part of these mental health and social services.

Among the crisis intervention approaches and settings encompassed in this continuum, consultation and education come under the general umbrella of primary prevention and enhancement. Twenty-four–hour crisis services can also be seen as primary prevention, depending on the precrisis state of the individual in crisis. Emergency mental health is most closely related to traditional psychiatry and the management of behavioral emergencies in hospital settings (Bellak & Siegel, 1983; Kravis, et al., 1993), which ideally should be linked to crisis and suicide prevention agencies. Outpatient care, partial hospital care, and twenty-four–hour inpatient care (residential) services should include crisis intervention. These elements of care are primarily concerned with underlying emotional and mental problems, which are the focus of secondary and tertiary prevention. The application of crisis intervention in these settings is illustrated further in Chapters Eight and Eleven.

To underscore the social and cultural concepts central to the Crisis Paradigm presented here, to redress the relative inattention to community-based crisis intervention, and to illustrate the economy of a comprehensive approach in terms of family stability and prevention of costly institutionalization, we will now consider crisis intervention practice in homes, natural settings, and peer group situations.

Natural and Peer Group Settings

Once health care or other human service workers become enculturated into mini-societies such as hospitals and other bureaucratic agencies, they may easily forget that others experience culture shock when entering them—not unlike the shock an anthropologist or tourist may feel when entering a foreign country. This point is illustrated by the comment of a visitor to a nursing home: "I couldn't stand the smells." For a person already in crisis, admission to a hospital for the purpose of receiving help during the crisis can itself be a hazardous event. Polak (1967) outlined this fact in his study of 104 men admitted to a psychiatric hospital in Scotland. Polak found that these men or their families had typically requested psychiatric hospital admission following previous unresolved crises around separation, physical illness, death, and migration. However, while offering temporary relief, admission also was frequently the occasion for another crisis because family patterns of interaction were disrupted, and the patient and his or her family often had disturbing and unrealistic fantasies and expectations about the purpose and meaning of hospitalization. Now, with some premature insurance-driven discharges, other crises are precipitated (Johnson, 1990).

Hansell (1976) notes how inviting a hospital environment seems to a person deprived of normal community supports. Hospitalization can also be misused by families who lack personal and social resources for relating to disturbed members. Hansell suggests that crisis can just as well lead to improved friendships as to "asylum."

Research thus not only supports the hazards of being uprooted from natural social settings but also provides a sober reminder of this social reality: agencies are indeed subcultures of the larger society in which crisis intervention by family members, friends, and neighbors is an everyday occurrence. This does not preclude the need for formal crisis intervention by persons specially trained for this task. Rather, it highlights the fact that the prospects for positive crisis resolution by individuals, families, and peer groups are enhanced and negative complications are reduced when crisis management and intervention occur as close as possible to natural settings. These points are illustrated in the following account of a counselor doing crisis work in a home.

CASE EXAMPLE: RAY

Last week, another counselor and I made a home visit to a family that was very upset because the parents thought their 22-year-old son Ray had "flipped out" on drugs. The parents had called with the express purpose of getting their son into a psychiatric hospital, even though he had refused to go before. I had said when they called that we would not automatically put Ray in the hospital but that we would come over to assess the situation and help the entire family through the crisis. We worked out a strategy for telling Ray directly and clearly the reasons for our visit. Ray had refused to come to the phone, shouting, "They're the people who will take me to the hospital in an ambulance." When we got there, a family session revealed that Ray was the scapegoat for many other family problems. We worked out a crisis service plan, and Ray started to show some trust in us after about two hours with the whole family. He could see that we didn't just come to whisk him off to a mental hospital. In the end, even Ray's family was relieved that he didn't have to go to the hospital. Before our home visit, they had seen no other way out. They had talked with several therapists before, but no one had ever come to the house or worked with the whole family.

The diversity and merits of innovative approaches can be illustrated further by the following example of crisis intervention by a volunteer in a peer group setting.

CASE EXAMPLE: RAMONA

Ramona was one of a group of eight bat-tered women in a shelter with no overnight staffing. This shelter, like most, screens its residents for acute suicidal tendencies, addic-tions, and mental disturbance. Nevertheless, Ramona became suicidal, and one night she locked herself in the parlor to protect herself from acting on her suicidal tendencies with kitchen knives. When she slept, she did so on the office sofa so she would not have to be alone. Ramona had not told her fellow house members why she did these things, although the other women did know that she was sui-cidal. Tension among the residents grew be-cause they did not understand Ramona's behavior. They were afraid that if they asked about it, she would become more suicidal (see Chapter Six regarding this popular myth). One of the residents said she would leave the house if the staff didn't get rid of Ramona.

Assessing the total situation, Diane, a volunteer staffer who was also a registered nurse trained in crisis intervention, called a meeting to discuss the problem. She ex-plained to Ramona that other residents were worried about her and asked, "Are you will-ing to meet with them and explain what's happening with you?" Ramona replied, "Sure," and eagerly jumped off the sofa. The volunteer added that she had experience with suicidal people and was not afraid to discuss suicide. This brought a sigh of relief and a "Thank God!" from Ramona. (Ramona was on the waiting list for admission to a local hospital psychiatric unit for treatment of other problems.)

Ramona explained her behavior as self-protection, not hostility, as her fellow resi-dents had perceived. She told the group that she had felt most protected and least suicidal when another resident had gone for a walk with her. Ramona also reassured everyone that in the event she hurt herself or died, that was her responsibility, not theirs. All resi-dents expressed relief at having the problem out in the open and agreed to keep future communication open with Ramona instead of trying to second-guess her.

These examples illustrate the need for more widespread attention to the basic principles of suicide prevention, crisis management, and standards for crisis ser-vice delivery. Later chapters discuss further the benefits of using peer support and home settings for crisis intervention.

Basic Steps of Crisis Management

As we have observed, crisis resolution will occur with or without the assistance of others, while crisis intervention can be carried out in a variety of settings, some natural, some institutional. Regardless of the context or variations in personal style, the probability of positive crisis outcomes is greatly enhanced by attention to the basic steps of crisis management. These steps include the following:

1. Psychosocial assessment of the individual or family crisis including evaluation of victimization trauma and the risk of suicide or assault on others[3]
2. Development of a plan with the person or family in crisis
3. Implementation of the plan, drawing on personal, social, and material resources
4. Follow-up and evaluation of the crisis management process and outcomes

Broadly, these steps correspond to the problem-solving process used in medical, nursing, and social work practice, as well as in other human service protocols. The basic steps can be followed in natural situations or in a formal, structured process. For example, people in natural settings frequently make assessments of suicidal and assault risks. Similarly, everyone recognizes when someone is "crazy," that is, not acting according to commonly accepted social norms. In the case discussed earlier, the family's assessment of their crisis was that Ray had "flipped out," that he needed psychiatric hospitalization, and that they were unable to handle the crisis alone. They managed the crisis by calling for and cooperating with professional helpers.

A focus on prevention would include providing the average person, through public education programs, with more skills in detecting victimization and suicide or assault potential, as well as in assessing the advantages and limits of psychiatric hospitalization. Professional helpers would then be less likely to simply discount what people in crisis say. After all, professional assessments must in the end rely on data presented by the traumatized, suicidal, or disturbed person, his or her family, police, and other lay persons (Atkinson, 1978). Figure 1.3 illustrates the link between natural and formal crisis management, as introduced in the Crisis Paradigm. The details of formal crisis assessment and management strategies (as practiced by the counselor in Ray's case) are discussed throughout the remainder of the book.

National Standards for Crisis Services

The importance of basic principles of crisis management was highlighted in 1976 by the launching of a program in the United States to certify comprehensive crisis services, including community-based agencies and programs in hospitals or community mental health centers. This program was developed and is directed by the American Association of Suicidology (AAS), a national standard-setting body for suicide prevention and crisis services. Certification is intended to assure people in crisis that the services provided by a certified crisis program meet the

[3]Some health professionals may wish to include a diagnosis following this step. See Chapter Three on diagnosis and labeling theory.

FIGURE 1.3. NATURAL AND FORMAL CRISIS MANAGEMENT.

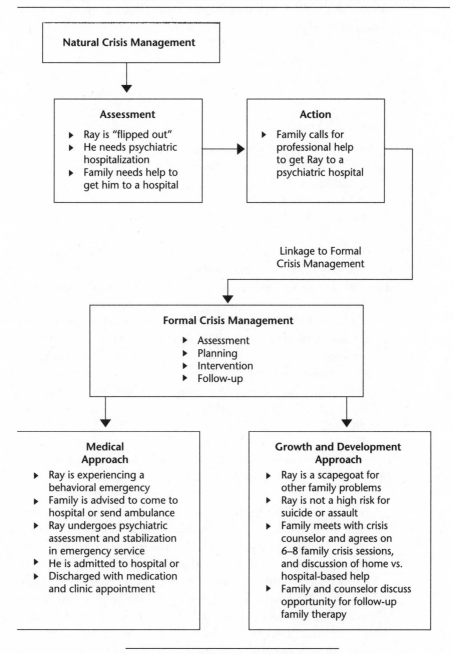

The medical approach is compared to the growth and development approach to formal crisis management.

minimum standards of service performance and program administration recommended by the AAS. In an age when consumers are increasingly conscious of the
quality of service they receive, certification is a step in the direction of assuring
such quality (Hoff & Miller, 1987).

Briefly, the AAS certification process includes evaluation of a crisis program
in seven areas (Hoff & Wells, 1989):

1. Administration
2. Training procedures
3. General service delivery systems
4. Services in life-threatening crises
5. Ethical issues
6. Community integration
7. Program evaluation

Programs are evaluated by examination of written materials describing the center's operation. Two regional certification committee members make a site visit.
The evaluation team rates the program on a scoring sheet according to predefined
standards. Data are gathered about the program and form the basis for evaluation.

The certification process does more than give a stamp of approval to acceptable or high-quality programs. The process also helps agencies improve services
if they do not meet minimum standards. Consultation for program upgrading is
available through the certification committee and other members of the AAS. Recently, the AAS also developed a certification process for individual crisis workers.
Following specific crisis training and experience, a worker can sit for an
examination.[4]

The relevance of these standards to the interagency coordination needed for
high-quality comprehensive crisis programs is illustrated by the following case excerpt from the 1989 edition of the *Certification Standards Manual:*

> At 11 P.M. a police officer calls the 24-hour telephone crisis service. A team of
> professional crisis workers—a psychiatric nurse with a master's degree and a
> volunteer with a B.A. in psychology—makes an outreach visit to the home of
> David Jones, whom the police and the Jones family believe to be acutely suici-
> dal, noncooperative, and in need of assessment for possible involuntary hospi-
> talization. Mr. Jones has refused police and family recommendations for
> treatment. The outreach team spends one and one-half hours interviewing Mr.
> Jones and his family in their home. Mr. Jones finally agrees to go to the emer-
> gency department of a community hospital, where he will be examined by psy-

[4]Information about these certification programs is available at the AAS Central Office: 4201
Connecticut Ave. NW Suite 310, Washington, D.C. 20008. Telephone (202) 237–2280. Fax:
(202) 237-2282.

chiatric liaison staff for possible hospitalization. Following assessment of Mr. Jones and his family situation, he remains overnight in the emergency department holding bed. The following morning, outpatient therapy for Mr. Jones and his family takes place at the community mental health center, where the hospital has an interagency service contract for follow-up of such mental health emergency cases. The family is also given the telephone number of the 24-hour telephone and outreach crisis program where the police had originally called on behalf of the family. (Adapted from Hoff & Wells, 1989, p. 3.)

This example highlights the comprehensive approach to crisis management that is developed in the remaining chapters.

Summary

The development of crisis theory and practice has sprung from diverse sources in the health field and social sciences. Approaches to crisis intervention vary with the needs of the person in crisis and the training and experience of helpers. Preventing crises, especially the negative outcomes of crises, is central to the approach of this book. Formal crisis management consists of four steps: assessment, planning, intervention, and follow-up, carried out in a psychosociocultural framework. The development of national standards for crisis service providers and workers attests to the growing maturity of formal crisis intervention as a recognized field grounded in knowledge and practice.

References

Action for mental health. (1961). Report of the Joint Commission on Mental Illness and Health. New York: Basic Books.

Aguilera, D. C. (1989). *Crisis intervention* (5th ed.). St. Louis: Mosby.

Antonovsky, A. (1980). *Health, stress, and coping.* San Francisco: Jossey-Bass.

Antonovsky, A. (1987). *Unraveling the mysteries of health.* San Francisco: Jossey-Bass.

Atkinson, J. M. (1978). *Discovering suicide: Studies in the social organization of sudden death.* Pittsburgh: University of Pittsburgh Press.

Barney, K. (1994). Limitations of the critique of the medical model. *The Journal of Mind and Behavior, 15*(1,2), 19–34.

Bellak, L., & Siegel, H. (1983). *Handbook of brief and intensive emergency psychotherapy.* Larchmont, NY: CPS.

Bertalanffy, L. von. (1968). *General systems theory* (Rev. ed.). New York: Braziller.

Bograd, M. (1984). Family systems approaches to wife battering: A feminist critique. *American Journal of Orthopsychiatry, 54*(4), 558–568.

Boston Women's Health Book Collective. (1992). *The new our bodies, ourselves.* New York: Simon & Schuster.

Broderick, C., & Smith, J. (1979). The general systems approach to the family. In W. Burr, et al. (Eds.), *Contemporary theories about the family.* New York: Free Press.

Brown, G. (1993). Life events and affective disorder: Replications and limitations. *Psychosomatic Medicine, 55*(3), 248–259.

Burstow, B. (1992). *Radical feminist therapy: Working in the context of violence.* Newbury Park: Sage.

Buss, A. R. (1979). Dialectics, history, and development: The historical roots of the individual-society dialectic. *Life-span Development and Behavior, 2,* 313–333.

Cade, B., & O'Hanlon, W. H. (1993). *A brief guide to brief therapy.* New York & London: W. W. Norton.

Caplan, G. (1964). *Principles of preventive psychiatry.* New York: Basic Books.

Caplan, G. (1974). *Support systems and community mental health.* New York: Behavioral Publications.

Caplan, G. (1981). Mastery of stress: Psychological aspects. *American Journal of Psychiatry, 138*(4), 413–420.

Caplan, G., & Grunebaum, H. (1967). Perspectives on primary prevention: A review. *Archives of General Psychiatry, 17,* 331–346.

Chandler, S. (1990). *Competing realities: The contested terrain of mental health advocacy.* New York: Praeger.

Cloward, R. A., & Piven, F. F. (1979). Hidden protest: The channeling of female innovations and resistance. *Signs: Journal of Women in Culture and Society, 4,* 651–669.

Danish, S. J., Smyer, M. A., & Nowak, C. A. (1980). Developmental intervention: Enhancing life-event processes. *Life-Span Development and Behavior, 3,* 339–366.

Ehrenreich, J. (Ed.). (1978). *The cultural crisis of modern medicine.* New York: Monthly Review Press.

Erickson, E. (1963). *Childhood and society* (2nd ed.). New York: W.W. Norton.

Ewing, C. P. (1978). *Crisis intervention as psychotherapy.* New York: Oxford University Press.

Fiedler, J. L., & Wight, J. B. (1990). *The medical offset effect and public health policy.* New York: Praeger.

Freidson, E. (1970). *Profession of medicine: Study of the sociology of applied knowledge.* New York: Harper & Row.

Friedman, S., & Fanger, M. T. (1991). *Expanding therapeutic possibilities: Getting results in brief psychotherapy.* Lexington, MA: Lexington Books.

Fromm, E. (1941). *Escape from freedom.* New York: Holt, Rinehart & Winston.

Fuchs, V. (1974). *Who shall live?* New York: Basic Books.

Gerhardt, U. (1979). Coping and social action: Theoretical reconstruction of the life-event approach. *Sociology of Health and Illness, 1,* 195–225.

Glass, A. T. (1957). Observations upon the epidemiology of mental illness in troops during warfare. Symposium on Prevention and Social Psychiatry. Washington: Walter Reed Army Institute of Research and The National Research Council.

Golan, N. (1978). *Treatment in crisis situations.* New York: Free Press.

Greenspan, M. (1983). *A new approach to women and therapy.* New York: McGraw-Hill.

Hallowitz, D. (1975). Counseling and treatment of the poor black family. *Social Casework, 56,* 451–459.

Hansell, N. (1976). *The person in distress.* New York: Human Sciences Press.

Hoff, L. A. (1990). *Battered women as survivors.* London: Routledge.

Hoff, L. A. (1983). Interagency coordination for people in crisis. *Information and Referral, 5*(1), 79–89.

Hoff, L. A. (1993). Review essay: Health policy and the plight of the mentally ill. *Psychiatry, 56*(4), 400–419.

Hoff, L. A., & Miller, N. (1987). *Programs for people in crisis: A guide for educators, administrators, and clinical trainers.* Boston: Northeastern University Custom Book Program.

Hoff, L. A., & Wells, J. O. (Eds.). (1989). *Certification standards manual* (4th ed.). Washington, D.C.: American Association of Suicidology.

Illich, I. (1976). *Limits to medicine.* Middlesex, England: Penguin.

Jacobson, G. F. (1980). Crisis theory. *New directions for mental health services: Crisis intervention in the 1980s, 6,* 1–10.

Jacobson, G. F., Strickler, M., & Morley, W. (1968). Generic and individual approaches to crisis intervention. *American Journal of Public Health, 58,* 338–343.

Janosik, E. H. (1984). *Crisis counseling.* Monterey, CA: Wadsworth.

Johnson, A. B. (1990). *Out of bedlam: The truth about deinstitutionalization.* New York: Basic Books.

Kalafat, J. (1984). Training community psychologists for crisis intervention. *American Journal of Community Psychology, 12*(2), 242–251.

Kaseje, D.C.O., & Sempebwa, E.K.N. (1989). An integrated rural health project in Saradidi, Kenya. *Social Science and Medicine, 28*(10), 1063–1071.

Kessler, R. C., & McLeod, J. D. (1984). Sex differences in vulnerability to undesirable life events. *American Sociological Review, 49*(Oct), 620–631.

Kravis, T. C., et al. (Eds.). (1993). *Emergency medicine* (3rd ed.). Germantown, MD: Aspen Systems Corporation.

Leff, J. (1990). Maintenance (management) of people with long-term psychotic illness. In I. Marks & R. Scott (Eds.), *Mental health care delivery: Innovations, impediments, and implementation* (pp. 17–40). Cambridge: Cambridge University Press.

Levine, M. (1981). *The history and politics of community mental health.* New York and Oxford: Oxford University Press.

Levine, S., & Kozloff, M. A. (1978). The sick role: Assessment and overview. *Annual Review of Sociology, 4,* 317–343.

Lindemann, E. (1944). Symptomatology and management of acute grief. *American Journal of Psychiatry, 101,* 101–148. Also reprinted in H. J. Parad (Ed.), *Crisis intervention: Selected readings* (1965). New York Family Service Association of America.

Marks, I. (1985). Controlled trial of psychiatric nurse therapists in primary care. *British Medical Journal, 290,* 1181–1184.

Marks, I., & Scott, R. (Eds.). (1990). *Mental health care delivery: Innovations, impediments, and implementation.* Cambridge: Cambridge University Press.

Maslow, A. (1970). *Motivation and personality* (2nd. ed.). New York: Harper & Row.

Mawby, R. I., & Walklate, S. (1994). *Critical victimology.* London: Sage.

McGee, R. K. (1974). *Crisis intervention in the community.* Baltimore: University Park Press.

McKinlay, J. B. (1990). A case for refocusing upstream: The political economy of illness. In P. Conrad & R. Kern (Eds.), *The sociology of health and illness: Critical perspectives* (3rd ed., pp. 502–516). New York: St. Martin's Press.

McNamee, S., & Gergen, K. J. (Eds.). (1992). *Therapy as social construction.* London: Sage.

Mirkin, M. P. (Ed.). (1994). *Women in context: Toward a feminist reconstruction of psychotherapy.* New York: Guilford.

Morley, W. E. (1980). Crisis intervention with adults. *New directions for mental health services: Crisis intervention in the 1980s 6,* 11–22.

Mosher, L. R., & Burti, L. (1989). *Community mental health: Principles and practice.* New York: W.W. Norton.

Pan American Health Organization (1993, November 16–17). Inter-American Conference on Society, Violence, and Health. Washington, D.C.

Panchuck, P. (1994). *The midlife experience of contemporary women: Views along the midway.* Unpublished doctoral dissertation. Boston: Leslie College.

Parsons, T. (1951). Social structure and the dynamic process: The case of modern medical practice. In *The social system,* (pp. 428–479). New York: Free Press.

Paykel, E. (1990). Innovations in mental health care in the primary care system. In I.M. Marks & R. Scott (Eds.), *Mental health care delivery: Innovations, impediments, and implementation* (pp. 69–83). Cambridge: Cambridge University Press.

Perlmutter, R. A., & Jones, J. E. (1985). Assessment of families in psychiatric emergencies. *American Journal of Orthopsychiatry, 55*(1), 130–139.

Polak, P. (1967). The crisis of admission. *Social Psychiatry, 2,* 150–157.

Putting people first: The reform of mental health services in Ontario. (1993). Toronto: Ministry of Health.

Rieker, P. P., & Carmen, E. H. (Eds.). (1984). *The gender gap in psychotherapy: Social realities and psychological processes.* New York: Plenum.

Robinson, D. (1971). *The process of becoming ill.* London: Routledge & Kegan Paul.

Scheper-Hughes, N., & Lovell, A. M. (1986). Breaking the circuit of social control: Lessons in public psychiatry from Italy and Franco Basaglia. *Social Science and Medicine, 23*(2), 159–178.

Schulberg, H. C., & Sheldon, A. (1968). The probability of crisis and strategies for preventive intervention. *Archives of General Psychiatry, 18,* 553–558.

Smith, L. (1978). A review of crisis intervention theory. *Social Casework, 59,* 396–405.

Smith, W. G. (1975). Evaluation of the clinical services of a regional mental health center. *Community Mental Health Journal, 7,* 47–57.

Stanko, E. A. (1990). *Everyday violence: How women and men experience sexual and physical danger.* London: Pandora.

Taplin, J. R. (1971). Crisis theory: Critique and reformulation. *Community Mental Health Journal, 7,* 13–23.

Thomas, J. (1992). The Cocoanut Grove inferno. *Boston Sunday Globe,* Nov. 22, 1, 38–39.

Turner R. S., & Avison, W. R. (1987). Gender and depression: Assessing exposure to life events in a chronically strained population. Paper presented at the Annual Meeting of the American Public Health Association, New Orleans.

Tyhurst, J. S. (1957). The role of transition states—including disasters—in mental illness. Symposium on Preventive and Social Psychiatry. Washington: Walter Reed Army Institute of Research and the National Research Council.

Urban, H. B. (1978). The concept of development from a systems perspective. *Life-Span Development and Behavior, 1,* 45–83.

Walsh, M. R. (1987). *The psychology of women: Ongoing debates.* New Haven: Yale University Press.

CHAPTER TWO

UNDERSTANDING PEOPLE IN CRISIS

Understanding people in crisis is the foundation for the assessment, planning, intervention, and follow-up—steps intrinsic to the crisis management process. A recurring problem in the social sciences is that theories are often formulated without sufficient grounding in reality (Bernstein, 1978). On the other hand, practitioners frequently do not study the values and theoretical assumptions implicit in research (Hoff, 1990; Roberts, 1981). For example, census figures reveal that mothers are awarded custody of their children in most cases. If fathers are routinely denied custody without comparing the parenting abilities of each parent, a belief in biological determinism (e.g., women are naturally better parents) is implied. In another example, the use of tranquilizers predominantly with women in crisis suggests theoretical assumptions about the nature of crisis and the people receiving the drugs (Boston Women's Health Book Collective, 1992; Corea, 1985). Also, crisis theories may rely too exclusively on the experience of ill rather than healthy individuals. As Antonovsky (1980, pp. 35–37) suggests, the crucial question may be, Why do people stay healthy? (salutogenesis) rather than, What makes them sick? (pathogenesis).

Understanding requires an examination of the central concepts of crisis theory. These concepts provide the building blocks for understanding the crisis experience and its resolution. They help answer the following questions about theory-based crisis management:

1. What are the origins of crisis?
2. How are the origins related to prediction and management of crisis?
3. How is crisis related to stress and illness?

4. How does the crisis state develop and how is it manifested?

5. How do different people resolve crises?

6. How does the interaction between natural and formal crisis management work to produce positive crisis outcomes?

In Chapter One, crisis was broadly linked to stress, emergencies, and emotional and mental disturbance. This chapter shows how these distressing situations are related and addresses the questions just listed.

The Origins of Crisis

The importance of examining the origins of crisis is based on the assumption that insight into how a problem begins enhances our chances of dealing with it effectively. Here, the term *origin* is used in the sense of the root source or beginning of a phenomenon—in this case, crisis. Considerations of origins may or may not include speculation about causes, because such an examination is associated with the so-called hard determinism found in the natural sciences. A search for cause-and-effect laws seems questionable in a humanistic framework (Brim & Ryff, 1980, pp. 383–387). This interpretation of origin also suggests that instead of asking what causes crisis, one would examine other matters, such as how some people respond to stressful events by going into crisis and others do not, or the reasons some people resolve crises by problem-solving and growth, some by suicide, and others by chronic emotional illness (Vaillant, 1993). The following discussion clarifies the relationships among crisis origins, risk factors, manifestations, and management strategies, in terms of origins and development. Broadly speaking, crisis origins fall into three categories: *situational* (traditional term: unanticipated); *transitional state* (traditional term: anticipated); and *cultural/social-structural*.

Situational Origins

Crises defined as situational originate from three sources: (1) material or environmental (e.g., fire or natural disaster); (2) personal or physical (e.g., heart attack, diagnosis of fatal illness, loss of limb or other bodily disfigurement from accidents or disease); and (3) interpersonal or social (e.g., death of a loved one or divorce (see Figure 2.1, upper circle, Box 1). Such situations are usually unanticipated. Since the traumatic event leading to possible crisis is unforeseen, one generally can do nothing to prepare for it except in an indirect sense: careful driving habits can reduce the risk of accident; changing risky lifestyle practices such as smoking can reduce the risk of heart attack or cancer; open communication may lessen the chance of divorce; a change in sexual behavior can reduce the risk of contracting AIDS. Crises arising from such cases originate, at least indirectly, from personal life choices. For example, keeping in good physical and psychological health, nurturing a social support system, and avoiding too many changes at one time prepares one indirectly to better handle unforeseen events (Turner & Avison, 1992). In other cases, such as loss of a child by sudden infant death syndrome (SIDS), the origin is simple rather than multifaceted, so if there is inappropriate self-blame in the crisis response, crisis counseling and grief work will usually result in a positive outcome (unless psychopathology was present before the crisis or the death is mistakenly attributed to parental abuse). In crises originating from complex social/cultural or interrelated sources, the implications for intervention are also more complex. At the other end of the spectrum, the stress and possible

FIGURE 2.1. CRISIS PARADIGM.

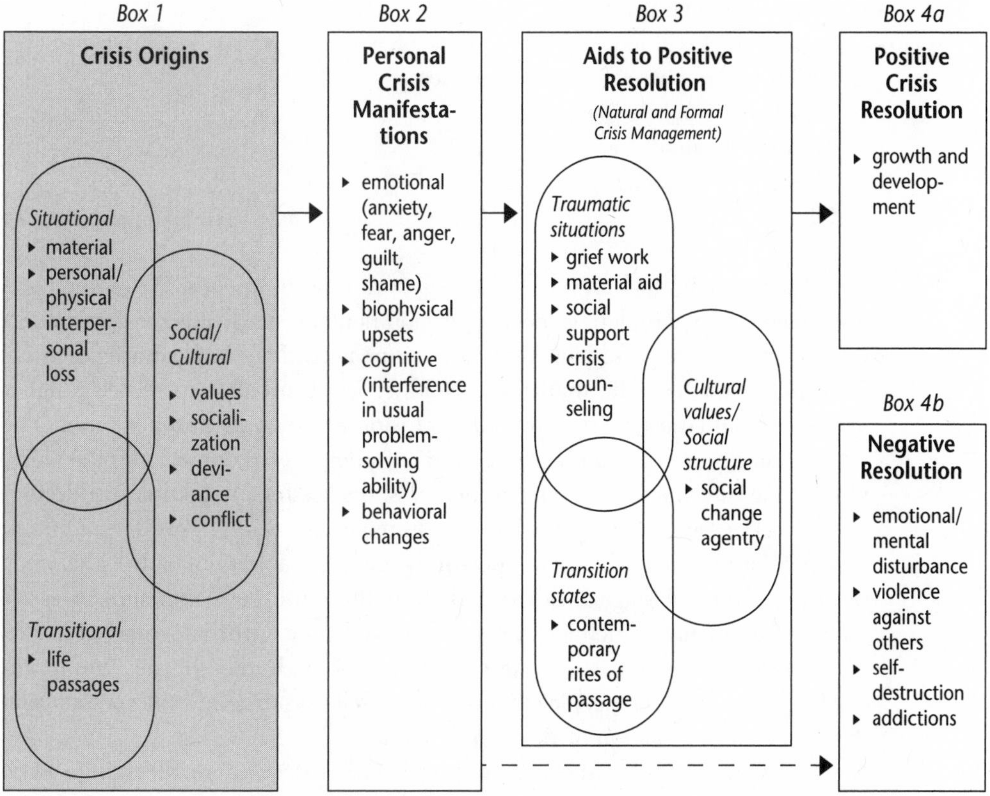

Crisis origins, manifestations, and outcomes, and the respective functions of crisis management have an interactional relationship. The intertwined circles represent the distinct yet interrelated origins of crisis and aids to positive resolution, even though personal manifestations are often similar. The arrows pointing from origins to positive resolution illustrate the *opportunity for growth and development* through crisis; the broken line at bottom depicts the potential *danger of crisis* in the absence of appropriate aids.

crisis originating from a natural event such as being struck and injured by lightning might be the easiest of all to handle, depending on the degree and type of physical injury.

Transition State Origins

The next broad category of crisis origins, transition states, consists of two types: (1) *universal:* life-cycle or normal transitions consisting of human development phases from conception to death, and (2) *nonuniversal:* passages signaling a shift in social status (see Figure 2.1, lower circle, Box 1). The first type of transition state is universal in that no one escapes life passages, at least not the first and last phases. Erickson (1963) and other developmental psychologists have identified human transition states as follows:

- Prenatal to infancy
- Infancy to childhood
- Childhood to puberty and adolescence
- Adolescence to adulthood
- Maturity to middle age
- Middle age to old age
- Old age to death

During each phase, a person is subject to unique stresses. He or she faces the challenge of completing specific developmental tasks. Failure to do so stunts human growth; the personality does not mature according to its natural potential. And while growth toward maturity is exciting, people usually experience a higher level of anxiety during developmental transition states than at other times. The natural change in roles, body image, and attitudes toward oneself and the world may create internal turmoil and restlessness. Successful completion of developmental tasks requires energy as well as nurturance and social approval from others.

With appropriate support, a person is normally able to meet the challenge of growth from one stage of life to another. In this sense, developmental crises are considered normal (Panchuck, 1994) and thus can be anticipated and prepared for. Developmental transition states need not be nightmarish; they can be rewarding times in which people enjoy a sense of self-mastery and achievement from the successful completion of developmental tasks.

Stress and turmoil can occur during periods of developmental change when the individual does not receive the normal social supports needed for the process of maturation. And each successive stage of development is affected by what took place in the previous phase. For some, the challenge of human growth is indeed a nightmare; life's turning points become crises with destructive effects rather than normal periods of change and challenge. Some people greet adolescence, middle age, and old age with suicide attempts, depression, or withdrawal to a closed, more secure, and familiar world. They approach life with a deep rejection of self and suspicion of the surrounding world.

The unique challenge in life is to move forward, not to stagnate or regress. For some, however, various situational factors make this a seemingly impossible task. Developmental challenges are particularly acute for young people today who are growing up in violent communities where economic security and other dreams are never born or are quickly dashed by multiple stressors and tragic events.

The other category of transition states—nonuniversal—includes turning points such as the change from student to worker or worker (including homemaker) to student. Migration and retirement are other examples. Crises originating from such sources differ from situational crises. Like the developmental transition states, nonuniversal passages are usually anticipated and people can prepare for them. Unlike developmental transitions, however, everyone does not experience them. And some transitions, such as relocation because of refugee status in a war-torn country, are complicated by cultural and economic factors. The transition states (universal and nonuniversal) from which some crises stem can be seen not only as markers along life's pathway but as processes that can develop in positive or negative directions (Danish, Smyer, & Nowak, 1980, p. 342; see Chapter Thirteen).

Crises developing from situational and transitional states are the easiest to understand and to handle successfully. The personal values involved in resolving such crises generally do not clash with common interpretations of life's experiences. For example, if one loses precious possessions and is left homeless by a fire caused by arson, one's ability to handle the stress involved is generally assisted by a knowledge of laws designed to bring the arsonist to justice and by insurance, which may partially compensate for the material loss. To summarize, situational crises and crises arising from transition states are distinct yet related. An individual in a major transition state is usually vulnerable. When the stress of an unanticipated traumatic event is added, however, the person is even more likely to experience a crisis since his or her coping capacity may be strained to the limit by these combined stressors.

To illustrate, let us consider Carol and Jim, who demonstrate a capacity for growth and development around divorce.

CASE EXAMPLE: CAROL AND JIM

Carol, age thirty-eight, and Jim, age thirty-six, decide mutually to obtain a divorce. They have been married thirteen years and have two children: Dean, age twelve, and Cindy, age nine. Together, they work out a custody and visiting agreement, satisfying their desires and taking the children's wishes into consideration. Carol and Jim had essen-tially untroubled childhoods and feel secure and confident as individuals. They can, therefore, avoid the common tactic of using their children as weapons against each other. The divorce is decidedly a source of stress to Dean and Cindy, but neither of the children experiences it as a crisis. Both parents are mature in their marital and parental roles;

thus, Carol and Jim do not deny their children the nurturance they continue to need
from each of them. Nor is the divorce a crisis
for either spouse. In fact, both saw their mar-

riage as limiting their personal growth. The
decision to divorce is not a crisis; rather, as
Maslow (1970) shows, it is an occasion for
further self-actualization or growth.

Many divorces, however, are more tumultuous than this couple's; many are
tragic. For example, in an abusive marriage, a man may greet the news of divorce
with a threat to kill first his wife and then himself (see Chapters Eight and Nine).
These cases, in their contrasting manifestations, illustrate (1) the highly subjective
nature of the crisis experience; (2) the various factors that influence the development of a crisis state; and (3) the intrinsic relationships among transitional, situational, and sociocultural influences on the crisis experience.

Cultural/Social-Structural Origins

Crises arising from cultural values and the social structure include job loss stemming from discrimination on the basis of age, race, gender, disability, or sexual
identity. In contrast, job loss from illness or poor personal performance can be
viewed as a result of a prior crisis or illness (see Figure 2.1, right circle, Box 1). Job
loss occurring from discriminatory treatment in the work force is rooted in cultural values about the diversity issues noted above—values that are embedded in
the social structure. Also in this category are crises resulting from deviant acts of
others, behavior that violates accepted social norms: robbery, rape, incest, marital infidelity, physical abuse. Crises from these sources are never truly expected;
there is something shocking and catastrophic about them. Yet in a sense they are
predictable. An older, infirm woman living in a high-crime area is more likely to
be attacked than a stronger and younger person. Other examples of cultural/
social-structural crises include the institutionalization of older people if motivated
by ageism and values about the nuclear family structure; violence against children
and women (related to values about discipline, women, and social-structural factors in the family); and residential dislocation (related to economic, class, and ethnic issues such as gentrification—the displacement of the poor by those better off
economically— during the renovation of urban centers).

In general, crises originating from sociocultural sources are less amenable to
control by individuals than crises arising from personal action. Thus, a person in
a racial minority group facing a housing crisis due to suspected discrimination and
a woman in job crisis due to alleged gender discrimination must be prepared to
confront the bureaucratic justice system. To avoid the downward spiral to be
discussed later in this chapter (see Figure 2.2), *social* factors should not be mis-
construed as *personal* liabilities producing crises. Consider the challenge of resolving a crisis that originates from the following twist in justice: a woman is
brutally beaten and threatened with her life; she and her children are left home-

less, while the man who has committed these crimes against her enjoys the comfort and security of the marital dwelling. This example of battering also illustrates the interrelationships among crisis origins. That is, an abused woman may suffer physical injury and loss of home (situational events) and be forced into a status change from married to single (transitional), but the *primary* origin of her crisis can be traced to cultural values about women, the socialization of boys and men toward aggression, and a widespread cultural climate approving of violence in the form of war, capital punishment, and pornography (Hoff 1990). Therefore, intervention strategies focused only on the upper and lower circles (see Figure 2.1, Box 3) without attention to social change strategies and public compensation for the woman's injuries usually will not be sufficient. Interrelated crisis origins are also apparent in the high suicide rates of gay, lesbian, and bisexual youth, and in people with AIDS, their families, and caretakers.

To illustrate further, note the difference in the element of control in the following crisis situations: (1) a heavy cigarette smoker with full knowledge of the evidence linking smoking to lung cancer receives a diagnosis of lung cancer; more than likely, insurance benefits will be available even though the illness results from a self-chosen high-risk lifestyle; (2) a Japanese-American survivor of the nuclear bomb blast at Hiroshima receives a diagnosis of leukemia; the victim is refused insurance coverage for the required medical care by private insurers and the United States government (*Survivors*, 1982, pp. 17–18).

A more complex example of crisis from these sociocultural sources involves the perpetrators of deviant acts. Here social and personal elements are intertwined. For example, the parents of an infant they have abused and brought to a hospital for treatment will probably be in crisis, as will a mother who loses custody of her children because of drug abuse. Such child abuse and neglect may be rooted in cultural values about physical discipline, mothers (as opposed to mothers and fathers together) as primary child rearers, and socioeconomic factors. Even though such deviance may be strongly influenced by social and cultural factors, individual perpetrators of violence against others need to be carefully considered for personal liability.

These illustrations provide a preview of the relationship between origins of crisis and strategies of intervention (to be discussed in detail in later chapters). For example, it seems ironic that tranquilizers, grief work, or psychotherapy might be considered the treatment of choice for Hiroshima survivors in crisis over the news of their nuclear-induced cancers; as will be shown in Chapter Ten, political action is more appropriate since the source of the crisis is political.

In short, whenever a crisis originates outside an individual, it is usually beyond the power of the person alone to gain control and manage successfully (Baum, Cohen, & Hall, 1993; Cloward & Piven, 1979; Gerhardt, 1979). Thus, the person is usually more vulnerable and has greater difficulty making sense of the traumatic event and avoiding negative coping strategies than when origins are situational or transitional (Perloff, 1983; Ryff & Essex, 1992; Sales, Baum, & Shore,

1984; Silver, Boon, & Stones, 1983). Therefore, public, social strategies should accompany any individual interventions on behalf of people whose crises originate in the sociocultural milieu.

Interrelationships Between Crisis Origins and Development

Identifying the origins of a crisis, important as that is, is only one step in the crisis management process. Various situational, developmental, and sociocultural factors do not in themselves constitute a crisis state. The factors placing people at risk vary and interact to produce a crisis that is manifested in emotional, cognitive, behavioral, and biophysical responses to traumatic life events (see Figure 2.1, Box 2).

Developmentalists Danish, Smyer, and Nowak (1980, pp. 342–345) cite several factors that affect how a person responds to events:

- *Timing:* For example, a first marriage at age sixteen or forty may be more stressful than at other times.
- *Duration:* This factor highlights the process aspect of life events such as pregnancy or retirement.
- *Sequencing:* For example, the birth of a child before marriage is usually more stressful than after.
- *Cohort specificity:* For example, a man becomes a house-husband and a woman a corporate executive.
- *Contextual purity:* This refers to how the event relates to other events and the lives of other people.
- *Probability of occurrence:* For example, the majority of married women will become widows.

The clinical relevance of these factors can be seen in Schulberg and Sheldon's (1968, pp. 553–558) probability formulation for assessing which persons are most crisis-prone:

1. *The probability that a disturbing and hazardous event will occur:* Death of close family members is highly probable, whereas natural disasters are very improbable.
2. *The probability that an individual will be exposed to the event:* Every adolescent faces the challenge of adult responsibilities, whereas fewer people face the crisis of an unwanted move from their settled dwelling.
3. *The vulnerability of the individual to the event:* The mature adult can adapt more easily to the stress of moving than a child in the first year of school or a retired person who has lived a long time in one community.

In assessing risk, then, one should consider (1) the degree of stress stemming from a hazardous event; (2) the risk of people being exposed to that event; and (3) the person's vulnerability or ability to adapt to the stress (Schulberg & Sheldon,

1968). Such probability predictions are an important preliminary to the prevention and enhancement activities discussed in Chapter One.

CASE EXAMPLE: DOROTHY

Dorothy, age thirty-eight, has been treated for depression three times during the past nine years. Before her marriage and the birth of her three children, Dorothy held a job as a secretary and now works part-time. Dorothy's husband, a company executive, accepted a job transfer to a new location in another city. This city is known for its hostile attitudes toward African-American families like Dorothy's. Dorothy dreaded the move and considered joining her husband a few months later. She thought this would allow her some time to see whether her husband's job placement was permanent. However, she abandoned the idea because she dreaded being away from her husband that long. One month after the move, Dorothy made a suicide attempt, and her husband took her to a hospital psychiatric unit.

In this case, the initial probability of the occurrence of the hazardous event—the move—was small. The probability of Dorothy's exposure to the event was high, considering her marital status and her dependence on her husband. Her racial identity made her more vulnerable to stress from sociocultural sources such as housing discrimination. Her vulnerability, in view of her past history, was also very high. Taken together, these factors put Dorothy at great risk for crisis. Recent research on vulnerability to life events underscores the emotional cost of caring for women like Dorothy. That is, women are more exposed to acute life stresses because of nurturant role expectations and greater concern for events that happen to significant others in their social network, with a consequent increased risk of depression (Conger, et al., 1993; Kessler & McLeod, 1984; Turner & Avison, 1992). For women like Dorothy, the risk further increases if they are faced with a hazardous event such as the death of a husband.

In the Schulberg and Sheldon formulation, the probability factors that contribute to a favorable outcome of crisis include the following:

1. The person who encounters and resolves a great number and variety of difficult situations is less likely to experience a crisis in future hazardous circumstances.
2. The person who has, or thinks he or she has, the ability to resolve a problem, is likely to resolve that problem successfully.
3. The person who has strong social supports is very likely to resolve life crises successfully and without destructive effects.

In another example, George Sloan—the subject of an upcoming Case Example—is affected by the concurrence of crisis with his son's school problem and his wife's menopause. Also, if Deborah and her family, who were discussed in

Chapter One, are from a racial minority group, the chance is increased that racially related stress on the job contributed to her heart attack; risk for future job-related crises is also increased due to her position in the social structure based on race.

The case of a family in crisis as a result of a teenager's suicide attempt also suggests the interactional aspect of crisis origins. While the teenager's crisis may stem directly from personal feelings of failure and worthlessness and indirectly from family conflict, the family's crisis of dealing with a suicidal member is usually affected by the culturally situated stigma still attached to self-destructive behavior (see Chapter Six).

These illustrations link the origins of crisis to life events, sociocultural factors, and personal values that influence the development and subjective manifestations of crisis in different individuals. This discussion highlights the need to identify specific crisis origins during assessment and to tailor intervention strategies to distinctive or interrelated origins. Appropriate strategies will increase the probability of positive crisis resolution and growth (see Figure 2.1, Box 3). Details of such assessment and intervention strategies are presented in the remainder of the book.

Stress, Crisis, and Illness

Theories and research on stress and coping occupy a prominent position in the literature of psychology, sociology, nursing, medicine, and epidemiology (Bebbington, et al., 1993; Brown, 1993; Brown & Harris, 1978; Dohrenwend & Dohrenwend, 1984; Hurwicz, et al., 1992; Killeen, 1990; Levine & Scotch, 1970). The issue of coping with stressful life events often revolves around the relationship between stress and illness; virtually all authorities agree that stress and illness are related. The questions for this book are as follows:

- Do stressful life events cause illness, and if so, what is the process involved?
- Do sick people experience more stressful life events than healthy people?
- To what extent do social and psychological resources buffer the impact of stressful life events?
- What effect, if any, do "resistance resources" (Antonovsky, 1980) have on stress arising from the social structure, that is, from race, class, gender, or age disparity?
- What is the relationship between stress and the concept and experience of crisis?

Imprecise definitions can create problems with these questions; sometimes the concepts of stress, crisis, and illness are used interchangeably. The following definitions may clarify the discussion:

Stress is described by Selye (1956, p. 15) as a specific syndrome that is nonspecifically induced. Stress can also be viewed as a relationship between the person and the environment (McElroy & Townsend, 1985). Ramsey (1982, p. 30) notes that the word *stress* has an indefinite meaning and that it symbolizes different things to people of various disciplines. For this book, stress is defined as the discomfort, pain, or troubled feeling arising from emotional, social, or physical sources and resulting in the need to relax, be treated, or otherwise seek relief. Stress is of two types: (1) *acute stress* is brief in duration and occurs with fairly predictable manifestations and results, one of which may be crisis; (2) *insidious stress* is longer in duration (weeks, months, or years) with less awareness by the person experiencing it and with long-range cumulative but less clearly certain effects, which may include burnout and disease (Landy, 1977, p. 311). Stress is inherent in the fact of living and may be experienced from any source: invasion of the body by organisms, internal psychological turmoil, cultural values, and social organization.

Burnout is a fairly recent concept. Spaniol and Caputo (1979, p. 2) define burnout as "the inability to cope adequately with the stresses of our work or personal lives." Freudenberger and Richelson (1980, p. 2) refer to burnout as a "malaise . . . a demon both of the society and times we live in and our ongoing struggle to invest our lives with meaning." It is manifested in physical signs and symptoms, feelings of cynicism, anger, and resentment, and poor social performance at home and work. Cherniss (1980) discusses the issue of burnout for staff in the human services. Burnout is distinguished from crisis by its chronic rather than acute character. Also, people suffering from burnout often are not aware of the connection between their feelings, their behavior, and the chronic stress they are under.

Disease is a pathological concept describing a condition that can be objectively verified through clinical observation and various laboratory tests (Foster & Anderson, 1978, p. 40). Such objective organic lesions or behavioral disturbances are observable by others regardless of the "diseased" person's awareness of them (Dubos, 1977, p. 32).

Illness is related to disease but is distinguished by its subjective character. It is a cultural concept that implies the social recognition that one cannot carry out expected social roles (Foster & Anderson, 1978, p. 40). For instance, a person may have an early cancerous lesion but not feel ill. Once the lesion is diagnosed as cancer, though, the person is considered ill and the social, psychological, and cultural dimensions of the disease surface: stigma, denial, fear of death. Illness may be claimed subjectively as a reason for inability to perform normally. For example, a person may say, "I don't feel well . . . I have a backache" (a condition not easily diagnosed), although no objective indicators of disease may be present. Thus, illness can be seen as

- *Punishment,* for example, "What did I do to deserve cancer?"
- *Deviance,* such as Parsons's (1951) concept of the "sick role"
- *An indicator of social system performance,* for example, absenteeism due to "illness," although the real reason is job dissatisfaction
- *A social control device,* for example, attaching a psychiatric label to battered women

- *A response to stress* from physical, environmental, social, psychological, or cultural sources (Foster & Anderson, 1978, pp. 145–153; Lieban 1977, pp. 24–27; McElroy & Townsend, 1985, pp. 268–325)

Emotional breakdown is an inability to manage one's feelings to the point of chronic interference in normal functioning; it is manifested in depression, anger, fear, and so on.

Mental breakdown is a disturbance in cognitive functioning manifested in the general inability to think and act normally. It progresses to the point of interference in the expression of feelings, everyday behavior, and interaction with others.

Crisis is an acute emotional upset affecting one's ability to cope emotionally, cognitively, or behaviorally and to solve problems by usual devices.

Research on stress, crisis, and emotional and mental breakdown reveals a lack of integration between clinical and social science insights (Pearlin & Schooler 1978). There is a need to correct the imbalance between clinical and developmental/social analysis of coping with stressful life events (Brim & Ryff, 1980, pp. 376–377; Gerhardt, 1979, p. 196; Pearlin & Schooler, 1978, p. 2). Researchers trained clinically and in social science may be able to bridge some of these gaps. However, the influence of medicalization and causal scientific models in all branches of human service practice has pervaded the stress research field.

A noted example of stress research that excludes personal meaning is the Holmes and Rahe (1967) Social Readjustment Rating Scale, designed to predict one's risk of illness or accident based on a cumulative stress score from life events. The scale is useful in sensitizing people to the various events in their lives that might be sources of stress, potential crisis, illness, or accidents. The assumption here is that awareness of potentially hazardous events enhances the possibility of constructive preventive action by the individual, as discussed in Chapter One. However, the scale omits the individual's interpretation of events, which influences whether the experience of stress is positive or negative. Sarason, Johnson, and Siegel, in a revised scale (1978), have reduced the deficiency of the Holmes and Rahe scale by providing an opportunity to evaluate various events in positive or negative terms.

Conclusions from much of the research on stress point to the limitations of causal models in the analysis of stress (Brim & Ryff, 1980, pp. 383–387). Increasing attention, however, is being directed to studying the process of stress and its relationship to hazardous events, illness, coping, and social support (Caplan, 1981; Hoff, 1990; Kessler & McLeod, 1984; Pearlin, et al., 1981).

Overly simplistic psychological accounts of stress and illness are not the only problem in the crisis intervention field. Durkheim's (1951) notion that people's positions in the social structure—lack of social integration and a sense of attachment to society—are causes of anomic and egoistic suicides is a prime example of sociological reductionism; it fails to account for differences in the way individuals interpret and cope with stressful life events from various sources. While cause-and-effect laws certainly operate with regard to the physical stressors of a gunshot wound to the heart or repeated inhalation of carcinogens—these stressors do cause death or lung cancer, respectively—*social action* such as suicide or violence against others cannot be explained within the same causal framework (Cicourel, 1964; Hoff, 1990; Louch, 1966). What is the relevance of reductionist causal reasoning to crisis response and management?

Acute or chronic stress does not automatically lead to emotional imbalance or mental incompetence, abuse of alcohol and other drugs, suicide, or assault on others. If it did, humans, who by nature are rational, conscious, and responsible for their behavior could routinely attribute their behavior to causes external to themselves and be excused from accountability. This, in fact, is the case in certain instances where mitigating circumstances allow an excuse for some behaviors that might otherwise be punishable. In general, however, responses to stress vary. Maslow's (1970) research, for example, underscores the apparent growth-promoting function of high-stress situations for achieving self-actualization, not destruction of self and others. Antonovsky's (1980) cross-cultural research on concentration camp survivors and women in menopause suggests similar conclusions. He proposes the concept of "resistance resources" (pp. 99–100)—including social network support and a "sense of coherence" (SOC)—as intervening variables in stressful situations. Such resources can make the difference between positive or negative responses to developmental transitions or to extreme stress (which a clinician might define as crisis) such as that experienced by concentration camp survivors. Research with battered women (Hoff, 1990) supports these views and the position taken in this book: stress, crisis, and illness (physical, emotional, and mental) are interactionally, not causally, related.

The Crisis/Psychiatric Illness Interface

Another argument about the relationship between stress, crisis, and illness concerns the traditional belief that crises of violence against women are precipitated by a woman's provocative behavior, presumably arising from her own emotional or mental disturbance. There is little evidence to support such a blame-the-victim conclusion (Hilberman, 1980; Ryan, 1971). The work of Rieker and Carmen (1986) and Hoff (1990), for example, reveals that the women's emotional symptoms do not *cause* battering, but rather, they occur almost invariably *after* the women have been victimized, both physically and psychologically.

Figure 2.2 illustrates this process in the downward spiral toward illness, a process which, for assault victims especially, usually begins with the misassignment of responsibility for the violence and abuse. Such a descent toward maladaptation can also occur in cases of oppression and discrimination based on race or sexual identity, for example. Key to this downward, possibly self-destructive or violent course is the process of *internalizing* blame or oppression originating from socio-

FIGURE 2.2. ABUSE, THE DOWNWARD SPIRAL, AND ALTERNATIVE PATH.

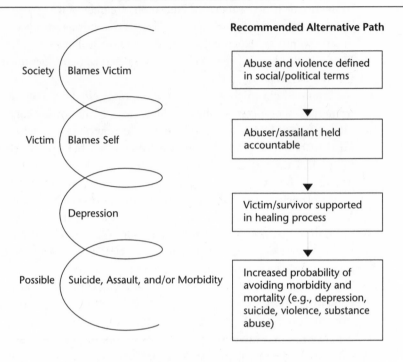

Recommended Alternative Path

Society | Blames Victim

Abuse and violence defined in social/political terms

Victim | Blames Self

Abuser/assailant held accountable

Depression

Victim/survivor supported in healing process

Possible | Suicide, Assault, and/or Morbidity

Increased probability of avoiding morbidity and mortality (e.g., depression, suicide, violence, substance abuse)

Primary prevention is ideal, but intervention at
Secondary and *Tertiary* levels can also
prevent morbidity and save lives.

cultural sources. Once a person or group inappropriately absorbs blame for others' actions and takes on the identity of victim, helplessness and/or horizontal violence—venting rage on people of one's own group, as in black-on-black violence—may prevent the proper channeling of anger toward personal healing and social change (see Figure 2.1, Box 3).

Thus, it is crucial to simultaneously acknowledge the pain of victimization and oppression but not lose sight of the fact that a downward spiral is not inevitable. Most important, then, for survival and growth beyond victimhood are social support and education toward a perspective that envisions the possibility of action and social change (Hoff, 1990; Wendell, 1990). Note that Figure 2.2 includes these alternatives to the downward spiral.

One of the most popular notions surrounding women's crises stemming from violence is that the violent man is under high stress. To the extent that this explanation is accepted, the person's violence is excused on the basis of presumed mental incompetence. While it is true that the extreme stress and anxiety associated with a crisis state can distort cognitive functions such as memory and decision making, mental incompetence would not be assumed if history revealed that the perpetrator's mental faculties were intact *before* the crisis (see Chapter Three). Thus, a person's decision to hit or kill his or her spouse during the high tension of a marital fight is neither wise nor excusable. Most social research (e.g., Gelles, 1974) supports the proposition that temporary insanity claims are really excuses used to evade responsibility for one's violent behavior. Another excusing claim is that the woman "asked for it." This does not negate recognition that some crimes are committed by people who are diagnosed as mentally ill according to commonly accepted criteria such as having delusions, hallucinations, or exhibiting bizarre behavior. Some recent jury acquittals of women who killed their husbands suggest that these women were not viewed as mentally ill; rather, the stress and danger of their circumstances after years of abuse were considered sufficient grounds for acquittal. Similarly, many men are excused from their battering, while some are convicted. One of the most striking findings of Hoff's (1990) research with battered women was the women's tendency to excuse their *husbands'* violence but not their *own* retaliatory violence, even if the wives were under the influence of drugs or alcohol. When women are convicted of murdering their husbands, however, research suggests gross discriminatory practices (Browne, 1987; Jones, 1980).

There is a remarkable similarity between these findings and those in Erich Lindemann's classic study (1944): survivors of the Cocoanut Grove disaster might have been spared the negative experience of serious psychopathology if they had had assistance, such as with grief work, at the time of the crisis. Battered women without resources and assistance for constructive crisis resolution may start the downward course and become suicidal, homicidal, addicted, or emotionally disturbed, especially after repeated abuse (see Chapter Eight). The reciprocal relationship between stress, crisis, and illness is observed further in the multifaceted stressors a battered woman must deal with while in crisis after a violent attack: physical injury, psychological upset, and change in her social situation (e.g., disrupted marriage or loss of residence or financial support). This relationship is illustrated in Figure 2.3. Similarly, the crisis-illness relationship can be observed among the homeless. When considering how basic home and shelter are for all, the most remarkable evidence of human resilience is the survival of so many people against the greatest of odds and continuing stressors, even with the burden of serious mental disturbance (Hoff, 1993).

In a scientific sense, then, concepts of crisis, stress, and illness are imprecise and complexly associated with the political economy, a medicalized approach to people in distress, social inequality, and dominant values about people and illness in the cultural milieu. Research, however, supports the view of an interactional, rather than causal, relationship between stress, crisis, and illness. What simplistic models miss is the influence of an individual's experience of stress, crisis, and illness. Table 2.1 illustrates the distinctions and relationships between these concepts. It also links the concepts with their origins, providing a preview of the next section and remaining chapters.

FIGURE 2.3. INTERACTIVE RELATIONSHIP BETWEEN *STRESS, CRISIS,* AND POSSIBLE *ILLNESS* IN A BATTERING SITUATION.

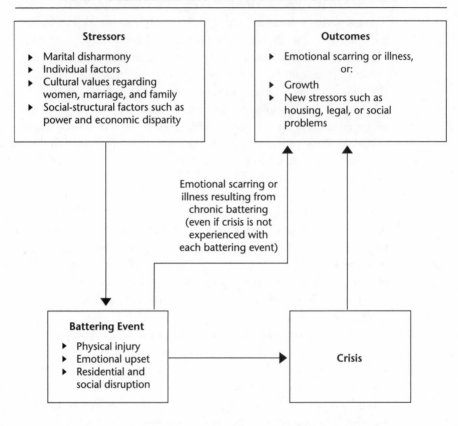

Stressors	**Outcomes**
▸ Marital disharmony ▸ Individual factors ▸ Cultural values regarding women, marriage, and family ▸ Social-structural factors such as power and economic disparity	▸ Emotional scarring or illness, or: ▸ Growth ▸ New stressors such as housing, legal, or social problems

Emotional scarring or illness resulting from chronic battering (even if crisis is not experienced with each battering event)

Battering Event	**Crisis**
▸ Physical injury ▸ Emotional upset ▸ Residential and social disruption	

The arrows suggest the interactional relationship between *stress, crisis,* and *illness.* Trouble and stressors in a marriage can lead to positive or negative outcomes through several different routes, depending on personal, social, and economic circumstances.

Development and Individual Manifestations of Crisis

We have seen how crisis originates from physical, material, personal, social, and cultural sources, as well as how it fits into the larger picture of life's ups and downs. Let us now consider the experience of crisis at the individual, personal level.

Why People Go into Crisis

People in crisis are, by definition, emotionally upset; they are unable to solve life's problems in their usual way. A happy, healthy life implies an ability to solve problems effectively. It also implies that basic human needs are fulfilled. Our basic needs include a sense of physical and psychological well-being, a supportive network of friends, family, and associates, and a sense of identity and belonging to one's society and cultural heritage. Hansell (1976, pp. 31–49) describes our essential needs as the "seven basic attachments." All of us have a stable arrangement of transactions between ourselves and our environment. According to Hansell, we are essentially attached to:

1. Food, oxygen, and other physical supplies necessary to life
2. A strong sense of self-identity
3. At least one other person in a close, mutually supportive relationship
4. At least one group that accepts us as a member
5. One or more roles in which we feel self-respect and can perform with dignity
6. Financial security or a means of participating in an exchange of the goods and services we need and value
7. A comprehensive system of meaning, that is, a set of values that help us to set goals and to understand ourselves and the world around us

People in crisis suffer a sudden loss or threat of loss of a person or thing considered essential and important. One or several of their basic attachments are severed or are at risk of being severed (Hansell, 1976). For example, the shock of the unexpected death of a loved one by car accident or heart attack can leave a person feeling incomplete and at a loss about what to do, where to turn. The individual's familiar source of support and comfort disappears without warning, with no time to adjust to the change. Similar shock occurs in response to the suicide of a friend, threat of divorce, diagnosis of a terminal illness such as AIDS, or an operation such as a mastectomy, which mutilates one's body. A person with AIDS for example, not only loses health and faces the probability of a drastically shortened life cycle but also may be abandoned by friends and family and scorned by would-be helpers.

CASE EXAMPLE: EDWARD

Edward, age forty-five, has been an outstanding assistant director of his company. When he is promoted to the vacated position of executive director, he becomes depressed and virtually nonfunctional. Edward, in spite of external signs of success, lacks basic self-confidence; he cannot face the challenge of the new job. The possibility of failure in his new position is unbearable. His anxiety about success prevents him from achieving the success he desires. Edward is one of the many people who, with the help of family and friends, and perhaps a crisis counselor, can avoid possible failure and depression. He has his whole past career, including many successes, to draw on profitably in his present job. With help, he might see that failure in his present position need not mean the end of a happy and productive life.

TABLE 2.1. DISTRESS DIFFERENTIATION.

Type of Distress or Problem	Origins	Possible Manifestations
Stress (acute)	Hazardous life events (such as heart attack, accident, death of loved one, violent attack, sudden job loss, natural disaster)	Emotional crisis General Adaptation Syndrome
	Invasion by microorganisms	General Adaptation Syndrome Disease process
	Man-made disaster	Annihilation of present civilization
Stress (chronic)	Strain in social relationships (such as marriage)	Burnout
	Position in social structure (age, sex, race, class)	Psychosomatic or stress-related illness
	Socioeconomic problems (such as unemployment)	Emotional or mental breakdown
	Chronic ill health	
	Developmental transition states	
Crisis	Traumatic situations (material, personal/physical, interpersonal)	Emotional Behavioral Cognitive Biophysical $\Big\}$ Changes
	Transition states (developmental and other)	
	Cultural values, social structure	
Emotional or mental breakdown	Failure of positive response to acute stress and/or crisis Continuation of chronic stress from various sources	Neurotic and/or psychotic symptoms (such as learned helplessness or self-denigration of a battered woman)

    Shock and a resulting crisis state can also occur at the time of normal role transitions. For example, Mary, age nineteen, relied very heavily on her mother for advice and support in all aspects of her life. One month after her honeymoon and the move into an apartment with her husband, she became depressed and sui-

Possible Responses		
Positive	**Negative**	**Duration**
Grief work	Failure to ask for and accept help	Brief
Adaptation, emotional and social growth through healthy coping	Suicide, assault, addiction, emotional/mental break-down	
Medical treatment, rest, exercise	Refusal of treatment, complications, possible premature death	
Prevention: Political action	Denial of possibility	
Life-style changes (such as diet, rest, exercise, leisure)	Exacerbation of burnout	Weeks, months, years, or lifetime
Social change strategies	All of the above, and mystification by and response to symptoms vs. sources of chronic stress	
Transition state preparation	Inability to accomplish new role tasks	
Grief work	Same as for acute stress	Few days to 6 weeks
Crisis coping and management by use of personal, social, and material resources		
Prevention: Education about sources of crisis and appropriate preventive action (such as contemporary rites of passage, action to reduce social disparities)		
Reorganization or change of ineffective emotional, cognitive, and behavioral responses to stress and crisis (usually with help of therapy)	Same as all of above, and increased vulnerability to crisis and inability to cope with acute and chronic stress	Weeks, months, years, or lifetime
Action to change social sources of chronic stress		

cidal and was unable to function at home or at work. Mary was obviously not ready for the move from adolescence into the more independent role of a young adult.

Caplan (1964) and Tyhurst (1957) note that for some people a crisis is trig-

CASE EXAMPLE: JOAN

Joan, age nineteen, is another person who cannot meet the challenge of increasing her personal and social resources; she cannot obtain a college credential for teaching and she worries about coming out as a lesbian. She is paralyzed by her fear of the responsibilities involved in a teaching career. At examination time, she is unable to study and fails over half of her college courses. The challenge to increase her "supplies" in preparation for an adult teaching responsibility is more than she can face without additional resources.

gered when they face a particularly challenging psychosocial event. A crisis for such individuals represents a call to new action that they cannot face with their present resources.

How a Crisis Develops

A crisis does not occur instantaneously. There are identifiable phases of development—psychosocial in character—that lead to an active crisis state. These phases were first described by Tyhurst (1957) in his study of individual responses to community disaster. Survivors experience three overlapping phases: (1) a period of impact, (2) a period of recoil, and (3) a post-traumatic period. This breakdown of phases applies most appropriately to crises originating from catastrophic, shocking events such as rape and other violent attacks, the death of a child from sudden infant death syndrome, or sometimes the news of the diagnosis of a terminal disease. (See "Individual Responses to Disaster" in Chapter Ten for a detailed description of these phases.)

Caplan (1964) describes four phases in the development of extreme anxiety and crisis. His description of phases is applicable to crises occurring in a more gradual process from less catastrophic stressors. Recognizing these phases of crisis development helps us to prevent stressful life events from becoming crises.

Phase One. A traumatic event causes an initial rise in one's level of anxiety. The person is in a predicament and responds with familiar problem-solving mechanisms to reduce or eliminate the stress and discomfort stemming from excessive anxiety. For example, John, age thirty-four, is striving toward a career as an executive in his company when he receives a diagnosis of multiple sclerosis. His wife Nancy is very supportive. He adjusts to this unexpected, disturbing event by continuing to work as long as he can. John also has the advantage of the most advanced medical treatment available for multiple sclerosis. In addition, John's physician is skillful in applying his knowledge of the emotional impact of John's diagnosis. At this stage, John's traumatic event does not result in a crisis for him.

Phase Two. In this phase, the person's usual problem-solving ability fails, and the stimulus that caused the initial rise in tension continues. To continue with the illustration of John's case: the disease process is advancing despite excellent medical treatment. John's wife begins to participate less in some of her own activities—including volunteer work—so she can spend more time with her husband. The accumulating medical expenses and loss of work time strain the family's financial resources. John and Nancy receive a report from school that their son Larry, age fourteen, is having behavioral problems. At this stage, since there is greater stress, the possibility of a crisis state for John increases, but a crisis is not inevitable. Whether it occurs or not depends on what happens next in John's life.

Phase Three. In this phase, the individual's anxiety level rises further. The increased tension moves the person to use every resource available—including unusual or new means—to solve the problem and reduce the increasingly painful state of anxiety. In John's case, he fortunately has enough inner strength, confidence, and sensitivity to recognize the strain of his illness on his wife and child. He looks for new ways to cope with his increasing stress. First, he confides in his physician, who responds by taking time to listen and offer emotional support. His physician also arranges for home health services through a visiting nurse agency. This outside health assistance frees Nancy from some of her steadily increasing responsibilities. The physician also encourages John and Nancy to seek help from the school guidance counselor regarding their son, Larry, which they do.

Another way to prevent a crisis state at this phase is to redefine or change one's goals. This means of avoiding crisis is not usually possible for someone who is emotionally isolated from others and feels locked into solving a problem alone. With the help of his physician, John could accept his illness as something that changed his capacity to function in predefined, expected ways. However, he does not have to alter his fundamental ability to live a meaningful, rewarding life because of illness. As John's illness progresses, it becomes necessary to change his role as the sole financial provider in the family. John and Nancy talk openly with each other about the situation. Together, they decide that Nancy will take a job to ease the financial strain. They also ask the nursing agency to increase the home health services, as Nancy is beginning to resent her confinement to the house and the increasing demands of being nurse to her husband.

Phase Four. This is the state of active crisis that results when

- Internal strength and social support are lacking
- The person's problem remains unresolved
- Tension and anxiety rise to an unbearable degree

An active crisis does not occur in John's case because he is able to respond constructively to his unanticipated illness. John has natural social supports and is able to use available help, so his stress does not become unbearable. The example of John illustrates how a full-blown crisis (phase four) can be avoided by various decisions and actions taken during any one of the three preceding phases.

   The following example of George Sloan is in sharp contrast to that of John. George's case will be continued and discussed in subsequent chapters.

CASE EXAMPLE: GEORGE SLOAN—PHASES OF CRISIS DEVELOPMENT

George Sloan, age forty-eight, works as a machinist with a construction company. Six evenings a week he works a second job as a taxi driver in a large metropolitan area. His beat includes high-crime sections of the city. He has just come home from the hospital after his third heart attack. The first occurred when he was forty-four and the second when he was forty-seven.

Phase One: George is advised by his physician to cut down on his work hours. Specifically, the doctor recommends that he give up his second job and spend more time relaxing with family and friends. George's physician recognizes his patient's vulnerability to heart attacks, especially in relation to his lifestyle. George rarely slows down. He is chronically angry about things going wrong and about not being able to get ahead financially. He receives his physician's advice with mixed feelings. On the one hand, he sees the relationship between his heavy work schedule and his heart attacks; on the other hand, he resents what he acknowledges as a necessary change to reduce further risk of death by heart attack.

   In any case, George's health and financial problems markedly increase his usual level of anxiety. He talks superficially to his wife, Marie, about his dilemma but receives little support or understanding from her; their marital relationship is already strained. Marie suggests that in place of George's second job, she increase her part-time job to full-time. George cannot accept this because of what it implies about his image of himself as the chief provider.

   George's discouragement and anger about not getting ahead are aggravated by Marie's complaints of never having enough money for the things she wants. George also resents what he perceives as the physician's judgment that he is not strong enough to do two jobs. At this stage, George is in a precrisis state with a high degree of stress and anxiety.

   Phase Two: George fails to obtain relief from his anxiety by talking with his wife. He does not feel comfortable talking with his physician about his reluctance to cut down the work stress as advised. When he attempts to do so, he senses that the physician is rushed. So he concludes that his doctor is only concerned about giving technical advice, not about how George handles the advice. The prospect of quitting his second job and bringing home less money leaves George feeling like a failure as a supporter of his family. His initial conflict and the rise in tension continue. If he quits his second job, he cannot preserve his image as an adequate family provider; yet he cannot reduce the risk of death by heart disease if he continues his present pace. Help from other resources seems out of his reach.

Phase Three: George's increased anxiety moves him to try talking with his wife again. Ordinarily, he would have abandoned the idea based on the response he had received earlier. Thus, this action constitutes an unusual effort for him, but he fails again in getting the help he needs. To make matters worse, George and Marie learn that their sixteen-year-old son, Arnold, has been suspended from school for a week due to suspected drug involvement. This leaves George feeling like even more of a failure, since he is seldom home during normal family hours. Also, Marie nags him about not spending enough time with the children. George's high level of anxiety becomes so obvious that Marie finally suggests, "Why don't you talk to the doctor about whatever's bothering you." George knows that this is a good idea but cannot bring himself to do it. He had been brought up to believe that somehow it is unmanly to get outside help to solve one's problems. His image of himself as the strong, masculine supporter of the family makes it impossible for him to give up his second job, although he knows the risks involved in continuing. For the same reason, he cannot bear the thought of his wife's working full-time, though she herself has proposed the idea several times. Personality and social factors block him from redefining or changing his goals as a means of problem resolution and crisis prevention. Financial concerns, along with the new problem of his son, further increase his anxiety level. George is in a predicament he does not know how to resolve.

Phase Four: George is at a complete loss about how to deal with all the stress in his life—the threat to his health and life if he continues his present pace, the threat to his self-image if he quits the second job, the failure to communicate with his wife, and the sense of failure and guilt in his role as a parent. His anxiety increases to the breaking point:

- He feels hopeless.
- He does not know where to turn.
- He is in a state of active crisis.

George's case illustrates situational (heart disease), maturational (adolescent changes), and sociocultural (sex-role stereotyping) factors in the development of life crises. It also highlights the subjective elements that contribute to a crisis state at different times in people's lives. George's heart disease was clearly an unanticipated, stressful event. His son Arnold's threat of suspension was unanticipated and a source of added stress. Yet, Arnold's adolescence was anticipated as a normal phase of human development. If George's heart disease had developed at a time when his marriage was less strained, he might have received more help and support. Also, Arnold might have made it through adolescence without school suspension if there had been regular support from both parents. As it turned out, George and Marie had their first report of Arnold's behavior problems in school shortly after George's first heart attack four years earlier. They were advised at that time to seek family or marital counseling; they did, but only for a single session. Finally, socialization of George and Marie to stereotypical male and female roles was an added source of stress and a barrier to constructive crisis resolution.

For another person, such as John in the previous case, or for George at another time of life, the same medical diagnosis and the same advice could have had an altogether different effect. This is also true for Arnold. A different response from his parents when he gave his first signals of distress, or a more constructive approach from school officials and counselors, might have prevented the additional stress of Arnold's school suspension. Or, different cultural expectations for husbands and wives could have altered each person's interpretation of the stressful situation.

The Duration and Outcomes of Crisis

People cannot stay in crisis forever. The state of crisis and the accompanying anxiety are too painful. There is a natural time limitation to the crisis experience because the individual cannot survive indefinitely in such a state of psychological turmoil. The emotional discomfort stemming from extreme anxiety moves the person toward action to reduce the anxiety to an endurable level as soon as possible. This aspect of the crisis experience underscores the *danger* and the *opportunity* that crisis presents.

Experience with people in crisis has led to the observation that the acute emotional upset lasts from a few days to a few weeks. The person must then move toward some sort of resolution; this is often expressed in terms such as: "I can't go on like this anymore"; "Something has got to give"; "Please, tell me what to do to get out of this mess—I can't stand it"; or "I feel like I'm losing my mind."

What, then, happens to the person in crisis? Several outcomes are possible:

1. The person can return to his or her precrisis state. This happens as a result of effective problem solving, made possible by internal strength, values, and social supports. Such an outcome does not necessarily imply new psychological growth as a result of the experience; the person simply returns to his or her usual state of being.
2. The person may not only return to the precrisis state but can grow from the crisis experience through discovery of new resources and ways of solving problems. These discoveries result from the crisis experience itself. John's case is a good example of such growth. He took advantage of resources available to him and his family, such as his physician and the school guidance counselor. He found new ways of solving problems. The result for John was a process of growth: (a) His concept of himself as a worthwhile person was reinforced in spite of the loss of physical integrity from his illness. (b) He strengthened his

marriage and ability to relate to his wife regarding a serious problem. This produced growth for both of them. (c) He developed in his role as a father by constructively handling the problem with his son in addition to his own personal stress.

3. The person responds to his or her problem by lapsing into neurotic, psychotic, or destructive patterns of behavior. For example, the individual may become very withdrawn, suspicious, or depressed. His or her distorted perception of events may be exaggerated to the point of blaming others inappropriately for the misfortunes experienced. Others in crisis resolve their problems, at least temporarily, by excessive drinking or other drug abuse, or by impulsive disruptive behavior. Still others resort to more extreme measures by attempting or committing suicide or by abusing or killing others.

All of these negative and destructive outcomes of the crisis experience occur when the individual lacks constructive ways of solving life's problems and relieving intolerable anxiety. George, for example, came to the conclusion in his despair that he was worth more dead than alive. Consequently, he was brought to the hospital emergency department after a car crash. George crashed his car deliberately but did not die as he had planned. This was his chosen method of suicidal death, which he thought would spare his family the stigma of suicide. He felt that he had already overburdened them. George's case will be continued in Chapters Three and Four with respect to his treatment in the emergency service and his follow-up care.

Considering all of the possible outcomes of a crisis experience, it becomes obvious that helpers should have the following goals:

- To help people in crisis at least return to their precrisis state
- To do everything possible to help people grow and become stronger as a result of the crisis and effective problem solving
- To be alert to danger signals in order to prevent negative, destructive outcomes of a crisis experience

The last goal is achieved by recognizing that negative results of crisis are often not necessary; they occur because of insensitivity and a lack of appropriate resources and crisis management skills in the human service sector (see Figure 2.1, Boxes 4a and 4b).

The Sociocultural Context of Personal Crisis

The contrasting cases of John (with multiple sclerosis) and George (with a heart attack) illustrate both the success and limitations of individual approaches to life crises. Let us suppose that John and George each had identical help available from human service agencies. If George's crisis response is rooted partially in social and cultural sources—as seems to be the case—then intervention must address these factors in order to be successful. Otherwise, unattended social and cultural issues can form a barrier to a strictly psychological crisis counseling approach. They also underscore McKinlay's (1990) argument about downstream versus upstream endeavors and link individual crisis management efforts to complimentary preventive strategies and social change action.

Preventive strategies were discussed in the previous chapter. Individual and social network crisis intervention approaches are considered in detail in the remaining chapters. Social action ideas are incorporated in relevant cases throughout the book. The social change aspects of comprehensive crisis work belong to the *follow-up* phase of the total process. In the Crisis Paradigm, such social change strategies are illustrated in the right circle of Box 3, corresponding to sociocultural crisis origins in Box 1. However, the foundation for such action is laid in one of the cognitive aspects of healthy crisis resolution, that is, in *understanding* the traumatic event, its sources, and how it affects the way one feels during crisis. For example, a rape victim can be helped to understand that she feels guilty and dirty about being raped, not because she is in fact guilty and dirty, but because of the widely accepted social value that women are responsible if they are raped because they dress provocatively, hitchhike, or in a similar way allegedly provoke the attack (see Figure 2.2).

The tradition among human service workers of claiming "value-neutrality" may cause some to object to including social change strategies as a formal part of service. Yet to offer only short-term crisis counseling or psychotherapy for problems stemming from cultural and social origins is value-laden in itself; that is, it suggests that the person adjust to a disadvantaged position in society rather than develop and act on an awareness of the underlying factors contributing to depression or suicidal feelings (e.g., Burstow, 1992; Chesler, 1972; Cloward & Piven 1979; Kessler & McLeod 1984; McNamee & Gergen, 1992). As Johnson (1990, p. 230) points out, professionals who focus solely on purportedly neutral "clinical" material and avoid "this policy stuff" shortchange themselves and clients whose crises are linked to various policy issues. Thus, it is not a question of whether crisis workers are value-free, since such work is almost inevitably affected by our values. Rather, values should be made explicit so that clients can make their own choices (such as accepting or acting on their disadvantaged position) from a more enlightened base.

Social Change Strategies in Comprehensive Crisis Approaches

Since readers are perhaps less familiar with social change strategies than with other aspects of crisis management follow-up such as psychotherapy for underlying personality problems, the following summary is offered. It highlights the principles of social change agentry as presented in the Crisis Paradigm and is adapted from the work of Chin and Benne (1969). These strategies are central to positive crisis resolution, particularly those crises originating from sociocultural sources.

Strategies Based on Reason and Research

Foremost among these strategies are research findings, new concepts, and the clarification of language to more closely represent reality as experienced by people, not as theorized by academics. These strategies rest on the assumption that people are reasonable and that, when presented with evidence, they will take appropriate action to bring about needed change. However, this strategy alone is usually not enough to move people toward change.

Strategies Based on Reeducation and Attitude Change

These approaches to change are based on the assumption that people are guided by internalized values and habits and that they act according to institutionalized roles and perceptions of self. For example, some parents remain in unhappy marriages for the sake of the children. This group of strategies includes an activity central to contemporary crisis theory: fostering learning and growth in the persons who make up the system to be changed. This includes people who are in crisis because of greater vulnerability stemming from a disadvantaged position in society. This change strategy is also relevant to people whose usual coping devices leave something to be desired, such as people with learned helplessness, those who drink excessively, or those who abuse others (see Figure 2.2). Prominent illustrations of this strategy include (1) the mediation and nonviolent conflict resolution programs being instituted to stem the tide of youth violence (Jenkins & Bell, 1992; Kottler, 1994); (2) reclaiming values such as respect for persons, the environment, and people different from ourselves (e.g., the Teaching Tolerance program of the Southern Poverty Law Center). Through such programs, the psychic pain of the crisis experience—in contrast to violence or chronic unhealthy coping—often moves people to learn new ways of coping with life's problems.

Power-Coercive Approaches

The emphasis in these strategies is on political and economic sanctions in the exercise of power, along with such moral power moves as playing on sentiments of guilt, shame, and a sense of what is just and right. It is assumed that political action approaches will probably not succeed apart from reeducation and attitude change. New action, such as a strike by nurses who have been socialized to a subservient role in the health care system, by ethnic minorities demanding an end to housing and job discrimination, or gays protesting increased harassment and violence since the AIDS crisis, usually requires "new knowledge, new skills, new attitudes, and new value orientations" (Chin & Benne, 1969, p. 42; Hoff, 1990; Holland, 1994).

In a similar view, Marris (1987, pp. 156–164) proposes that new formulations of social meaning should accompany struggles to assert the ideals of society and to implement social justice policies. This presumes collective planning by people concerned with those who are distressed or in crisis because of discrimination and repressive policies: feminists; racial equity groups; gay, lesbian, and bisexual activists; the disabled, and others.

The incorporation of these social change strategies into a comprehensive approach to crisis prevention and management underscores the suggestions of social analysts to consider intervention strategies that correspond to the origins of stress and crisis as illustrated in the Crisis Paradigm. Also, Cloward and Piven (1979), in their discussion of female deviance, claim that women's coping through depression, passive resistance, and lower rates of violence is related to the source of their stress. Many women have been socialized to accept the view that women's stress is determined biologically and stems from natural psychic weakness (Sayers, 1982). Thus, women may expect to simply *endure* what nature offers—not unlike the survivors of natural disaster. However, social sources of stress can be *resisted*—as can the threat of man-made disaster (Lifton, 1967). These ideas support the importance of consciousness-raising in the civil rights and women's movements. It is now common for health and mental health professionals to refer battered women or rape victims to women's support groups that sensitize survivors to these kinds of social and political issues.

Table 2.2 illustrates how these ideas are encompassed in a comprehensive crisis management approach with respect to the various elements of the crises experienced by George Sloan and his family and by Ramona, a battered woman (see Chapter One). The approaches can be grouped as follows: preventive/enhancement, immediate or short-term, and long-range (follow-up). This diagram suggests that primary prevention and enhancement activities can abort a destructive crisis outcome like premature death. It demonstrates, too, the interactions and relationship (not necessarily an orderly sequence) between strategies, as well as the fact that various elements of comprehensive crisis management may be included in a single encounter with a person in crisis. The diagram reveals that it is never too late to consider preventive/enhancement approaches (such as those at secondary and tertiary levels), even if a suicide attempt has been made; nor is it ever too late to learn from the experiences of others (Hoff & Resing, 1982).

The case of George suggests the intersection of responses relevant to crises originating from two sources: traumatic personal situations and transition states. Ramona's case reveals the interaction of crises from three sources: a traumatic event, life-cycle development, and social/cultural factors. These illustrations also underscore the point made in the last chapter that people will resolve their crises with or without the help of significant others. People rich in personal, social, and material resources are often able to resolve crises positively in a natural (as op-

TABLE 2.2. COMPREHENSIVE CRISIS MANAGEMENT.

Crisis Element	Approaches to Crisis Management and Resolution		
	Preventive/ Enhancement	Immediate or Short-term	Long-range (Follow-up)
George			
Heart attack	Life-style factors (such as diet, exercise, relaxation)	Life-support measures	Life-style factors
Marital strain	Marriage preparation Communication	Marriage counseling	Normative reeducative change
Midlife change and marital strain	Rites of passage (such as a support group)*	Women's support group Men's support group	Normative reeducative change strategies
Arnold's school suspension	Rites of passage (such as adolescent support group)	Family and social network crisis counseling	Family counseling or therapy
George's suicide attempt	Family support and normative reeducative change following first heart attack	Individual and family crisis counseling	Family counseling Normative reeducative change Life-style factors
Ramona†			
Threat to life, homelessness	Women's support group Normative reeducative change	Physical refuge and peer support in shelter Crisis counseling (personal, legal, residential focus)	Political/coercive and normative reeducative change strategies
Self-blame, depression	Same as above	Counseling, peer support, or psychotherapy	Same as above, as well as possible psychotherapy

*Contemporary substitutes for traditional "Rites of Passage" are discussed in Chapter Thirteen.
†Ramona is discussed in Chapter One.

posed to institutional) context with the help of family, friends, and neighbors. Many, however, lack such resources, or for personal, cultural, and political reasons, the resources cannot be successfully mobilized during crisis. In these instances, help in the form of crisis intervention is needed to manage the crisis and promote positive crisis resolution (see Figure 2.1, Box 4a). The rest of this book is devoted to the principles and strategies necessary for effective crisis intervention—assessment, planning, implementation of plan, follow-up—the formal aspects of crisis management.

Summary

Success in crisis assessment and intervention depends on understanding (1) the origins of crisis, (2) how crisis differs from stress and illness, and (3) the developmental and individual manifestations of crisis. Regardless of the origin of crisis, people in crisis have a number of characteristics in common. The probability of preventing negative outcomes for these people is increased by helpers' sensitivity to the origins of crisis and the application of appropriate intervention strategies in distinct sociocultural contexts. These concepts are illustrated in the Crisis Paradigm, which provides the theoretical framework of this book.

References

Antonovsky, A. (1980). *Health, stress, and coping.* San Francisco: Jossey-Bass.

Baum, A., Cohen, L., & Hall, M. (1993). Control and intrusive memories as possible determinants of chronic stress. *Psychosomatic Medicine, 55*(3), 274–286.

Bebbington, P., Wilkins, S., Jones, P., Foerster, A., Murray, R., Toone, B., & Lewis, S. (1993). Life events and psychosis: Initial results from the Camberwell Collaborative Psychosis Study. *British Journal of Psychiatry, 162,* 72–79.

Bernstein, R. J. (1978). *The restructuring of social and political theory.* Philadelphia: University of Pennsylvania Press.

Boston Women's Health Book Collective. (1992). *The new our bodies, ourselves* (4th ed.). New York: Simon & Schuster.

Brim, O. G., & Ryff, C. D. (1980). On the properties of life events. *Life-Span Development and Behavior, 3,* 367–388.

Brown, G. W. (1993). Life events and affective disorder: Replications and limitations. *Psychosomatic Medicine, 55*(3), 248–259.

Brown, G. W., & Harris, T. (1978). *The social origins of depression.* London: Tavistock.

Browne, A. (1987). *When battered women kill.* New York: Free Press.

Burstow, B. (1992). *Radical feminist therapy: Working in the context of violence.* Newbury Park: Sage.

Caplan, G. (1964). *Principles of preventive psychiatry.* New York: Basic Books.

Caplan, G. (1981). Mastery of stress: Psychosocial aspects. *American Journal of Psychiatry, 138*(4), 413–420.

Cherniss, C. (1980). *Staff burnout.* Beverly Hills: Sage.

Chesler, P. (1972). *Women and madness.* New York: Doubleday.

Chin, R., & Benne, K. D. (1969). General strategies for effecting change in human systems. In W. G. Bennis, K. D. Benne, & R. Chin (Eds.), *The planning of change* (2nd ed.), pp. 32–57. New York: Holt, Rinehart & Winston.

Cicourel, A. V. (1964). *Method and measurement in sociology.* New York: Free Press.

Cloward, R. A., & Piven, F. F. (1979). Hidden protest: The channeling of female innovations and resistance. *Signs: Journal of Women in Culture and Society, 4,* 651–669.

Conger, R. D., Lorenz, F. O., Elder, G. H., & Simons, R. L. (1993). Husband and wife differences in response to undesirable life events. *Journal of Health and Social Behavior, 34*(1), 71–88.

Corea, G. (1985). *The hidden malpractice: How American medicine treats women* (Rev. ed.). New York: Harper Colophon Books.

Danish, S. J., Smyer, M. A., & Nowak, C. A. (1980). Developmental intervention: Enhancing life-event processes. *Life-Span Development and Behavior, 3,* 339–366.

Dohrenwend, B. S., & Dohrenwend, B. P. (Eds.). (1984). *Stressful life events and their context.* New Brunswick, NJ: Rutgers University Press.

Dubos, R. (1977). Determinants of health and disease. In D. Landy (Ed.), *Culture, disease, and healing: Studies in medical anthropology* (pp. 31–40). New York: Macmillan.

Durkheim, E. (1951). *Suicide.* New York: Free Press. (Original work published 1897)

Erickson, E. (1963). *Childhood and society* (2nd ed.). New York: W.W. Norton.

Foster, G. M., & Anderson, B. G. (1978). *Medical anthropology.* New York: Wiley.

Freudenberger, H. J., & Richelson, G. (1980). *Burnout.* Toronto: Bantam Books.

Gelles, R. A. (1974). *The violent home.* Beverly Hills: Sage.

Gerhardt, U. (1979). Coping and social action: Theoretical reconstruction of the life-event approach. *Sociology of Health and Illness, 1,* 195–225.

Hansell, N. (1976). *The person in distress.* New York: Human Sciences Press.

Hilberman, E. (1980). The 'wife-beater's wife' reconsidered. *American Journal of Psychiatry, 137,* 1336–1347.

Hoff, L. A. (1990). *Battered women as survivors.* London: Routledge.

Hoff, L. A. (1993). Review essay: Health policy and the plight of the mentally ill. *Psychiatry, 56*(4), 400–419.

Hoff, L. A., & Resing, M. (1982). Was this suicide preventable? *American Journal of Nursing, 82,* 1106–1111.

Holland, H. (1994). *Born in Soweto.* London: Penguin.

Holmes, T. H., & Rahe, R. H. (1967). The social readjustment rating scale. *Psychosomatic Medicine, 11,* 213–218.

Hurwicz, M. L., Durham, C. C., Boyd-Davis, S. L., Gatz, M., & Bengtson, V. L. (1992). Salient life events in three-generation families. *Journal of Gerontology, 47*(1), 11–13.

Jenkins, E. J., & Bell, C. C. (1992). Adolescent violence: Can it be curbed? *Adolescent Medicine: State of the Art Reviews, 3*(1), 71–86.

Johnson, A. B. (1990). *Out of bedlam: The truth about deinstitutionalization.* New York: Basic Books.

Jones, A. (1980). *Women who kill.* New York: Holt, Rinehart & Winston.

Kessler, R. C., & McLeod, J. D. (1984). Sex differences in vulnerability to undesirable life events. *American Sociological Review, 49*(Oct), 620–631.

Killeen, M. (1990). The influence of stress and coping on family caregivers' perceptions of health. *International Journal of Aging and Human Development, 30*(3), 197–211.

Kottler, J. (1994). *Beyond blame: A new way of resolving conflicts in relationships.* San Francisco: Jossey-Bass.

Landy, D. (Ed.). (1977). *Culture, disease, and healing: Studies in medical anthropology.* New York: Macmillan.

Levine, S., & Scotch, N. (1970). *Social stress.* Chicago: Aldine.

Lieban, R. W. (1977). The field of medical anthropology. In D. Landy (Ed.), *Culture, disease, and healing: Studies in medical anthropology* (pp. 13–31). New York: Macmillan.

Lifton, R. J. (1967). *Death in life.* New York: Simon & Schuster.

Lindemann, E. (1944). Symptomatology and management of acute grief. *American Journal of Psychiatry, 101,* 101–148.

Louch, A. R. (1966). *Explanation and human action.* Berkeley: University of California Press.

Marris, P. (1987). *Meaning and action: Community action and conceptions of change* (2nd ed.). London: Routledge & Kegan Paul.

Maslow, A. (1970). *Motivation and personality* (2nd ed.). New York: Harper & Row.

Mawby, R. I., & Walklate, S. (1994). *Critical victimology.* London: Sage.

McElroy, A., & Townsend, P. K. (1985). *Medical anthropology in ecological perspective.* Boulder, Colo.: Westview Press.

McKinlay, J. B. (1990). A case for refocusing upstream: The political economy of illness. In P. Conrad & R. Kern (Eds.), *The sociology of health and illness: Critical perspectives* (pp. 502–516). New York: St. Martin's Press.

McNamee, S., & Gergen, K. J. (Eds.). (1992). *Therapy as social construction.* London: Sage.

Panchuck, P. (1994). The midlife experience of contemporary women: Views along the midway. Unpublished Ph.D. dissertation. Boston: Leslie College.

Parsons, T. (1951). Social structure and dynamic process: The case of modern medical practice. In *The social system.* Glencoe, IL: Free Press.

Pearlin, L. E., & Schooler, C. (1978). The structure of coping. *Journal of Health and Social Behavior, 19,* 2–21.

Pearlin, L. E. et al. (1981). The stress process. *Journal of Health and Social Behavior, 22*(4), 337–356.

Perloff, L. S. (1983). Perceptions of vulnerability. *Journal of Social Issues, 39*(2), 41–61.

Ramsey, J. M. (1982). *Basic paltophysiology: modern stress and the disease process.* Menlo Park, CA: Addison-Wesley.

Rieker, P., & Carmen (Hilberman), E. (1986). The victim-to-patient process: The disconfirmation and transformation of abuse. *American Journal of Orthopsychiatry, 56,* 360–371.

Roberts, H. (Ed.). (1981). *Doing feminist research.* London: Routledge & Kegan Paul.

Ryan, W. (1971). *Blaming the victim.* New York: Vintage Books.

Ryff, C. D., & Essex, M. J. (1992). The interpretation of life experience and well-being: The sample case of relocation. *Psychology & Aging, 7*(4), 507–517.

Sales, E., Baum, M., & Shore, B. (1984). Victim readjustment following assault. *Journal of Social Issues, 40*(1), 117–136.

Sarason, I. G., Johnson, J. H., & Siegel, J. M. (1978). Assessing the impact of life changes: Development of the life experiences survey. *Journal of Consulting Psychology, 46,* 932–946.

Sayers, J. (1982). *Biological Politics.* London: Tavistock.

Schulberg, H. C., & Sheldon, A. (1968). The probability of crisis and strategies for preventive intervention. *Archives of General Psychiatry, 18,* 553–558.

Selye, H. (1956). *The stress of life.* New York: McGraw-Hill.

Silver, R. L., Boon, C., & Stones, M. H. (1983). Searching for meaning in misfortune: Making sense of incest. *Journal of Social Issues, 39*(2), 81–102.

Spaniol, L., & Caputo, J. J. (1979). *Professional burnout.* Lexington, Mass.: Human Service Associates.

Survivors. (1982). A public television documentary. Boston: WGBH Educational Foundation.

Turner, R. J., & Avison, W. R. (1992). Innovations in the measurement of life stress: Crisis theory and the significance of event resolution. *Journal of Health and Social Behavior, 33*(1), 36–50.

Turner, R. J., & Avison, W. R. (1987). Gender and depression: Assessing exposure and vulnerability to life events in a chronically strained population. Paper presented at the annual meeting of the American Public Health Association, New Orleans.

Tyhurst, J. S. (1957). The role of transition states—including disasters—in mental illness. Symposium on Preventive and Social Psychiatry. Washington: Walter Reed Army Institute of Research and The National Research Council.

Vaillant, G.E. (1993). *The wisdom of the ego: Sources of resilience in adult life.* Cambridge, Mass.: Harvard University Press.

Wendell, S. (1990). Oppression and victimization: Choice and responsibility. *Hypatia: A Journal of Feminist Philosophy, 5*(3), 15–46.

CHAPTER THREE

IDENTIFYING PEOPLE IN CRISIS

We know, generally, how crises originate, and we know how to predict and prevent crises and destructive crisis outcomes in large population groups. This general knowledge, however, must be made accessible for use with individuals in actual or potential crisis. Crises from some sources are predictable and thus more easily prepared for; preparation helps reduce the risk of crisis as well as the possibility of destructive crisis outcomes. Common sources of predictable crises are developmental states and the role changes marking adolescence, adulthood, marriage, midlife, retirement, and old age. Typically, a person may first be a student, then get a job, marry, become a parent, and reach the age of retirement. Since role changes usually are anticipated, precautions can be taken to avoid crisis. But some people do not, or cannot, prepare themselves for these events; the possibility of crisis for them is increased. For example, a young person whose parents have been overly indulgent and inconsistent in their responses will find it difficult to move from adolescence into adulthood. Overprotective parents stifle a child's normal development, and thus the move to adulthood becomes a risk and a hazard rather than an opportunity for further challenge and growth. Also, a person need not rush into marriage but can thoughtfully consider the possibility and the related role changes. Yet many do rush, and crises result.

Another factor affecting these predictable role changes is the element of timing (see Chapters Two and Thirteen). For example, a man or woman marrying for the first time at age forty may have planned very carefully for this life change, but altering an established pattern of living alone and being independent may still lead to unanticipated stress. Also, parental and other social supports for newlyweds are less likely to be available in later marriages. On the other hand, while a planned event such as a return to school at midlife can be hazardous due to atypical timing, an older student may be less vulnerable to crisis. That is, the more mature student or marriage partner often has the advantage of experience, financial security, and clear-cut goals—valuable resources that younger people may possess in lesser measure.

Another aspect of a potentially hazardous role transition, even if prepared for, is its timing with other life events—or what Danish, Smyer, and Nowak (1980) call its "contextual purity." Many of the life changes on the Holmes and Rahe (1967) Social Readjustment Rating Scale are within a person's control (e.g., marriage or returning to school in midlife), while others are not (e.g., menopause or death of an elderly parent). By careful planning and by delaying controllable changes, a person can lower his or her cumulative stress score and reduce the hazards of crisis, illness, and accidents.

Other life events are less predictable: the sudden death of a loved one; serious physical illness; urban dislocation; personal and financial loss through flood, hurricane, or fire; or the birth of a premature infant. When these unanticipated events occur during transition states or when they originate from cultural values or one's disadvantaged social position, the probability of crisis is increased.

These examples and the interactive nature of crisis origins (discussed in Chapters One and Two) underscore the subjective nature of the crisis experience and the need to identify *individuals* at risk. Regardless of how predictable crisis responses might be for groups, *general* risk factors must be translated into an assessment of the issues and problems faced by *this* person or family at *this* particular time. Such an assessment—and assistance based on it—implies the need for precise information about individuals and families who might be in crisis. For example:

1. In what developmental phase is the person or family?
2. What recent hazardous events have occurred in the life of this person or family?
3. How has this person or family interpreted these events?
4. Is there actual or potential threat to life? How urgent is the need for intervention?
5. What is the sociocultural milieu in which all of this is happening?

The ramifications of these and related questions form the basis for this discussion of identifying and assessing people in crisis, the focus of Box 2 in Figure 3.1, Crisis Paradigm.

The Importance of Crisis Assessment

The crisis worker must consider life events, transition states, and hazardous sociocultural factors when assessing whether or not a person is in crisis. Observers

FIGURE 3.1. CRISIS PARADIGM.

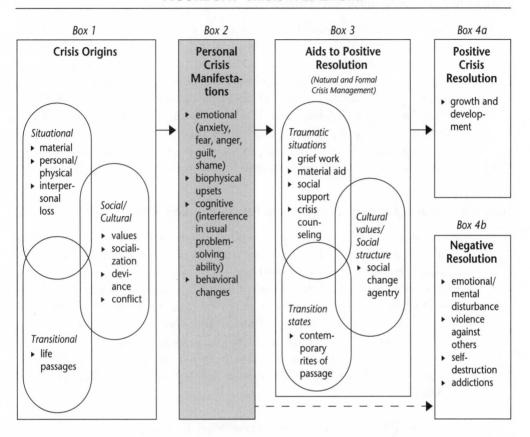

Crisis origins, manifestations, and outcomes, and the respective functions of crisis management have an interactional relationship. The intertwined circles represent the distinct yet interrelated origins of crisis and aids to positive resolution, even though personal manifestations are often similar. The arrows pointing from origins to positive resolution illustrate the *opportunity for growth and development* through crisis; the broken line at bottom depicts the potential *danger of crisis* in the absence of appropriate aids.

may think that a person who is emotionally upset is obviously in a state of crisis. This is not necessarily so; a thorough assessment should precede such a judgment. Still, an untrained observer may quickly dismiss the need for assessment in order to proceed to a seemingly more urgent task—to *help* the individual. Such well-intended help sometimes has the opposite effect, however. This is most likely to happen if the urge to help springs from a helper's excessive need to be needed, thus obscuring the distressed person's need for mastery and self-determination. One way to avoid misplaced helping is for potential helpers to be aware of and not indulge in "rescue fantasies." Another is to identify people who are at risk through a careful process of assessment.

Impediments to Adequate Assessment

Assessment can be impeded by the very nature of the crisis intervention process—a humane function that is growing in popularity. Helping people in crisis is immediate and often highly rewarding. However, human service workers who are most inclined to action and who are involved in obtaining immediately observable results often do not take time to study and evaluate their own work (Hoff & Miller, 1987; Schulberg & Sheldon, 1968). When the challenge of self-review is combined with the difficulty of evaluating any helping process objectively, it is easy to see how crisis intervention can flounder. Without a sound theoretical base and established techniques, there is little to distinguish it from intuitive first aid.

Hazards of Inadequate Assessment and Psychiatric Labeling

The failure to assess before helping is often responsible for the misapplication of the crisis model. In the human service field, it is particularly unfortunate to misjudge a person in crisis by poor observation and inadequate assessment. Ultimately, these errors result in a failure to help that can have lifelong, destructive effects. Successful crisis prediction and assessment increases the possibility of preventive intervention and makes hospital admission (and its attending risks) less likely (see "Preventing Crisis" and "Promoting Growth" in Chapter One).

The importance of assessment and the resolution of crisis as an alternative to psychiatric hospitalization is further highlighted by what happens after admission:

> The admission itself tends to promote denial of the social forces in the family and community that have produced it [the admission]. The patient may then emerge as the scapegoat for these family and community problems, and psychiatric assessment [vs. crisis assessment] after admission tends to focus on the patient's symptomology [vs. strengths and problem-solving ability] as the major cause of admission (Polak, 1967, p. 153).

Institutionalization is certainly more expensive than community-based crisis intervention, but that is not the only consideration. The institutionalization of an upset person can possibly make matters worse—and certainly more complicated. After diagnosis, the person takes on the identity of a patient and falls into roles expected by the institution (Becker, 1963; Goffman, 1961; Lemert, 1951). Essentially the same thing happens to an adolescent confined to a detention home and to an old person placed in a nursing home. But some families do institutionalize disturbed or aggressive people when they can no longer care for them at home. They find managing behavior that falls outside "normal" limits to be very difficult, and in certain cases impossible.

Every society has social norms, that is, expectations of how people should interact with others. When people deviate from these norms, sanctions are applied or stigmas attached to pressure the deviant member to return to acceptable behavior, suffer the consequences of their deviance, or behave according to their stigmatized status. Thus, deviance can be considered from three perspectives as illustrated in the following examples:

1. In Western societies, a widow may be socially ostracized if she mourns the loss of her husband longer than the generally acceptable few weeks. If she does so, she deviates from the expected norm for grief and mourning in a death-denying society.
2. A person who is caught and convicted of stealing a car or molesting a child has engaged in behavior that is explicitly forbidden in most societies. While these are clear-cut examples of deviance, the results of such violations vary. For example, an African American is more likely to be apprehended and judged harshly for a car theft than is a white person in the United States. One factor influencing such variance is "police discretion" (Bittner, 1967), which, in turn, is influenced by racial climate. Another is the "social construction of reality" (Berger & Luckmann, 1967; Daniels, 1978).
3. Some people are considered deviant not for particular actions but for some aspect of their being. Thus, a gay person, a woman in menopause, an old person, or a handicapped individual carries a "mark" and can be stigmatized as a result of a physical, social, or mental attribute. The physical or social mark (difference) may become indistinguishable from the person's identity. Goffman (1963) refers to this as "spoiled identity." Thus, a person does not *suffer* from paraplegia or schizophrenia but *is* a paraplegic or schizophrenic; the person who takes his or her own life does not just *commit* suicide but *is* a suicide. The person's identity becomes encompassed in a particular behavior or physical or mental characteristic.

Labeling theory—a controversial topic in social science—has been the subject of lively debate for years (Gove, 1975; Scheff, 1975). Briefly, labeling theory proposes the concepts of primary and secondary deviance in an interactive relationship as illustrated in Figure 3.2. The argument between advocates and critics of labeling theory centers around this question: Would secondary deviance occur if the person who is labeled did not experience both an altered self-concept and a change in the way others perceive him or her? An extreme view is that primary deviance could virtually be dismissed except for the detrimental effects of labeling and the secondary deviance following it. In contrast, Gove (1978) suggests that the higher rates of depression among women have nothing to do with the labeling of mental illness. Rather, he says, it is related to their disadvantaged position in society. This may be true if, as Cloward and Piven (1979) suggest, women are indeed socialized to *endure* rather than *resist* oppression. Each of these positions has implications for crisis assessment. That is, certain personal attributes

FIGURE 3.2. RELATIONSHIP BETWEEN PRIMARY AND SECONDARY DEVIANCE.

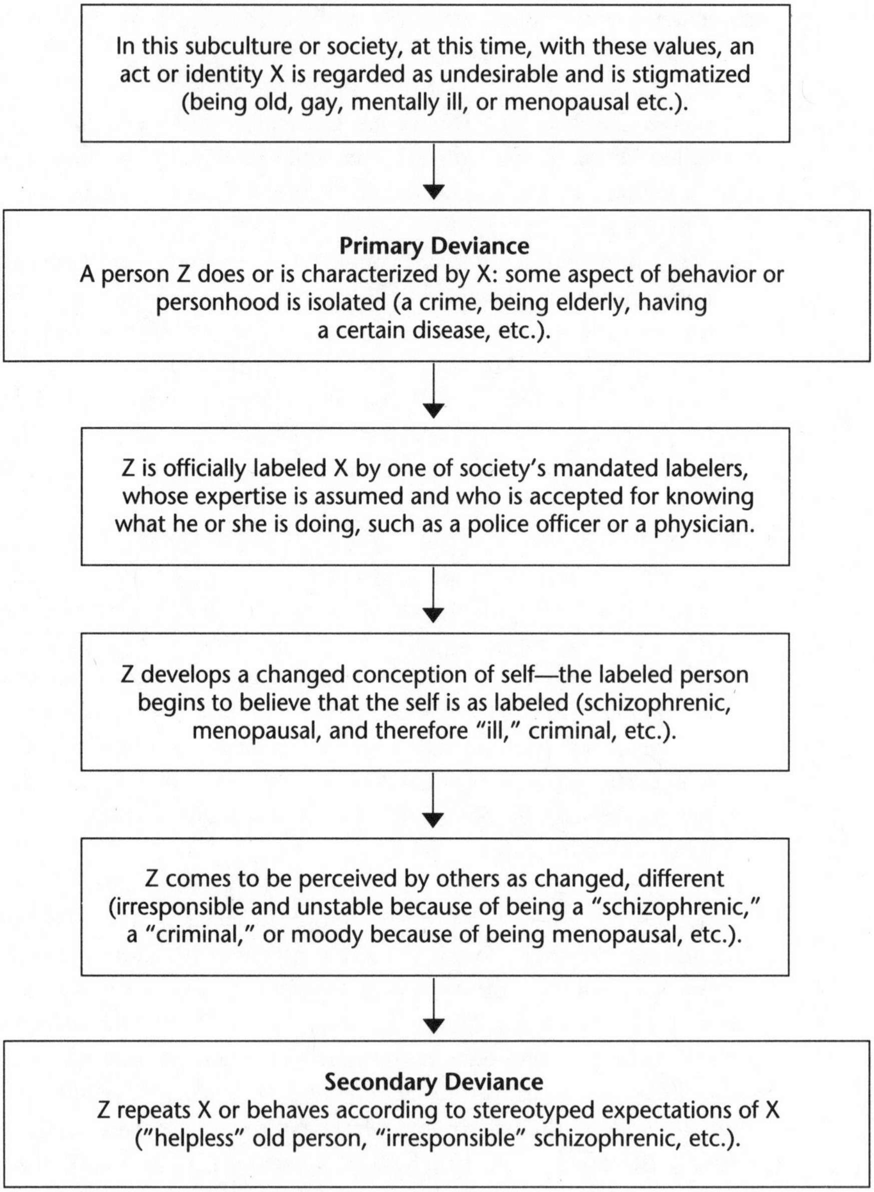

In this subculture or society, at this time, with these values, an act or identity X is regarded as undesirable and is stigmatized (being old, gay, mentally ill, or menopausal etc.).

↓

Primary Deviance
A person Z does or is characterized by X: some aspect of behavior or personhood is isolated (a crime, being elderly, having a certain disease, etc.).

↓

Z is officially labeled X by one of society's mandated labelers, whose expertise is assumed and who is accepted for knowing what he or she is doing, such as a police officer or a physician.

↓

Z develops a changed conception of self—the labeled person begins to believe that the self is as labeled (schizophrenic, menopausal, and therefore "ill," criminal, etc.).

↓

Z comes to be perceived by others as changed, different (irresponsible and unstable because of being a "schizophrenic," a "criminal," or moody because of being menopausal, etc.).

↓

Secondary Deviance
Z repeats X or behaves according to stereotyped expectations of X ("helpless" old person, "irresponsible" schizophrenic, etc.).

X = A deviant act or identity
Z = A particular person labeled as deviant

(Thanks to John McKinlay for his ideas about representing labeling theory in this format.)

or behaviors do not fall into the range of behavior and conditions commonly accepted as normal and desirable. This is primary deviance, which exists whether or not it is identified with a label. For example, some people break social rules even though they are not always caught and identified as rule breakers.

There are distinct disadvantages for those who are labeled because of widespread gender, sexual identity, or other bias (Holden, 1986; Rabin, Keefe, & Burton, 1986). People may try to "pass" or hide their identities because of the prejudices of others. For example, gay and lesbian people are very careful about coming out; many women will not reveal their age, or they become avid consumers of beauty aids for keeping a youthful appearance; people with a psychiatric problem may not wish to reveal the diagnosis, as they often experience prejudice in the job market; women (many of whom have been abused) are more likely than men to be diagnosed with borderline personality disorder. Alternatively, people may feel compelled to act as others expect. For example, misbehaving children who are inappropriately labeled as disabled refer to their social security disability checks as "crazy" money; convicted law breakers often repeat their offenses; or a person diagnosed as schizophrenic may say, "How do you expect me to succeed in this job? I'm a schizophrenic." Diagnostic labeling has also been critiqued for its inappropriate application cross-culturally (Hagey & McDonough, 1984) and for ethical implications (Mitchell, 1991). In cases of domestic abuse, it can obscure the primary *social* issue of violence (Hoff, 1990).

Labeling theory is particularly relevant in crisis assessment practice and in the relationship of crisis to illness. If crisis is viewed as an opportunity for change and growth rather than as an illness or an occasion for social or psychiatric labeling, assessment can be an important step toward growth. But crisis assessment should not be confused with traditional psychiatric diagnosis; psychiatry is not highly scientific and diagnoses can often be contradictory. An example of this is the contradictory evidence presented by psychiatrists representing the defense and the prosecution in criminal cases with insanity pleas. The trial of John W. Hinckley, who attempted to assassinate President Reagan, is a case in point. This does not mean that efforts to improve the objectivity of psychiatric diagnostic procedures should stop. Nor does it deny the fact that some people in crisis are also mentally disturbed and thus diagnosable in a psychiatric framework. It simply means that a crisis experience should be assessed and managed in a crisis—not an illness—framework, so that negative outcomes such as illness are avoided. If illness was present before the crisis, the chances of its recurrence are reduced. Crisis assessment and intervention should not be cast in a medical framework because this currently accessible, humane approach to helping distressed people might then become as bureaucratic and inaccessible as some aspects of the traditional health care system (Warshaw, 1989). In short, one might ask: Why attach a diagnostic label that is actually or potentially damaging when illness may not be the central issue and when the person's subjective meaning system is central to the crisis resolution process?

The negative results of inadequate assessment and psychiatric patient identity are dramatically revealed in a study by Rosenhan (1973). The study uncovered the destructive effects of placing disturbed people in psychiatric hospitals and
labeling them with a psychiatric diagnosis such as schizophrenia. Rosenhan
demonstrated that the professional psychiatric helpers charged with the admission
and diagnosis of those regarded as insane could not distinguish between pseudopatients and the truly disturbed. This was so even when the professionals were
forewarned by the researcher that certain people presenting themselves for hospital admission would be pseudopatients. Once the pseudopatients were hospitalized, their subsequent behavior was interpreted within the framework of their
psychiatric label, although their behavior was normal. Consequently, they had a
difficult time getting released from the hospital even though they had no objective
signs of mental illness. The study supports Polak's (1967) observations that psychiatric hospitalization

- Is a crisis in itself
- Is the direct result of previously undetected and unresolved crisis
- Should be avoided whenever possible
- Should be used only as a last resort when all other efforts to help have failed
- Should be substituted, whenever possible, with accurate crisis assessment and
  intervention in the person's natural social setting

Now that psychiatric hospitalization is less common and thousands are discharged without housing or adequate community support, mentally disturbed people nevertheless endure similar biases and burdens in life on the streets (Hoff, 1993;
Johnson, 1990).

This discussion supports the earlier recommendations about assessment and
intervention in natural settings (see "Natural and Peer Group Settings" in Chapter One). It is not that psychiatrists and other mental health professionals do not
understand the difference between crisis and mental illness; but once a patient is
admitted to a medical or hospital facility, it is difficult to avoid diagnosing them,
regardless of what individuals may think about the practice. And when diagnoses
identify psychological and social states, objectivity is reduced, and the potential
for damaging results increases. Capponi (1992), for example, describes the challenges faced by "psychiatric survivors" of the system purportedly designed to help
them. In sum, the person in crisis and the family should be advised that there
are many constructive ways of resolving life's crises (Breggin, 1992; Hansell, l976;
Polak, 1976). Alternatives to hospitalization will be discussed in subsequent
chapters.

Inadequate assessment of crisis has another negative result. When there is
only the *appearance*—not the reality—of crisis, an ill-advised response might reinforce crisis-like behavior as well as the notion that the only way to get help is to

convince potential helpers that there is a crisis. Increasingly, this pattern is observed in calls to hotlines from discharged mental patients or chronically ill people who lack the longer-term treatment and support their condition requires. The complexity and danger of this situation is discussed further in Chapter Six.

The Distinctiveness of Crisis Assessment

The ability to discriminate, then, between a crisis and a noncrisis state requires prediction and assessment skills. Good intentions are not enough. The development of assessment skills does not take years of intensive study and training. It does require the ability to combine what is known from observing and helping people in crisis with the natural tendency to help someone in trouble. Teachers, parents, nurses, police officers, physicians, and clergy are in the front lines where most life crises occur. In these roles, people can do a great deal to help others and prevent unnecessary casualties, especially when formal training is added to a natural crisis-management ability (Hoff, 1995; Hoff & Miller, 1987; McCarthy & Knapp, 1984; Walfish, 1983).

Ivan Illich (1976) asserts that the bureaucratization of medicine has deprived ordinary people of helping tools they could readily use on behalf of others if the system allowed their use. His point is consistent with the current emphasis on primary care and responsibility for one's own health. Bureaucracies jeopardize the human aspect of the crisis intervention approach, the very quality that has made it an accessible, inoffensive way for distressed people to receive help. Similarly, the pervasiveness of individualism and the power of the medical model (Barney, 1994) present a temptation to medicalize the crisis assessment and intervention process. As many tools as possible should be available to people who are willing and able to help others (Illich, 1976). By sharpening the assessment and helping techniques that people have always used, frontline workers become particularly suited for the prevention of acute crises, or what Jacobson, Strickler, and Morley (1968) call "anticipatory intervention." When a full-blown crisis is in progress, frontline workers usually must collaborate creatively with counselors and mental health professionals who are trained to do a more comprehensive crisis assessment (Stein & Lambert, 1984). The different levels of assessment are discussed in the next section. Thus, the crisis approach can be grounded in theory and sound principles of practice without taking on the disadvantages of elitism among human service workers. The distinctiveness of crisis assessment can be summarized as follows:

1. The crisis assessment *process,* unlike traditional psychiatric diagnosis, is intricately tied to crisis *resolution.* Besides the issues already discussed, this is another compelling reason why assessment in comprehensive crisis management cannot

be overstressed. For example, if an individual learns during assessment that the fear of "going crazy" is a typical crisis response, fear is relieved, and he or she is already helped along the path of positive crisis resolution.

2. Crisis assessment occurs immediately rather than days or weeks later as in traditional psychiatric practice.

3. The focus in crisis assessment is on immediate, identifiable problems rather than on personality dynamics or presumed coping deficits.

4. Historical material is dealt with in a special way in crisis assessment. Probing into psychodynamic issues such as unresolved childhood conflicts and repressed emotions is inappropriate. In contrast, it is not only appropriate but necessary to obtain a person's history of solving problems, resolving crises, and dealing with stressful life events. Such information is vital for assessing and mobilizing the personal and social resources needed to effect positive crisis outcomes. It can be obtained by asking, for example, "What have you done in the past that has worked for you when you're upset?"

5. Crisis assessment is not complete without an evaluation of risk to life (see Chapters Six, Eight, and Nine).

6. Crisis assessment is not something done *to* a person but is a process carried out *with* a person; assessment must be carried out in active collaboration with significant others. Thus, a service contract is a logical outcome of appropriate crisis assessment.

7. Social and cultural factors and community resources are integral to a comprehensive crisis assessment, since the origins and manifestations of crisis are social as often as they are individual.

The Assessment Process

Knowledge of probability factors about crisis guides us in assessing particular individuals in possible crisis. However, health and human service workers encountering someone in distress may still have many questions: What do I say? What questions should I ask? How do I find out what's really happening with someone who seems so confused and upset? How do I recognize a person in crisis? If the person in crisis is not crazy, what distinguishes him or her from someone who is mentally disturbed but not in active crisis? What do the family and community have to do with the person in crisis? In short, human service workers need a framework for the assessment process.

Distinguishing Levels of Assessment

Two levels of crisis assessment should be completed by the crisis worker. The following questions must be asked at each level:

Level One: Is there an obvious or potential threat to life, either the life of the individual in crisis or the lives of others? In other words, has the person been abused? And what are the risks of suicide, assault, and homicide?

Level Two: Is there evidence that the person is unable to function in his or her usual life role? Is the person in danger of being extruded from his or her natural social setting? What are the psychological, socioeconomic, and other factors related to the person's coping with life's stressors?

Level One assessment should be done by everyone. This includes people in their natural roles of friend, neighbor, parent, and spouse, as well as people in various professional positions: physicians, teachers, nurses, police officers, clergy, welfare workers, and prison officials. This level of assessment is critical. It has life and death dimensions and forms the basis for mobilizing emergency services on behalf of the person, family, or community in crisis.

Every person in crisis should be assessed regarding victimization and danger to self and others (Hoff & Rosenbaum, 1994). (Techniques for assessment of suicidal danger are presented in detail in Chapter Six. Assessment for victimization trauma is presented in Chapter Eight. Assessing the risk of assault or homicide is discussed in Chapter Nine.) Here, a key facet of crisis work is emphasized: *No crisis assessment is complete without inquiring directly about victimization and the danger of suicide and assault or homicide.*

If a layperson or a professional without crisis training suspects that a person is at probable risk for abuse, suicide, assault, or homicide, an experienced professional crisis worker should be consulted. Some life-threatening situations must be approached collaboratively with the police or forensic psychiatry specialists (see Chapter Nine). Crisis centers certified by the American Association of Suicidology have such collaborative relationships for handling high-risk crises (Hoff & Wells, 1989).

Level Two assessment involves considering personal and social characteristics of the distressed person and his or her family. This is usually done by a trained crisis counselor or mental health professional. Level Two assessment is comprehensive and corresponds to the elements of the total crisis experience:

1. *Identification of crisis origins.* What hazardous events occurred? Was there transition-state turmoil? What sociocultural factors are involved?
2. *Development of crisis.* Is the person in the initial or acute phase of crisis? (See "How a Crisis Develops" in Chapter Two).
3. *Manifestations of crisis.* How does the person interpret hazardous events, and what are the corresponding emotional, cognitive, behavioral, and biophysical responses to them? Are the events perceived as threat, loss, or challenge? Does the person deal with the accompanying stress effectively?

4. *Identification of* personal, family, interpersonal, and material *resources.*
5. *Determination of the sociocultural milieu* of the person or family in crisis.

All professional human service workers should acquire skill in this kind of assessment if they do not already have it. Close friends and family members are often able to make such an assessment as well. The chances for their success depend on their personal level of self-confidence, general experience, and previous success in helping others with problems. In general, however, a person unaccustomed to dealing with people in crisis or with no special training in crisis intervention should consult experienced professional crisis counselors. This is especially important in assessing people in complex, life-threatening, or catastrophic situations. The different focuses and performances of Level One and Two assessments are summarized in Table 3.1. Let us now consider the assessment process in detail.

Identifying Origins and Phases of Crisis Development

A basic step in crisis assessment is identification of the events or situations that led to the person's distress. Sifneos (1960, p. 177) and Golan (1969) elaborate on Caplan's concept of crisis development in phases. They differentiate between the hazardous event and the precipitating factor, which, along with the person's vulnerability, constitute the components of the crisis state. As noted in Chapter Two, stressful and shocking events can arise from personal or material sources, transition states, or sociocultural situations.

The *hazardous event* is the initial shock or situation that sets in motion a series

TABLE 3.1. CRISIS ASSESSMENT LEVELS.

	Focus of Assessment	Assessment Done By
Level One	Risk to life • Victimization • Self (suicide) • Assault/homicide (child, partner, parent, mental health or community worker, police officer)	Everyone (natural and formal crisis managers) • Family, friends, neighbors • Hotline workers • Frontline workers: clergy, police officers, nurses, physicians, teachers • Crisis and mental health professionals
Level Two	Comprehensive psychosocial aspects of the person's life pertaining to the hazardous event, including assessment of chronic self-destructiveness	Counselors or mental health professionals specially trained in crisis work (formal crisis managers)

of reactions culminating in a crisis (Golan, 1969). If the event is not already apparent, the helping person should ask directly, "What happened?" Sometimes people are so upset or overwhelmed by a series of things that they cannot clearly identify the sequence of events. In these instances, it is helpful to ask when the person began feeling so upset. Simple, direct questions should be asked about the time and circumstances of all upsetting or dangerous events. Putting events in order has a calming effect; the person experiences a certain sense of self-possession in being able to make some order out of confusion. This is particularly true for the person who is afraid of losing control or "going crazy."

The experience of stressful, hazardous events is not in itself a crisis. It is one of several components of the crisis state. After all, the process of living implies the everyday management of stressful life events. Research with battered women, for example, reveals them to be capable survivors despite daunting odds (Hoff, 1990). The question is, how is *this* particular event unusual in terms of its timing, severity, danger, or the person's ability to handle it successfully? This component of crisis corresponds to Caplan's first phase of crisis development, which may or may not develop into a full-blown crisis, depending on personal and social circumstances (see the example of John, Chapter Two). People who seek help at the beginning stage of crisis development may avoid an acute crisis by early prevention and strategic intervention (Rapaport, 1965, p. 30).

Since hazardous events alone are insufficient to constitute a crisis state, the assessment process must also focus on the *immediacy* of the person's stress—the precipitating factor. This is the proverbial straw that broke the camel's back—the final, stressful event in a series of such events that pushes the person from a state of acute vulnerability into crisis. The precipitating event is not always easy to identify, particularly when the presenting problem seems to have been present for a long time (Golan, 1969).

The precipitating factor is often a minor incident. Nevertheless, it can take on crisis proportions in the context of other stressful events and the person's inability to use usual problem-solving devices. In this sense, it resembles Caplan's third phase of crisis development, following the failure of ordinary problem solving (the second phase). It corresponds to what Polak (1967) calls the final event that moves a family to bring a member to a psychiatric hospital for admission after a series of antecedent crises. In a series of crises experienced by the same person, the precipitating factor in one crisis episode may be the hazardous event in the next. Thus, in real life—as opposed to theoretical discussion and models—hazardous events or situations and precipitating factors may be hard to distinguish. Yet, determining the mutual presence of these two components is useful in the assessment process, especially for distinguishing between *chronic stress* and an *acute crisis state*. For example, a chronic problem rather than a crisis is suggested in this interchange: *Question:* What brought you here *today*—since these problems have been with you for some time now? *Response:* I was watching a television program on depression and finally decided to get help for my problems.

Assessing Individual Crisis Manifestations

In crisis assessment, the identification of hazardous events or situations and the precipitating factor must be placed in meaningful context. This is done by ascertaining the subjective reaction of the person to stressful events. Sifneos (1960) and Golan (1969) refer to this component of crisis assessment as the "vulnerable state." It corresponds to Caplan's second and fourth phases of crisis development. Its focus is on the emotional, biophysical, cognitive, and behavioral *responses* the person makes to recent stressful events. A person's subjective response can be elicited by questions such as those illustrated in Table 3.2. The answers to questions like these are important for several reasons:

TABLE 3.2. ASSESSING PERSONAL RESPONSES.

Sample Assessment Questions	Possible Verbal Responses	Interpretation in Terms of Personal Crisis Manifestations (Emotional, Cognitive, Behavioral)
How do you feel about what happened? (for example, divorce or rape)	*Divorce:* I don't want to live without her... If I kill myself she'll be sorry.	Feelings of desperation, acute loss, revenge (emotional)
(Or, if the feelings have already been expressed spontaneously), I can see you're really upset.	*Rape:* I shouldn't have accepted his invitation to have a drink... I suppose it's my fault for being so stupid.	Guilt, self-blame (emotional, cognitive)
What did you do when she told you about wanting a divorce?	I figured, good riddance. I only stayed for the kids' sake. But now that she's gone, I'm really lonely and I hate the singles' bar scene.	Relief, ambivalence (emotional, cognitive)
	Or: I went down to the bar and got drunk and have been drinking a lot ever since.	Unable to cope effectively, desire to escape loneliness (emotional, behavioral)
How do you usually handle problems that are upsetting to you?	I generally talk to my closest friend or just get away by myself for a while to think things through.	Generally effective coping ability (behavioral, cognitive)
Why didn't this work for you this time?	My closest friend moved away and I just haven't found anyone else to talk to that I really trust.	Realization of need for substitute support (cognitive, behavioral)

- They provide essential information to determine whether or not a person is in crisis.
- They suggest whether the person's usual coping devices are, for example, healthy or unhealthy, and how these ways of coping are related to what Caplan calls the personal, material, and sociocultural supplies needed to avoid crisis.
- They provide information about the meaning of stressful life events to various people and about the individual's particular definition of the situation, which is essential to a personally tailored intervention plan.
- They link the assessment process to intervention strategies by providing baseline data for action and learning new ways of coping.

The relationship between hazardous events, people's responses to these events (their vulnerability), and the precipitating factor is illustrated in Figure 3.3.

The answers to our assessment questions provide a broad picture of what Hansell (1976) calls "crisis plumage," the distinguishing characteristics of a person in crisis compared to one who is not. This plumage consists of distress signals that people send to others when they experience a loss or a threat of loss, are abused or in danger, or are challenged to increase their "supplies"—their basic needs or life attachments. Signals of distress include the following:

1. Difficulty in managing one's feelings
2. Suicidal or homicidal tendencies
3. Alcohol or other drug abuse
4. Trouble with the law
5. Inability to effectively use available help

These signals usually indicate that a person is coping ineffectively with a crisis and needs assistance to forestall negative crisis outcomes. In short, people proceed through life with material, personal, and sociocultural resources, as well as problem-solving devices for dealing with various stressors. When these resources are intact, people generally avoid the possible negative outcomes of stressful life events. For example, in assessing the vulnerability of an assault victim, careful attention must be paid to the circumstances of victimization. In contrast, if the attack is linked to the victim's character traits, we are very close to victim-blaming, which hampers the person's recovery (Sales, Baum, & Shore, 1984, pp. 132–133), and may contribute to the downward spiral depicted in Figure 2.2. When psychosocial resources are wanting, the person in crisis usually seeks help from others to compensate for a temporary inability to deal constructively with life's stressors. The help received is crisis intervention. If the help obtained is from human service institutions or professionals, it is known as formal crisis manage-

FIGURE 3.3. COMPONENTS OF THE CRISIS STATE.

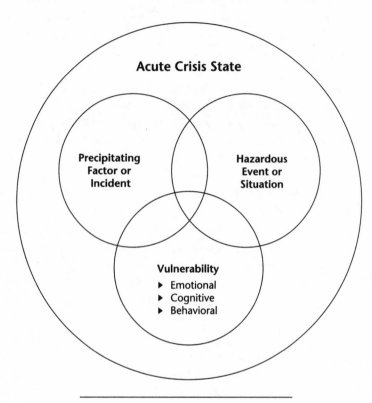

The components in the intertwining circles represent the interactional
process that characterizes the crisis experience.

ment, as distinguished from natural crisis management. However, in order to be
part of the crisis solution rather than the problem, crisis workers must assess in
greater detail the parameters of an individual's vulnerability. To do so requires
understanding the emotional, biophysical, cognitive, and behavioral responses
to hazardous events. Let us consider, then, the characteristics of crisis plumage—
how people in crisis feel, think, and act (see Figure 3.1, Box 2).

Feelings and Biophysical Response. People in crisis experience a high degree of
anxiety and tension. Another common theme is a sense of loss or emptiness. This
feeling springs directly from an actual or threatened loss in self-esteem, material
goods, social relationships, or a failure to reach a life goal such as promotion or
retirement. Other feelings frequently experienced are fear, shock, anger, guilt, em-

barrassment, or shame. Fear is often expressed in terms of losing control or not understanding why one is responding in a certain way. Anger is directed inward for not being able to manage one's life, or at a significant other for leaving, dying, or inflicting physical abuse. Guilt and embarrassment often follow anger that does not seem justified. How can one be angry at a dead person when considering one's luck in being alive after an accident or disaster? People who are abused by someone they love often feel ashamed—an outcome of the victim-blaming legacy.

Of all feelings common to the crisis experience, anxiety is probably the most familiar. A certain degree of tension is a normal part of life; it serves to move us to make appropriate plans for productive action. Without it, we become nonproductive. For example, Terri, a student, has no anxiety about passing or failing a course. Therefore, she does not exert the effort required to study and achieve a passing grade. When a person is excessively anxious, however, negative results usually occur. A state of great anxiety is one of the most painful experiences a human being can have.

Anxiety is manifested in a number of ways. Some characteristics will be peculiar to the person concerned. Commonly experienced signs of anxiety are:

- Sense of dread
- Fear of losing control
- Inability to focus on one thing
- Physical symptoms: sweating, frequent urination, diarrhea, nausea and vomiting, tachycardia (rapid heartbeat), headache, chest or abdominal pain, rash, menstrual irregularity, and sexual disinterest

---

CASE EXAMPLE: DELAINE

Delaine, age forty-five, feels bereft after the recent death of her husband. Her friends have been supportive since his death from chronic heart disease. She chides herself and feels guilty about not being able to take the loss any better. She knew her husband's condition was precarious; nevertheless, she had depended on him as a readily available source of reassurance. Since she is basically a cheerful person, always on hand to support others in distress, she is embarrassed by what she perceives as weakness following her husband's death.

Because she cries more than usual, Delaine is afraid she may be losing control. At times, she even wonders whether she is going crazy. It is noteworthy that Delaine is

in a major developmental transition to middle age. Also, the oldest of her three children was recently married, leaving her with a sense of loss in her usual mothering role. An additional, but anticipated, loss is the recent news that one of her close friends will soon be leaving town. This threatens to further erode Delaine's base of support. She feels angry about all the losses in her life, asking, "Why does all this have to happen to me at once?" But she also feels guilty about her anger; after all, she thinks her friend deserves the opportunity that the move will afford her and her husband, and she knows her daughter has every right to get married and live her own life.

What Delaine does not acknowledge is that

- She also has a right to her feelings about these disturbing events.
- She has a right and a need to express those feelings.
- Her feelings of loss and anger do not cancel the good feelings and support she can continue to have from her daughter and friend, although in an altered form.

Were it not for these developmental and situational factors, Delaine might not have experienced her husband's death as a crisis. The stability of Delaine's life transactions was disrupted on several counts:

- Her role as wife changed to that of widow.
- Her role as mother of her oldest daughter was altered by her daughter's marriage.
- Her affectional attachment to her husband was completely severed.
- Affectional attachment to her friend will be altered in terms of physical distance and the immediacy of support.
- Her notion of a full life includes marriage, so she must adjust—at least temporarily—to a change in that perception.

Thoughts, Perceptions, and Interpretations of Events. Feelings—especially of high anxiety—have great impact on perceptions and thinking processes. In crisis, one's attention is focused on the acute shock and anguish being experienced and a few items concerning the crisis event. As a consequence, the person's usual memory and way of perceiving may be altered. He or she may have difficulty sorting things out. The relationship between events may not seem clear. People in crisis feel caught in a maze of events they cannot fit together. They often have trouble defining who they are and what their skills are. The state of anguish and resulting confusion can alter a person's ability to make decisions and solve problems—the very skills needed during a crisis. This disturbance in perceptual processes and problem-solving ability increases the individual's already heightened state of anxiety. Sometimes, the person fears losing control.

The distorted perceptual process observed in crisis states should not be confused with mental illness in which a person's *usual* pattern of thinking is disturbed. In a crisis state, the disturbance arises from and is part of the crisis experience. There is a rapid return to normal perception once the crisis is resolved.

CASE EXAMPLE: JOAN

Joan, age thirty-four, called a mental health center stating that her husband had just left the house with his rifle and that she did not know where he was going. She was afraid for her life as they had had an argument the night before during which she complained about his drinking, and he had threatened her. On further questioning, it turned out that Joan's husband had left the house at his usual time for work in a neighboring town.

Case Example, cont.

He had left with the rifle the previous evening after the argument, although on occasion he also took his gun along to work, as he explained it, in case he had a chance to go hunting. After three hours, he had returned, apparently calmed down, and put away the gun. The gun was still in the house when Joan called. There was nothing in the interaction to lead an observer to conclude that Joan's husband would not be home as usual after a day at work.

Noteworthy in this example is Joan's disturbed perceptual process. On questioning, she cannot recall certain details without help and cannot put all the facts into logical order. Joan is obviously very anxious about her safety. Complicating this feeling of anxiety is her sense of guilt about her role in precipitating the argument by mentioning her husband's drinking. Her anxiety is consistent with her perception—not necessarily the reality—of a threat to her safety. The determining factor is how she *perceives* the event. Nevertheless, marital discord and the presence of a gun underscore the importance of assessing thoroughly for a history of abuse and safety resources for a woman like Joan. One of the most common complaints from abused women and their advocates is that people do not believe them or take their stories seriously.

The feelings of people in crisis are usually consistent with their perception of the situation (Dressler, 1973). Recognition of this fact should decrease the possibility of casting people with similar problems into a common mold. The perception of the event is one of the factors that makes an event a crisis for one person but not for another.

Joan's case illustrates how excessive anxiety interferes with effective problem solving. If Joan were not so anxious, she would probably have arrived at an obvious way to ensure her immediate safety, that is, by removing the gun or leaving the house and seeking help. Joan probably knows that the use of weapons is intrinsically connected with their availability, but her anxiety prevents her from using that knowledge.

Other aspects of cognitive functioning spring from different socialization processes and value systems that influence how particular events are interpreted. Illness, for example, has a different meaning and crisis potential for various ethnic and religious groups (see Chapter Eleven and Zborowski, 1952). A state legislator who was jailed for a minor offense killed himself hours after being imprisoned. For this elected official, the transgression meant loss of reputation, whereas a person arrested for repeated drunken driving may interpret the event differently because he or she has less to lose. People socialized to feel incomplete without marriage will probably experience the loss of a spouse as an occasion of crisis, whereas others grow from the challenges of greater independence. These examples illustrate the importance of being culturally sensitive and not imposing our own values and behavior norms on others. No situation or disturbance affects two people alike, and the same person may respond differently to similar events at different times in life. Thus, varying and subjective interpretations of life events are integral aspects of a crisis response and must be assessed accordingly.

Behavior. Behavior usually follows from what people think and feel and from their interpretations of life events. If a person feels anxious and has a distorted perception of events, he or she is likely to behave in unusual ways. However, what may seem unusual, distorted, or "crazy" to an outsider may be considered normal behavior within certain cultural groups. In order to determine whether a person's behavior is normal or deviant, we need to start with *that* person's cultural definition of what is usual, not our own. This is particularly important if the crisis worker and person in distress are from different cultures, classes, or ethnic groups. If the distressed person is too upset to provide this kind of information, it should be elicited from family or friends whenever possible. Failing that, a consultation with someone of the person's ethnic or cultural group would be useful.

A significant behavioral sign of crisis is the individual's inability to perform normal vocational functions in the usual manner, for example, when a person cannot do necessary household chores, concentrate on studies, or work at an outside job. Another sign is a change in social behavior, such as withdrawing from friends, making unusual efforts to avoid being alone, or becoming clingy or demanding (Hansell, 1976). As social connections break down, the person may also feel detached or distant from others. Some people in crisis act on impulse. They may drive a car recklessly, attempt suicide, or attack others as a desperate means of solving a problem (see Chapters Six and Nine).

Some people will go out of their way to reject the assistance offered by friends. Often, this response arises out of a sense of helplessness and embarrassment at not being able to cope in the usual manner. The person fears that acceptance of help may be misinterpreted as a confirmation of weakness. To allay such fears, it is paramount that crisis workers examine their attitudes and any biases they may bring to the assessment milieu (Hoff, 1995). People in crisis may also behave in ways that are inconsistent with their thoughts and feelings. For example, a young woman witnessed a shooting accident that caused the death of her boyfriend. Initially, she was visibly upset by the event and was brought by her family to a mental health emergency clinic. During the interview with a counselor, she laughed inappropriately when talking about the shooting and death she had witnessed—a sign of very high anxiety. Another behavioral signal is atypical behavior, such as driving while intoxicated by a person with no previous record of such behavior.

In summary, when assessing vulnerability, it is important to find out how *this* particular person is reacting *here and now* to whatever happened. The simplest way to assess a person's vulnerability is to ask, How do you feel about what happened? What do you usually do when you're upset? and similar questions suggested in Table 3.2.

Family and Community Assessment

Our discussion of the assessment process thus far has focused primarily on techniques to determine the hazardous events or situations precipitating the crisis and the individual's response to these events: emotional, cognitive, behavioral, and biophysical. Crisis assessment, however, is incomplete without evaluating the person's social resources and cultural milieu (see Kaplan, Cassel, & Gore, 1977). This includes inquiring whether the person thinks his or her family and other social contacts are real or potential assets or liabilities. Asking whether network members are part of the problem or part of the solution is often the full extent of social assessment in much of crisis practice, in spite of a historic emphasis on sociocultural factors (Caplan, 1964). In this book, social assessment means that the person's social network members are deliberately—not just incidentally—included in the assessment process. This is not difficult to do, but it does require a worker's willingness to make the effort. Often, workers cite a lack of time or the inaccessibility of the family as reasons for emphasizing an individual approach to assessment. But this probably obscures their own lack of conviction or skills in the use of social approaches. In view of what is known about the social aspects of crisis responses, these issues should be examined in order to refine crisis assessment and intervention strategies.

Including a social approach in assessment reduces the chances of misidentifying who is in crisis. That is, sometimes the person who appears or is brought in for help may be upset but not in crisis. A complete assessment could reveal the entire family to be in crisis, as could happen, for example, when a teenager tries to commit suicide.

Evaluation of the sociocultural context and community resources is related to family assessment; the context may figure in the origin and resolution of crises, as illustrated in the Crisis Paradigm. Evaluation should include questions about whether the person has received necessary help from community resources, as well as inquiries about cultural and socioeconomic factors that may contribute to the person's vulnerability and ability to resolve crises constructively. For example, negative factors such as racial unrest or positive ones such as opportunities for welfare mothers to become economically self-sufficient should be considered. These aspects of comprehensive crisis assessment and their implications for intervention are elaborated further in Chapter Five.

The individual and sociocultural aspects of crisis assessment are summarized and illustrated with examples in Table 3.3. This diagram elaborates on the concept of healthy and unhealthy coping (Caplan & Grunebaum, 1967). It outlines the relationship between crisis origins and the personal manifestations of crisis (see Figure 3.1, Boxes 1 and 2). It also links the crisis assessment process to various intervention techniques. For example, if assessment reveals that a person is not coping well in general terms—emotional, biophysical, cognitive, and behavioral—the information received can be used to help the person cope more effectively.

TABLE 3.3. DIFFERENTIATION: EFFECTIVE AND INEFFECTIVE CRISIS COPING ACCORDING TO CRISIS EPISODE.

Crisis Episode			Crisis Coping	
Hazardous Event	Origin	Personal Manifestations	Ineffective	Effective
Loss of child by death	*Situational:* unexplained physical mal-functioning of child, for example, SIDS	Emotional Biophysical	Depression Stomach or other ailments	Grief work
		Cognitive	Conviction of having done something wrong to cause death of the child	Recognizing and accepting that there is nothing one could have done to prevent the death
		Behavioral	Inability to care for other chil-dren appro-priately (for example, over-protective)	Attendance of peer support group
Physical battering by partner	*Sociocultural:* values and other factors affecting relationships	Emotional	Crying, depres-sion, feelings of worthlessness, self-blame, and helplessness	Anger, shock (How could he do this to me?), outrage at the fact that it happened
		Cognitive	Assumption that the beating was justified: in-ability to decide what to do	Conviction of inappropriate-ness of violence between men and women; decision to leave and/or otherwise re-order one's life free of violence
		Behavioral	Alcohol abuse, abuse of chil-dren, excusing of partner's violence	Seek refuge in nonviolent shel-ter; initiate steps toward economic in-dependence; participate in peer group support and social change activities

On the other hand, careful assessment can show when not to intervene—in areas in which the person's coping is adequate, or the person feels help is not needed. Even a person who is acutely upset can be helped to realize that he or she is coping adequately in *some* aspects of life (e.g., at work but not at home or vice versa). In short, a skilled crisis worker supports healthy coping and, guided by assessment data, avoids doing either too little or too much.

The next section describes a structured approach to carrying out the assessment process, using the concepts discussed so far.

An Assessment Interview

An interview (see Table 3.4) with George Sloan, age forty-eight, is conducted by an emergency department nurse. George is brought to the hospital by police following an attempt to commit suicide by crashing his car. (This case illustration is continued from Chapter Two.)

Besides the technical aspects of asking clear, direct questions, this interview excerpt illustrates another important point. The nurse reveals an understanding of Mr. Sloan's problem and empathizes with the despair he must be feeling when she says:

- So, your car accident was really an attempt to kill yourself?
- Sounds like you've been having a rough time, George.
- I can see that your illness and all your other troubles have left you feeling pretty bad.
- George, I can see that you're feeling desperate about your situation.
- I'm glad your suicide attempt didn't work.

The nurse clearly comes through as a person with feelings and concern about a patient who is in despair. Concern is conveyed by a gentle tone of voice and an unstylized manner. Furthermore, the nurse expresses feelings without sounding sentimental and shocked, and apparently is not afraid to be with a person in crisis. As shown by this interview, effective assessment techniques are not highly complicated or veiled in mystery. The techniques require:

- A straightforward approach with simple, direct questions
- The ability to empathize, to appreciate the other person's perspective
- An ability to grasp the depth of another's despair and share the feelings this evokes
- The courage not to run away from frightening experiences like suicide attempts

The interview also shows that ascertaining suicide risk (Level One assessment) is an integral part of thorough crisis assessment. Parents, teachers, friends, and

TABLE 3.4. INTERVIEW EXAMPLE: GEORGE SLOAN.

Signals of Distress and Crisis to be Identified	Assessment Techniques
	Nurse: Hello, Mr. Sloan. Would you like to be called Mr. Sloan or George?
	George: George is fine.
	Nurse: Will you tell me what happened, George?
	George: I had a car accident. Can't you see that without asking? (Slightly hostile and seemingly reluctant to talk.)
	Nurse: Yes, I know, George. But the police said you were going the wrong way on the expressway. How did that happen?
Active Crisis State: Extreme anxiety to the breaking point	*George:* Yes, that's right—(hesitates). Well, I just couldn't take it anymore—but I guess it didn't work.
	Nurse: Sounds like you've been having a rough time, George. Can you tell me what it is you can't take anymore?
Hazardous Event Situation: Physical illness	*George:* Well, I've got heart trouble...
Vulnerable State: Loss of external social supports or inability to use them	It's gotten to be too much for my wife—I can't expect her to do much more....
Loss of personal coping ability	We're having trouble with our 16-year-old son, Arnold....
Inability to communicate stress to significant others	I just couldn't take it anymore. I figured I'd do everybody a favor and get rid of myself.
High-lethal suicide attempt	*Nurse:* So your car accident was really an attempt to kill yourself?
	George: That's right—that way, at least my wife wouldn't lose the insurance along with everything else she's had to put up with.
	Nurse: I can see that your heart trouble and all your other troubles have left you feeling pretty bad.
Depression	*George:* That's about it—too bad I came out alive. I really feel I'm worth more dead than alive.
	Nurse: I can see that you're feeling desperate about your situation. How long have you felt this way?

	George: I've had heart trouble for about four years. After my last heart attack, the doctor told me I had to slow down or it would probably kill me. Well, there's no way I can change things that I can see.
Precipitating Factor: Inability to perform in expected role as father	*Nurse:* What happened this past week that made you decide to end it all?
	George: Well, our kid Arnold got suspended from school—that did it! I figured if a father can't do any better with his son than that, what's the use?
	Nurse: I gather from what you say and feel that you just couldn't see any other way out.
State of Active Crisis: Vulnerability: Fixated on role expectations; inability to use outside helping resources	*George:* That's right—money is really getting tight; my wife was talking about getting a full-time job and that really bothers me to think that I can't support my family anymore. And if she starts working more, things might get even worse with Arnold. There was no one to talk to. Suicide's the only thing left.
	Nurse: With all these problems, George, have you ever thought about suicide before?
History of poor coping ability	*George:* Yes, once, after my doctor told me to really watch it after my last heart attack. I felt pretty hopeless and thought of crashing my car then. But things weren't so bad then between me and my wife, and she talked me out of it and seemed willing to stick with me.
	Nurse: I see—but this time you felt there was nowhere else to turn. Anyway, George, I'm glad your suicide attempt didn't work. I'd really like to help you consider some other ways to deal with all these problems.
	George: I don't know what they could be. I really feel hopeless, but I guess I could see what you've got to offer.
	Nurse: There are several things we can discuss.

(To be continued in Chapter 4, "Helping People in Crisis")

police can augment their natural tendencies to help by learning these assessment techniques. Failure to use the techniques can mean the difference between life and death for someone like Mr. Sloan. It is not uncommon for people in his condition to be treated medically or surgically without anyone finding out about his intention to commit suicide. If he receives only medical or surgical treatment and nothing else changes in his life, George Sloan will probably commit suicide within six to twelve months. He is already in a high-risk category (see Chapter Six).

Another objective of the initial interview is to provide the person in crisis with concrete help. If Mr. Sloan had not felt the nurse's acceptance and concern, he would not have dropped his initial resistance to sharing his dilemma. The nurse opened the discussion of alternatives to suicide.

Once an individual is identified as being in a state of crisis, the helping person proceeds to give or obtain whatever assistance is indicated. In complex situations or in circumstances involving life and death, the helper should engage the services of professional crisis workers (Hoff & Miller 1987; Hoff & Wells, 1989).

Once the state of crisis is ascertained, the professional crisis worker engages the person in a full-scale evaluation (Level Two assessment) of his or her problems. This involves the person's family and other significant people. Such assessment techniques are currently practiced in many crisis and counseling clinics and community mental health programs. A framework and sample tool from a comprehensive assessment protocol is discussed next.

Comprehensive Crisis Assessment

A well-organized worker uses tools that aid in assessment. If a crisis worker lacks direction and a sense of order, this adds to the confusion a person in crisis feels. While tools emphasize a structured approach to the process, no record-keeping system or mechanical tool such as computer analysis can substitute for the empathy, knowledge, and experience of a skilled clinician. Records are to complement, not displace, clinical judgment and expertise in the psychosocial interview process. Nor should record-keeping procedures be allowed to depersonalize interaction with a distressed person.

Philosophy and Context of Sample Record System

The framework and sample tool recommended to guide and record the crisis management process as conceived in this book was selected because it illustrates the principles that should guide any crisis-sensitive record system. The example presented here:

- Is based on the understanding of crisis in the psychosociocultural perspective emphasized in this text
- Is client-centered in that it includes the person's self-evaluation as an integral part of the assessment process
- Assumes that the client is a member of a social network—not simply an indi-

vidual in psychological disequilibrium—and that disruption or threat of disruption from essential social attachments is often the occasion of crisis

- Provides a structured, standardized framework for gathering data from the individual and significant others while including subjective, narrative-style information from the client
- Focuses on a view of the person in crisis as a human being functioning at varying degrees of adequacy or inadequacy, not merely as a diagnostic entity
- Assists in fostering continuity between the various steps of the crisis management process (assessment, planning, intervention, follow-up) by providing relevant, organized information so that the client's level of functioning, goals, and methods for attaining these goals can be sharply defined and used as a guide in the course of service
- Provides supervisory staff with information necessary to monitor service and assure quality care to clients on an ongoing basis
- Provides administrative staff the database needed for monitoring and evaluating service program outcomes in relation to stated objectives

The record system of which this sample tool is a part was developed by a special task force in the Erie County Mental Health System in Buffalo, New York. It is unique in that it incorporates crisis management principles into the assessment and record-keeping requirements of a state and county mental health department while retaining its client-centered focus. Clients at risk for crisis who were served in this mental health system included (1) people experiencing various unanticipated hazardous life events who therefore were at risk of extrusion from their natural social setting; (2) people vulnerable to crisis because of chronic mental or emotional disturbance, chemical dependence, or disadvantaged social circumstances. Some of the case examples cited in this book are drawn from people who requested service in this crisis-sensitive mental health system.

The record system was tested in the 1970s with crisis and mental health workers in the community mental health agencies that adopted the system. Included were the majority of publicly funded programs serving urban, suburban, and rural communities in a metropolitan area with a population of 1.25 million. Participants in testing the system also included people receiving service. A client was considered an active partner in developing the record and had full access to it. Examples of client feedback were:

- I'm not as bad off as I thought.
- This takes some of the mystery out of mental health.
- Getting help with a problem isn't so magical after all.
- Now I have a diary of how I worked out my problems and got better.

Staff members using the forms receive formal training in crisis intervention and in using the record system according to written specifications. Although the category "Violence Experienced" was added in 1982 and was published in two earlier editions of this text, recent research (Tilden, et al., 1994) documents that education and clinical application on this topic are far from routine (Hoff, 1995), despite growing public concern about violence and health professionals' roles in prevention and in the treatment of victims. (See Chapters Six, Eight, and Nine for a more detailed discussion of this topic, a suggested triage tool for use in all entry points to the health and social service system (Hoff & Rosenbaum, 1994), and an adaptation of the tool in instances of woman battering.

Service Forms

The following description for using the forms is excerpted from the complete specifications.[1] Because of their life and death implications, specifications and rating scales are included in this book for three of the seventeen items: *item 12,* victimization trauma; *item 13,* assessing risk of suicide; and *item 14,* assault/homicide—they are included in Chapters Eight, Six, and Nine, respectively. The forms included here illustrate assessment information with reference to the case example of George Sloan, which is continued from Chapter Two. The seventeen items in the Self-Assessment Worksheet illustrate the "Basic Life Attachments" (items 1–11) and "Signals of Distress" (items 12–17) discussed in this and the previous chapter. The same seventeen items are used for client assessment and program evaluation purposes at (1) completion of the service contract (discharge); and (2) periods designated for formal follow-up, especially of high-risk clients, for example, six or twelve months after discharge.

Initial Contact Sheet

This form (see Exhibit 3.1) is intended to provide basic demographic and problem information at the time the client requests service or is presented for service by another person or agency. This information should provide the worker with sufficient data to make several key decisions early in the helping process:

- How urgent is the situation?
- Who is to be assigned responsibility for proceeding with the next step?
- What type of response is indicated as the next step?

[1]For complete forms, specifications for their use, and information about reliability and validity studies, the reader is referred to the author, who can be contacted through the publisher.

This form is used chiefly by the worker designated to handle incoming calls and requests for service during a specified period of time, sometimes called a triage worker. The "Crisis Rating" section of the form should be completed according to the following guidelines:

Crisis Rating: How Urgent Is Your Need for Help?

> *Very Urgent:* Request requires an immediate response within minutes; crisis outreach; medical emergency requiring an ambulance (overdoses); severe drug reaction; or police needed if situation involves extreme danger or weapons.
>
> *Urgent:* Response should be rapid but not necessarily immediate—within a few hours. Example: low-to-moderate risk of suicide or mild drug reaction.
>
> *Somewhat Urgent:* Response should be made within a day (twenty-four hours). Example: planning conference in which key persons are not available until the following evening.
>
> *Slightly Urgent:* A response is required within a few days. Example: client's funding runs out within a week and she or he needs public assistance.
>
> *Not Urgent:* When a situation has existed for a long time and does not warrant immediate intervention, a week or two is unlikely to make any significant difference. Examples: A child with a learning disability; a couple that needs marital counseling.

Client Self-Assessment Worksheet

The Client Self-Assessment Worksheet (see Exhibit 3.2) can be used in two ways: (1) it can serve as an interview guide in a face-to-face session with the client; (2) the client (if not acutely upset) can be given the form to complete, after which the items are discussed in a face-to-face interview. Such use of this form assumes that "the record belongs to the client." This principle needs shoring up because psychiatric groups have used legal channels to keep mental health clients from gaining access to their records. A client-centered record reflects the view that clients are in charge of their lives and that the helping process should not be mysterious to them. The worksheet is *never* to be used without a personal interview. The "Significant Other Worksheet" and the "Child Screening Checklist" (see Exhibit 3.3) can be used in a similar fashion.

A cautionary note is in order here: forms can never substitute for rapport, time, and sensitivity to the unique needs of each distressed person. Clinicians bombarded with management information systems must be careful to avoid *recording* more and more about *doing* less and less.

EXHIBIT 3.1. INITIAL CONTACT SHEET.

Today's Date _1-15-95_   Walk-in _____   ID # _101_
    Time _5:30_ AM   Phone _____   SS # _123-98-456_
              (PM) Outreach _Police_   Welfare/
                    Written _____   Medicaid # _____

SERVICE REQUESTED FOR
Client's NAME _George_   _O._   _Sloan_
              First   Middle   Last   Permanent _✓_
Address _33 Random Avenue Middletown 01234 Central_ Temporary _____
         Street   City/Town   Zip County Catchment Area _3_
Phone # _123-0987_   Means of Transportation _Ambulance_
Directions to home (if outreach) _____
Sex: Male _✓_ Female ___ Date of Birth _1947_   Age _48_

SERVICE REQUESTED BY Name _____ Phone # _____
PRESENTING SITUATION/PROBLEM — What made you decide to seek help today?
   (use other side if needed)
George Sloan, 48, was brought to E.R. by police following a suicide attempt by car crash. His intention was to die as he saw no way out of his personal and family problems. Has had heart trouble for 4 years. Was urged to quit second job and take office job in Police Dept. His 16-yr. old son's suspension from school adds to his sense of failure. Feels he has no one to talk to. Had considered suicide after last heart attack but support from his wife prevented him then from crashing his car. While initially reluctant, Mr. Sloan now seems open to counseling assistance.

Have you talked with anyone about this?   Yes _____ Who? _____
Address _____   No _✓_ Phone # _____
                                     Date of last contact: _____
Are you taking ANY medication now? Yes _✓_ What? 1. _nitroglycerine_
(if more than 3 begin list on MH-2) No _____ 2._____
                                               3._____

CRISIS RATING How urgent is your need for help? | Comments
☒ Immediate (within minutes)   Recommend Mr. Sloan receive
☐ Within a few hours   ☐ Within a few days   full assessment and crisis
☐ Within 24 hours   ☐ Within a week or two counseling while being
DISPOSITION (Check all that apply)   treated for injuries from
☒ Crisis   suicidal car accident, plus
☒ Medical Emergency   follow-up with entire
☒ Assessment (specify) _Individual and Family_ family.
☐ Discharge Planning
☐ Expediting/Advocacy
☐ Other (explain) _____
☒ Referral made to: _Psychiatric Liaison Service_ Confirmed: Yes _✓_ No __ Date _1-15-95_
Date of Next Contact _____ Assigned to _John Doe, M.S.W._
Date of Assignment _____ Request taken by _Jane Doe, R.N._

                                                              MH-1

EXHIBIT 3.2. CLIENT SELF-ASSESSMENT WORKSHEET: GEORGE SLOAN.

Date *1-15-95*   Name *George Sloan*

1. <u>Physical Health</u>   Circle one for each question.
    How is your health?   Excellent
    Comments: *No problems except for heart.*   Good
    Feel OK except for chest pain, which is getting   (Fair)
    more frequent.   Poor
                                                                          Very Poor

2. <u>Self-Acceptance/Self-Esteem</u>
    How do you feel about yourself as a person?   Excellent
    Comments: *Not very good — especially when I think*   Good
    about my son's trouble that it's probably my   Fair
    fault. Seems like I'm no good at anything   (Poor)
    lately.   Very Poor

3. <u>Vocational/Occupational</u>
    (Includes student & homemaker)   Excellent
    How would you judge your work/school situation?   Good
    Comments: *I can still do patrol work, but the*   (Fair)
    doctor says I should slow down.   Poor
                                                                          Very Poor

4. <u>Immediate Family</u>
    How are your relationships with your family and/or spouse?   Excellent
    Comments: *Ever since my first heart attack*   Good
    we seem to be going from bad to worse,   Fair
    especially with our son Arnold.   (Poor)
                                                                          Very Poor

5. <u>Intimate Relationship(s)</u>
    Is there anyone you feel really close to and can rely on?   Always
    Comments: *Not really. Things used to be better*   Usually
    between my wife and me, but we seem   Sometimes
    to be drifting apart.   (Rarely)
                                                                          Never

6. <u>Residential</u>
    How do you judge your housing situation?   (Excellent)
    Comments: _____   Good
    _____   Fair
    _____   Poor
    _____   Very Poor

7. <u>Financial</u>
    How would you describe your financial situation?   Excellent
    Comments: *As long as I have my second job*   (Good)
    it's O.K., but I don't like the idea of my   Fair
    wife working full-time.   Poor
                                                                          Very Poor

8. <u>Decision-Making Ability</u>
    How satisfied are you with your ability   Always Very Satisfied
    to make life decisions?   Almost Always Satisfied
    Comments: *Mostly around the problems*   (Occasionally Dissatisfied)
    we have with Arnold.   Almost Always Dissatisfied
                                                          Always Very Dissatisfied

EXHIBIT 3.2., CONT.

Circle one for each question.

9. Life Philosophy/Goals

How satisfied are you with how your
life goals are working for you?

Comments: *I almost always felt
satisfied before the heart trouble
started 4 years ago.*

- Always Very Satisfied
- Almost Always Satisfied
- Occasionally Dissatisfied
- (Almost Always Dissatisfied)
- Always Very Dissatisfied

10. Leisure Time/Community Involvement

How satisfied are you with your
use of free time?

Comments: *I don't have much free time,
but I really like my work. I suppose
our whole family could use more time together.*

- Always Very Satisfied
- Almost Always Satisfied
- (Occasionally Dissatisfied)
- Almost Always Dissatisfied
- Always Very Dissatisfied

11. Feeling Management

How comfortable are you with
your feelings?

Comments: *Just during the last few
months I really started feeling
depressed. My wife says I bottle everything up.*

- Always Very Comfortable
- Almost Always Comfortable
- (Occasionally Uncomfortable)
- Almost Always Uncomfortable
- Always Very Uncomfortable

12. Violence Experienced

To what extent have you been troubled
by physical violence against you?

Comments: _____
_____
_____

- (Never)
- Once only
- Several times within 6 months
- Once or twice a month
- Routinely (every day or so)

13. Lethality (self)

Is there any current risk of
suicide for you?

Comments: *I still can't see any way
out except suicide, but right now I
feel a little better from talking with you.*

- No Predictable Risk of Suicide Now
- Low Risk of Suicide Now
- Moderate Risk of Suicide Now
- High Risk of Suicide Now
- (Very High Risk of Suicide Now)

14. Lethality (other)

Is there any risk that you might
physically harm someone?

Comments: _____
_____
_____

- (No Predictable Risk of Assault Now)
- Low Risk of Assault Now
- Moderate Risk of Assault Now
- High Risk of Assault Now
- Very High Risk of Assault Now

15. Substance Use (Drug and/or Alcohol)

Does use of drugs/alcohol interfere
with performing your responsibilities?

Comments: _____
_____
_____

- (Never interferes)
- Rarely interferes
- Sometimes interferes
- Frequently interferes
- Constantly interferes

16. Legal

What is your tendency to get in
trouble with the law?

Comments: _____
_____
_____

- (No Tendency)
- Slight Tendency
- Moderate Tendency
- Great Tendency
- Very Great Tendency

17. Agency Use

How successful are you at getting help
from agencies (or doctors) when you need it?

Comments: *I don't like going to doctors
and avoid it if at all possible.*

- Always Successful
- (Usually Successful)
- Moderately Successful
- Seldom Successful
- Never Successful

Any additional comments?   MH-6A

EXHIBIT 3.3. CHILD SCREENING CHECKLIST.

ID#
_____

Child's Full Name _____Sex___Birthdate_____

School Problems
a) poor grades__   d) suspended__
b) does not get along with students__   e) poor attendance__
c) does not get along with teachers__

Family Relationship Problems
does not get along with: father__ mother__ brothers__ sisters__
refuses to participate in family activities__
refuses to accept and perform family responsibilities__

Peer Relationship Problems
prefers to be alone__   prefers to be with adults__
does not associate with age mates__   not accepted by others__

Dissocial Behavior
excessive lying__ hurts others__ hurts self__ destructive__ runaway__
substance use__ court involvement__ other__

Personal Adjustment Problems
temper tantrums__ easily upset__ speech problems__ sleep disturbances__
nervous mannerisms__ eating problems__ fearful__ lacks self-confidence__
clinging and dependent__ wetting, soiling, retention__ other__

Medical and Developmental Problems
chronic illness__ allergies__ physical handicaps__ accident prone__
seizures__ physical complaints__ lengthy or frequent hospitalizations__
medication__ surgery__ MR__ other__

Development Milestones (Administer to all pre-schoolers. Check behaviors
present, up to and including present age.)

Age	Activity	Age	Activity
1	____ imitates speech sounds	2 1/2	____ climbs stairs,
1	____ feeds self with fingers		alternating feet
1	____ pulls self to feet	3	____ forms sentences
1 1/2	____ uses single words	3	____ dresses self--no fasten-
ers			
1 1/2	____ walks alone	4	____ recognizes three colors
2	____ understands simple directions	4	____ throws ball overhand
2	____ scribbles with pencil or crayon	5	____ speaks clearly
2 1/2	____ combines words into phrases	5	____ buttons clothing

In years or months, at what age do you think your child is functioning?____

Strengths and assets:

Comments:

Screened by   Date _____

Summary

Some people are at greater risk of crisis than others. Identifying groups of people who are most likely to experience a crisis is helpful in recognizing individuals in crisis. People in crisis have typical patterns of thinking, feeling, and acting. There is no substitute for a thorough assessment of whether a person is or is not in crisis. The assessment is the basis of the helping plan; it can save lives and reduce the occurrence of other problems, including the unnecessary placement of people in institutions.

References

Barney, K. (1994). Limitations of the critique of the medical model. *The Journal of Mind and Behavior, 15*(1, 2), 19–34.

Becker, H. S. (1963). *Outsider: Studies in the sociology of deviance.* New York: Free Press.

Berger, P. L., & Luckmann, T. (1967). *The social construction of reality.* New York: Anchor-Doubleday.

Bittner, E. (1967). Police discretion in the emergency apprehension of mentally ill persons. *Social Problems, 14*(3), 278–292.

Breggin, P. (1992). *Beyond conflict: From self-help and psychotherapy to peacemaking.* New York: St. Martin's Press.

Caplan, G. (1964). *Principles of preventive psychiatry.* New York: Basic Books.

Caplan, G., & Grunebaum, H. (1967). Perspectives on primary prevention: A review. *Archives of General Psychiatry, 17,* 331–346.

Capponi, P. (1992). *Upstairs in the crazy house.* Toronto: Penguin.

Cloward, R. A., & Piven, F. F. (1979). Hidden protest: The channeling of female innovation and protest. *Signs: Journal of Women in Culture and Society, 4,* 651–669.

Daniels, A.K. (1978). The social construction of military psychiatric diagnosis. In J. G. Manis & B. N. Meltzer (Eds.), *Symbolic interaction,* (3rd ed., pp. 380–392). Boston: Allyn Bacon.

Danish, S. J., Smyer, M. A., & Nowak, C. A. (1980). Developmental intervention: Enhancing life-event processes. *Life-Span Development and Behavior, 3,* 339–366.

Dressler, D. M. (1973). The management of emotional crises by medical practitioners. *Journal of American Medical Women's Association, 28*(12), 654–659.

Goffman, E. (1961). *Asylums.* New York: Doubleday.

Goffman, E. (1963). *Stigma.* Englewood Cliffs, NJ: Prentice-Hall.

Golan, N. (1969). When is a client in crisis? *Social Casework, 50,* 389–394.

Gove, W. (Ed.) (1975). *The labeling of deviance.* New York: John Wiley.

Gove, W. (1978). Sex differences in mental illness among adult men and women: An examination of four questions raised regarding whether or not women actually have higher rates. *Social Science and Medicine, 12,* 187–198.

Hagey, R., & McDonough, P. (1984). The problem of professional labeling. *Nursing Outlook, 32*(3), 151–157.

Hansell, N. (1976). *The person in distress.* Human Sciences Press.

Hoff, L. A. (1990). *Battered women as survivors.* London: Routledge.

Hoff, L. A. (1993). Review essay: Health policy and the plight of the mentally ill. *Psychiatry, 56*(4), 400–419.

Hoff, L. A. (1995). *Violence issues: An interdisciplinary curriculum guide for health professionals.* Ottawa: Health Canada, Health Services Directorate.

Hoff, L. A., & Miller, N. (1987). *Programs for people in crisis: A guide for educators, administrators, and clinical trainers.* Boston: Northeastern University Custom Book Program.

Hoff, L. A., & Rosenbaum, L. (1994). A victimization assessment tool: Instrument development and clinical implications. *Journal of Advanced Nursing, 20*(4), 627–634.

Hoff, L. A., & Ross, M. (1993). *Curriculum guide for nursing: Violence against women and children.* Ottawa: University of Ottawa, Faculty of Health Sciences.

Hoff, L. A., & Wells, J. O. (Eds.). (1989). *Certification standards manual* (4th ed.). Denver: American Association of Suicidology.

Holden, C. (1986). Proposed new psychiatric diagnoses raise charges of gender bias. *Science, 231,* 327–328.

Holmes, T. H., & Rahe, R. H. (1967). The social readjustment rating scale. *Psychosomatic Medicine, 11,* 213–218.

Illich, I. (1975). *Tools for conviviality.* Great Britain: Fontana/Collins.

Illich, I. (1976). *Limits to medicine.* Middlesex, England: Penguin.

Jacobson, G. F., Strickler, M., & Morley, W. (1968). Generic and individual approaches to crisis intervention. *American Journal of Public Health, 58,* 338–343.

Johnson, A. B. (1990). *Out of bedlam: The truth about deinstitutionalization.* New York: Basic Books.

Kaplan, B. H., Cassel, J., & Gore, S. (1977). Social support. *Medical Care, 15,* 47–58.

Lemert, W. M. (1951). *Social pathology.* New York: McGraw-Hill.

McCarthy, P. R., & Knapp, S. L. (1984). Helping styles of crisis interveners, psychotherapists, and untrained individuals. *American Journal of Community Psychology, 12*(5), 623–627.

Miller, T. W., Kamenchenki, P., & Krasniasnski, A. (1992). Assessment of life stress events: The etiology and measurement of traumatic stress disorder. *International Journal of Social Psychiatry, 38*(3), 215–227.

Mitchell, G. (1991). Nursing diagnosis: An ethical analysis. *Image: Journal of Nursing Scholarship, 23*(2), 99–103.

Polak, P. (1967). The crisis of admission. *Social Psychiatry, 2,* 150–157.

Polak, P. (1976). A model to replace psychiatric hospitalization. *Journal of Nervous and Mental Disease, 162,* 13–22.

Rabin, J., Keefe, K., & Burton, M. (1986). Enhancing services for sexual minority clients: A community mutual health approach. *Social Work,* July-August, 294–298.

Rapaport, L. (1965). The state of crisis: Some theoretical considerations. In H. Parad (Ed.), *Crisis intervention: Selected readings* (pp. 22–31). New York: Family Service Association of America.

Rosenhan, D. L. (1973). On being sane in insane places. *Science,* 179, 250–258. Also reprinted in H. D. Schwartz & C.S. Kart, *Dominant issues in medical sociology.* Addison-Wesley, 1978; and in P. J. Brink (Ed.), *Transcultural nursing.* Prentice-Hall, 1976.

Sales, E., Baum, M., & Shore, B. (1984). Victim readjustment following assault. *Journal of Social Issues, 40*(1), 117–136.

Scheff, T. J. (Ed.) (1975). *Labeling madness.* Englewood Cliffs, NJ: Prentice-Hall.

Schulberg, H. C., & Sheldon, A. (1968). The probability of crisis and strategies for preventive intervention. *Archives of General Psychiatry, 18,* 553–558.

Sifneos, P. E. (1960). A concept of "emotional crisis." *Mental Hygiene, 44,* 169–179.

Stark, E., Flitcraft, A., & Frazier, W. (1979). Medicine and patriarchal violence: The social construction of a "private" event. *International Journal of Health Services, 9,* 461–493.

Stein, D. M., & Lambert, M. J. (1984). Telephone counseling and crisis intervention: A review. *American Journal of Community Psychology, 12*(1), 101–126.

Tilden, V. P., Schmidt, T. A., Limandri, B. J., Chiodo, G. T., Garland, M. J., and Loveless, P. A. (1994). Factors that influence clinicians' assessment and management of family violence. *American Journal of Public Health,12*(4), 628–633.

Walfish, S. (1983). Crisis telephone counselors' views of clinical interaction situations. *Community Mental Health Journal, 19*(3), 219–226.

Warshaw, C. (1989). Limitations of the medical model in the care of battered women. *Gender & Society, 3*(4), 506–517.

Zborowski, M (1952). Cultural components in responses to pain. *Journal of Social Issues, 8,* 16–30. Also reprinted in P. Conrad & R. Kern (Eds.), (1981). *The sociology of health and illness: Critical perspectives.* St. Martin's Press.

Zealberg, J. J., Santos, A. B., & Fisher, R. K. (1993). Benefits of mobile crisis programs. *Hospital and Community Psychiatry, 44*(1), 16–17.

CHAPTER FOUR

HELPING PEOPLE IN CRISIS

Understanding the crisis model lays the foundation for assessing people at risk. The focus in this chapter is on the interpersonal context of crisis management and on specific strategies for assisting people who are acutely upset. Specifically, communication and rapport, planning, contracting, and working through the crisis toward a positive outcome will be discussed. The principles and techniques suggested can be applied in a wide variety of crisis intervention settings: homes, hospitals, clinics, hotlines, and alternative crisis services. While these principles and techniques can be varied and adapted according to professional training, personal preference, and setting, the fundamental ideas remain.

Communication and Rapport: The Immediate Context of Crisis Work

Crisis management strategies are not likely to work if a crisis worker has failed to establish rapport with the person in crisis. Just as assessment is part of the helping process (King, 1971), rapport and effective communication are integrated throughout all stages of crisis management: assessment, planning, intervention, and follow-up.

The Nature and Purpose of Communication

Human beings are distinguished from the nonhuman animal kingdom by our ability to produce and use symbols and to create meaning out of the events and circumstances of our lives. Through language and nonverbal communication, we let our fellow humans know what we think and feel about life and about each other. For example, a man might say, "Life is not worth living without her." He may be contemplating suicide after a divorce from his wife because he sees life without his cherished companion as meaningless. A rape victim or fatally ill woman might say, "What did I do to deserve this?" thus accounting for the situation by blaming herself. Communication is the medium through which

- We struggle to survive (for example, by giving away prized possessions or saying "I don't care anymore" as a cry for help after a serious loss)
- We develop meaningful human communion and maintain it (such as by giving and receiving support during stress and crisis)
- We bring stability and organization into our lives (such as by sorting out the chaotic elements of a traumatic event with a caring person)
- We negotiate social and political struggles at the national and international levels

When communication fails, a person may feel alone, abandoned, worthless, and unloved, or conflict and tension may be created in interpersonal relations. The most tragic result of failed communication is violence toward self and others; at the societal level, this translates into war. Such destructive outcomes of failed communication are more probable in acute crisis situations. Given the importance of communication in the development and resolution of crisis, let us consider some of the factors that influence our interactions with people in crisis.

Factors Influencing Communication

Many sources provide theoretical knowledge about human communication: psychology, sociology, cultural anthropology, ecology, and sociolinguistics (e.g., Dahnke & Clatterbuck, 1990; Hall, 1969; Pluckhan, 1978). These sources provide important insights into communication as it applies to crisis work.

Psychology. As noted in the previous chapter, cognitive functions are significant in crisis response and coping. The way a person perceives stressful events influences how that person feels about these events and communicates his or her feelings. When an event and a person's perception of the meaning of the event are incongruous, and thus lead to a culturally inappropriate expression of feelings, this may indicate mental impairment and greater vulnerability to stress. For example, a person who feels depressed and unworthy of help will usually have difficulty expressing feelings such as anger—feelings that might be appropriate after a traumatic event such as a violent attack. A worker who feels insecure with the crisis model of helping can have difficulty communicating effectively; the worker may talk too much or may fail to be appropriately active when the situation calls for worker initiative.

Sociology. Sociological factors affecting communication in crisis situations spring from society at large as well as from the subcultures of various crisis service delivery systems. These include status, role, and gender factors, and political and economic factors (Campbell-Heider & Pollock, 1987). For example, a nurse may not communicate concern to a person in the hospital who is suspected of being suicidal, assuming that assessment for suicide risk is someone else's responsibility. Or the policies and economics of insurance and hospital care may obscure the fact that community-based help is often more appropriate than hospital care. Similarly, the predominance of individualistic approaches may obscure the highly effective group medium of helping people in crisis.

Cultural Anthropology. Insights from cultural anthropology are pivotal in communication with people in crisis. Our sensitivity to another person's values and beliefs is crucial to understanding what life events mean to different people. Members of particular cultural groups are almost invariably characterized by a degree of ethnocentrism—the conviction that one's own value and belief system is superior. At its best, ethnocentrism is a necessary ingredient of cultural identity and a person's sense of belonging to a social group. At its worst, ethnocentrism can become exaggerated and destructive, for example, in resolving community problems among different ethnic groups. Members of a cultural group may impose their values on others, assume an attitude of superiority about their own customs, or be disdainful toward people unlike themselves. Pluckhan (1978, p. 117) refers to this as "internal noise," which interferes with effective communication.

It is important to remember in crisis work that, for many people, certain values are worth dying for. Needless to say, if an *imposed*—rather than a negotiated—crisis management plan contradicts dearly held values and threatens a person's sense of self-mastery, the chances of success are minimal. Examples of values that may be critical include a person's (1) idea of the meaning of death, illness, and health; (2) feeling about whether to seek and accept help; and (3) opinion about how help should be offered. For example, a person contemplating suicide but seeking one last chance to get help may interpret a prescription for sleeping pills as "an invitation to die" (Jourard, 1970). Crisis workers should also be aware that many human service professionals in the United States and other Western societies hold values of the white, middle-class majority.

Ecology. Environmental factors are intricately tied to cultural values regarding privacy. Examples from the previous chapters suggest that the environment in which crisis service is offered influences the outcome of the crisis. If a person lacks privacy, such as in a busy hospital emergency department, the likelihood of successful communication during crisis is reduced. Thus, a serious commitment to crisis service delivery in emergency settings would provide for separate rooms to facilitate the kind of communication necessary for people in crisis. A worker's skills are useless if staffing and material factors prevent the effective application of those skills (Hoff & Miller, 1987).

Similarly, in crisis work done by police officers and outreach staff, such as mediating a marital fight, spatial factors can be critical in saving lives. The expression, "A man's home is his castle," symbolizes a personalized and defended territory. Inattention to these unstated but culturally shared experiences can result in violent behavioral—that is, nonverbal—communication about this hidden dimension of public and private life (Hall, 1969). Police officers often refer to the "sixth sense" they develop through street experience and sensitivity to environmental factors related to crisis. Potential victims in high-crime areas should also sensitize themselves to elements in their environment that may signal a crisis of violence so they can protect themselves. Police or neighborhood associations are good sources of this kind of information.

Sociolinguistics. Sociolinguistics is the study of social theories of language. Scholars examine how social factors such as race, sex, class, region, and religion influence language and how language can both influence health status (Pennebaker, 1993) and condition thought and social action. Language is the common medium for verbal communication between particular linguistic communities and the most observable way to ascertain the ideas, beliefs, and attitudes of various cultural groups. Insensitivity to an individual's linguistic interpretation can reflect a lack of appreciation of cultural values. Effective crisis workers should have something in common linguistically with various ethnic groups if they are to serve people in the groups within the framework of their value systems.

Language, then, serves as an important link between individual and social approaches to crisis. For example, in *individual* crisis work with a victim of rape or racially motivated violence, a worker helps the person talk about the event, work through feelings, and develop a plan of action such as reporting to the police. The *sociocultural* element in this kind of crisis situation is the message to women and ethnic minority groups that they are responsible for their own victimization (Ryan, 1971). Such cultural messages are revealed in conversation: "Women and blacks are their own worst enemies," or "Why does she [a battered woman] stay?" Such messages influence how women and members of racial minorities respond emotionally, cognitively, and behaviorally to violent events.

The written word similarly conveys the beliefs and values of a cultural community. For example, you may have observed many pages ago that the language in this book is nonmedical and nonsexist. This usage is based on the recognition that language is a powerful conveyor of social and cultural norms governing social status and behavior. Relationships between women and men and the contrast between medical and developmental approaches to crisis intervention can be revealed through language (Vetterling-Braggin, Elliston, & English, 1977, pp. 105–170).

Crisis workers will discover other examples in which sensitivity in communication affects interactions with people in crisis. Communication is not only necessary for carrying out the crisis intervention process, it is also an integral aspect of the helping process itself.

Relationships, Communication, and Rapport

The most technically flawless communication skills are useless in the absence of rapport with the person in crisis. Conversely, if our values, attitudes, and feelings about a person are respectful, unprejudiced, and based on true concern, those values will almost always be conveyed to the person regardless of any *technical* errors in communication. This point cannot be overemphasized. For example, it is commonplace to hear the expression: "I thought he was suicidal, but I didn't say anything because I was afraid I'd say the wrong thing." This argument represents a gross misconception of the nature of language. If we truly are concerned about whether a person lives or dies, this concern will almost invariably be conveyed in what we say unless we

- Deliberately say the opposite of what we mean
- Are mentally disturbed, with an accompanying distortion and contradiction between thought and language
- Lack knowledge about suicidal people or feel anxious about how the person will respond to our sincere message and therefore fail to deliver it (see Chapter Six)

Thus, crisis workers must learn the technical aspects of skillful communication with people who are upset (Haney, 1991; Thompson, 1988). They must avoid asking why and refrain from asking questions that lead to yes or no answers; they must not make judgments or offer unrealistic reassurance. But it is equally important to establish rapport and foster the relationship necessary for a distressed individual to accept help. Truax and Carkhuff (1967) make this point by demonstrating that the *quality of the relationship* we establish is far more important than theoretical and technical knowledge in bringing about positive outcomes with people in crisis. In particular, this includes the worker's ability to convey empathy, caring, and sincerity (McGee, 1974, p. 274). Truax and Carkhuff (1967) also found that nonprofessional persons are highly capable of creating such relationships and that mental health professionals' demonstrations of empathy *decrease* as the length of time after their original training *increases*.

In our efforts to establish rapport, two objectives are central:

1. We should make the distressed person feel understood. We can convey understanding by using reflective statements such as, "You seem to be very hurt and upset by what has happened," and "Sounds like you're very angry." If our perception of what the person is feeling is incorrect, the words "seem to be" and "sounds like" provide an opening for the person to explain his or her perception of the traumatic event. The expression, "I understand" should generally be avoided, since it may be perceived as presumptuous; there is always the possibility that we do not truly understand. Parents who suffer the loss of a child say that no one but a similarly grieving parent can truly understand.
2. If we are unclear about the nature or extent of what the person feels or is troubled by, we should convey our wish to understand by asking, for example, "Could you tell me more about that?" or "How do you feel about what has happened?" or "I'm not sure I understand—could you tell me what you mean by that?"

Besides these techniques for establishing rapport, there are several other means of removing barriers to effective communication (Pluckhan, 1978, pp. 116–128):

1. Become aware of the internal and external noises that may inhibit our ability to communicate sincerely.
2. Avoid double messages. For example, we may convey concern at a verbal level but contradict our message by posture, facial gestures, or failure to give undivided attention. Traditionally, this is known as the "double bind" in communication (Bateson, 1958).
3. Avoid unwarranted assumptions about other people's lives, feelings, and values (Kottler, 1994).
4. Keep communication clear of unnecessary professional and technical jargon; when technical terminology is unavoidable, translate it.
5. Be aware of the trust-risk factor in communication. We must periodically examine whether we are trustworthy and what kind of social, cultural, and personal situations warrant the trust needed to accept help from another (Pluckhan, 1978, pp. 88–89). Also, keep in mind that some people are distrustful not because of us but because they have been betrayed by others they trusted.
6. Take advantage of opportunities to improve self-awareness, self-confidence, and sensitivity to factors affecting communication (human relations courses, biofeedback training, assertiveness workshops).

These suggestions represent a small part of the communication field as it pertains to crisis work. Since communication is inseparable from culture and human life, its importance in helping people in crisis can hardly be overestimated (Haley, 1963, 1987). Keeping in mind these contextual aspects of crisis work, let us pro-

FIGURE 4.1. CRISIS PARADIGM.

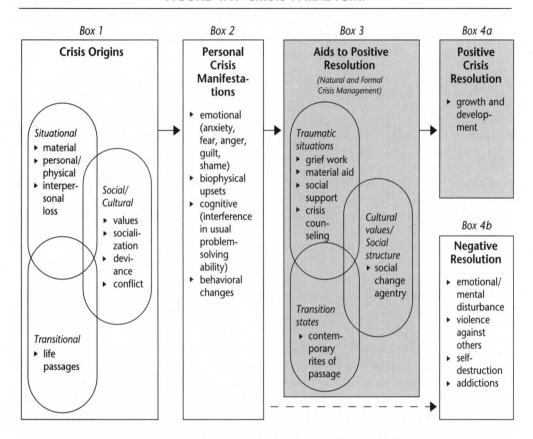

Crisis origins, manifestations, and outcomes, and the respective functions of crisis management have an interactional relationship. The intertwined circles represent the distinct yet interrelated origins of crisis and aids to positive resolution, even though personal manifestations are often similar. The arrows pointing from origins to positive resolution illustrate the *opportunity for growth and development* through crisis; the broken line at bottom depicts the potential *danger of crisis* in the absence of appropriate aids.

ceed to specific strategies of planning, intervention, and follow-up in the crisis management process. In the Crisis Paradigm, these steps are illustrated in the intertwined circles in Box 3 (see Figure 4.1).

Planning with a Person or Family in Crisis

There is no substitute for a good plan for crisis resolution. Without careful planning and direction, a helper can only add to the confusion already experienced by the person in crisis. Some may argue that in certain crisis situations there is no time to plan, as life and death issues may be at stake. Rather than excusing the need for planning, this only underscores its urgency. A good plan can be formulated in a few minutes by someone who knows the signs of crisis, is confident in his or her own ability to help, and is able to enlist additional, immediate assistance in cases of impasse or life and death emergency.

CASE EXAMPLE: ROBERT

A police officer was called to the home of Robert, who had recently been discharged from a hospital. He had angrily barricaded himself in the bathroom and was making threatening comments to his family. On arrival, the officer learned that a team consisting of a psychiatrist and a social worker was already at the home. They were frightened by Robert's threats and were unable to persuade him to unlock the door. The officer identified himself and asked Robert to open the door. He refused. The officer then forced the door open. There was no formal discussion between the officer and the mental health team. Robert became frightened and stabbed the officer in the shoulder with a kitchen knife.

This case illustrates several points:

1. Action occurred *before* planning. As a result, the resources of the professional mental health and police systems were not used to their fullest capacity.
2. When police officers and others are injured by mentally disturbed persons, the injury is often related to the worker's inadequate training in crisis intervention (see Chapter Nine). Bard (1972), in his action research in New York City, found that police deaths and injuries on the job were significantly reduced after officers received training in crisis intervention.
3. The time spent *planning*—even if it is only a few minutes—can prevent injuries and save lives.

Assessment and Planning Linkage

A useful plan consists of more than vague or haphazardly formulated intentions. Planning with a person for crisis resolution follows assessment that the person is in a crisis or precrisis state. The information needed for the plan is obtained from careful assessment. The following key questions, in the context of a skilled interview, represent a more general summary of the seventeen items included in the assessment forms presented in Chapter Three.

- To what extent has the crisis disrupted the person's normal life pattern?
- Is she or he able to go to school or hold a job?
- Can the person handle the responsibilities of daily life, for example, eating and personal hygiene?
- Has the crisis situation disrupted the lives of others?

- Has the person been victimized by crime?
- Is the person suicidal, homicidal, or both?
- Is the person coping through substance abuse?
- Does the person seem to be close to despair?
- Has the high level of tension distorted the person's perception of reality?
- Is the person's usual support system present, absent, or exhausted?
- What are the resources of the individual helper or agency in relation to the person's assessed needs?

The answers to such questions provide the worker with essential data for constructing the intervention plan. This involves first, thinking through the relationships between events and the way the person is thinking, feeling, and acting and then formulating some possible solutions with the person and his or her family (McGee, 1974).

To assure that the plan is specific to the person's crisis response and corresponding needs, a worker may set priorities by checking the assessment form for ratings of 3, 4, or 5 (the lower functional levels). The worker should then ask the person which problem or issue seems the most urgent, for example, "It seems there are a lot of things upsetting you right now. . . . Which of these is the most important for you to get help with immediately?"

Decision Counseling

Skill in decision counseling (Hansell, 1970) is intrinsic to the crisis assessment, planning, and intervention process. Decision counseling is cognitively oriented and allows the upset person to put distorted thoughts, chaotic feelings, and disturbed behavior into some kind of order. The person is encouraged to:

- Search for boundaries of the problem. ("How long has this been troubling you?" or "In what kind of situation do you find yourself getting most upset?")
- Appraise the meaning of the problems and how they can be mastered. ("How has your life changed since your wife's illness?")
- Make a decision about various solutions to the problem. ("What do you think you can do about this?" or "What have you done so far about this problem?")
- Test the solutions in a clear-cut action plan that is documented in a service contract.

In decision counseling, the crisis worker facilitates crisis resolution by helping the person decide

- What problem is to be solved? ("Of the things you are troubled by, what is it you want help with now?")
- How can it be solved? ("What do you think would be most helpful?")

- When should it be solved? ("How about coming in after school today with your husband and your son?")
- Where should it be solved? ("Yes, we do make home visits. Tell me more about your situation so we can decide if a home or office visit is best.")
- Who should be involved in solving it? ("Who else have you talked to about this problem who could be helpful?")

Decision counseling also includes setting goals for the future and forming an alternative action plan to be used if the current plan fails or goals are not achieved.

In decision counseling, the counselor must have thorough knowledge of the person's functional level and of his or her network of social attachments. Used effectively, this technique makes maximum use of the turmoil of crisis to: (1) assess current coping ability; (2) develop new problem-solving skills; (3) establish more stable emotional attachments; (4) improve the person's social skills; and (5) increase the person's competence and satisfaction with life patterns.

Developing a Service Contract

Once an action plan is agreed on by the person in crisis and the worker, it is important to confirm the plan in a service contract (see Exhibit 4.1). The nature of the contract is implied in the fact that the plan for crisis intervention is *mutually arrived at by the helper and the person in crisis.* If the person in crisis comes to the attention of professional crisis counselors or mental health professionals with training in crisis intervention, the service contract should be formalized in writing. It is implicit in the contract that:

- The person is essentially in charge of his or her own life.
- The person is able to make decisions.
- The crisis counseling relationship is one between partners.
- Both parties to the contract—the person in crisis and the crisis counselor—have rights and responsibilities, as spelled out in the contract.
- The relationship between the helper and person in crisis is complementary rather than between a superior person and a subordinate.

Institutional psychiatry and traditional mental health professions in North America have come under serious attack for violating civil rights (Breggin, 1991; Kelly & Weston, 1974; Szasz, 1970). Individuals have been locked up, medicated, and given electric shock against their will in mental institutions. Many human rights and consumer groups have protested such treatment (Capponi, 1992). Currently, groups like the Alliance for the Mentally Ill (AMI) and the Ontario Psychiatric Survivors Association (OPSA) do advocacy work around these issues. Protection of human rights has become an important public issue, which makes

EXHIBIT 4.1. SERVICE CONTRACT.

SERVICE CONTRACT

S=Satisfied U=Unsatisfied

Name _____ ID# _____

Significant Other _____

Case Manager _____

Back up _____

Code

1. Physical
2. Self-Acceptance
3. Vocational
4. Immediate Family
5. Intimate Relationship(s)
6. Residential
7. Financial
8. Decision Making
9. Life Philosophy
10. Leisure Time/ Community Involvement
11. Feeling Management
12. Lethality (self)
13. Lethality (other)
14. Substance Use
15. Legal
16. Agency Use
17. Violence Experienced

Code #	Date	Problem Statement	Method/Technique Tasks for achieved goals (include review date)	Expected Outcome (include date)	Goal Achieved	
					S or U	Date

drawing up contracts as safeguards against abuse of those rights more important than ever.

People have the right to either use or refuse services; the formal service contract protects that right. In addition, the contract establishes the following:

- What the client can expect from the counselor
- What the counselor can expect from the client
- How the two parties will achieve the goals on which they have agreed
- The target dates for achieving the goals defined in the contract

Nothing goes into a contract that is not mutually developed by client and counselor through decision counseling. Both parties sign the contract and retain copies. Receiving help on a contractual basis has these effects: (1) reducing the possibility that the helping relationship will degenerate into a superior/subject or rescuer/victim stance; (2) enhancing the self-mastery and social skills of the client; (3) facilitating growth through a crisis experience; (4) reducing the incidence of failure in helping a person in crisis. The example of a service contract is adapted from the record system described in Chapter Three.

Evaluating the Crisis Management Plan

If planning is as important as has been suggested, criteria by which to evaluate plans should be useful (Caplan & Grunebaum, 1967). A plan can be used in several ways: (1) as a self-evaluation tool; (2) as a checklist for evaluating what might be missing or determining why progress seems elusive; (3) as a means by which supervisors can monitor client service; (4) as data for consultants who are brainstorming with workers about complex or difficult crisis situations. A good plan should have the following characteristics:

1. *Developed with the person in crisis.* A good intervention plan is developed in active collaboration with the person in crisis and significant people in his or her life. The underlying philosophy is that people can help themselves with varying degrees of help from others. Doing things to, rather than with, a person in crisis can lead to failure in crisis intervention. If the goals for crisis intervention and problem solving are formulated by the helper alone, those goals are practically worthless—no matter how appropriate they appear. Inattention to this important element of the planning process is probably responsible for more failures in healthy crisis resolution than any other single factor. Making decisions *for* rather than *with* the person in crisis violates the growth and development concept that is basic to crisis intervention. If a worker takes over, this implies that the person cannot participate in matters of vital concern. The person in crisis may feel devalued. Also, when a counselor assumes control, other important characteristics of the plan may be overlooked, for example, attention to the person's cultural pattern and values.

2. *Problem-oriented.* The plan focuses on immediate, concrete problems that di-

rectly contribute to the crisis, that is, the hazardous event or situation and the precipitating factor. For example, a teenage daughter has run away, a woman gets a diagnosis of breast cancer, or a man learns he has AIDS. The plan should avoid probing into personality patterns or underlying psychological or marital problems contributing to the risk of crisis. These are properly the aim of psychotherapy or ongoing counseling, which the individual may choose after the immediate crisis is resolved. Exploration of previous successes and failures in problem solving is appropriate in the crisis model.

3. *Appropriate to a person's functional level and dependency needs.* The helper assesses how the person is thinking, feeling, and acting. If the individual is so anxious that he or she cannot think straight and make decisions (as assessed through decision counseling), the helper takes a more active role than might otherwise be indicated. In general, a crisis worker should never make a decision for another unless thorough assessment reveals that the person is unable to make decisions independently.

If the person is feeling pent up with emotion, the plan should include adequate time to express those feelings. It is legitimate to give directions for action if the person's behavior and thinking are chaotic. Success in this kind of action plan is based on the belief in a person's ability to help himself or herself once the acute crisis phase is over. A firm, confident approach, based on accurate assessment and respect for the person, inspires confidence and restores a sense of order and independence to the individual in crisis.

Success in this aspect of planning implies an understanding of human interdependence. Healthy *inter*dependence is keeping a good balance between dependence and independence needs. Some individuals are too dependent most of the time; others are too independent most of the time. The excessively independent person will probably have a hard time accepting the need for more dependence on others during a crisis. Asking for help is viewed as a loss of self-esteem. The very dependent person, on the other hand, will tend to behave more dependently during a crisis than the situation warrants.

These considerations underscore the need for thorough assessment of a person's strengths, resources, and usual coping abilities. A good rule of thumb is never to do something *for* a person until it is clear that the person cannot do it alone. We all resent extreme dependence on others, as it keeps us from growing to our full potential. It is equally important that helpers not fail to do for a person in crisis what assessment reveals he or she cannot do alone. The crisis intervention model calls for active participation by the worker. However, the crisis counselor needs to know when to let go so the person can once again take charge of his or her life. This is more easily done by workers who are self-aware and self-confident.

4. *Consistent with a person's culture and lifestyle.* Inattention to a person's lifestyle, values, and cultural patterns can result in the failure of a seemingly perfect plan. We must be sensitive to the person's total situation and careful not to impose our own value system on a person whose lifestyle and values are different. Various cultural, ethnic, and religious groups have distinct patterns of response to events such

as death, physical illness, divorce, and pregnancy out of wedlock. A sincere interest in people different from ourselves conveys respect, elicits information relevant to health, and curbs ethnocentric tendencies.

5. *Inclusive of the person's significant other(s) and social network.* If people in crisis are viewed as social beings, a plan that excludes their social network is incomplete. Since crises occur when there is a serious disruption in normal social transactions or a person's self-perception in interpersonal situations, planning must attend to these important social factors. This is true even when the closest social contacts are hostile and are contributing significantly to the crisis.

It is tempting to avoid dealing with family members who appear to want a troubled person out of their lives. Still, significant others should be brought into the planning, at least to clarify whether or not they are a future source of help. In the event that the person is no longer wanted (for example, by a divorcing spouse or parents who abandon their children), the plan will include a means of helping the individual accept this reality and identify new social contacts. A child not helped to face such harsh realities may spend years fantasizing about reuniting a broken family. Put another way, our plan should include information about whether the family (or other significant person) is part of the problem or part of the solution. (See Chapter Five.)

6. *Realistic, time-limited, and concrete.* A good crisis intervention plan is realistic about needs and resources. For example, a person who is too sick or who has no transportation or money should not be expected to come to an office for help. The plan should also contain a clear time frame. The person or family in crisis needs to know that actions A, B, and C are planned to occur at points X, Y, and Z. This kind of structure is reassuring to someone in crisis. It provides concrete evidence that:

- Something definite will happen to change the present state of discomfort.
- The seemingly endless confusion and chaos of the crisis experience can be handled in terms familiar to the person.
- The entire plan has a clearly anticipated ending point.

For the person who fears going crazy, is threatened with violence, or who finds it difficult to depend on others, it is reassuring to look forward to having events under control again within a specified time.

An effective plan is also concrete in terms of place and circumstances. For example: family crisis counseling sessions will be held at the crisis clinic at 7 P.M. twice a week; one session will be held at daughter Nancy's school and will include her guidance counselor, the school nurse, and the principal. Or, police will provide transportation for a victim of violence.

7. *Dynamic and renegotiable.* A dynamic plan is not carved in marble; it is alive, meaningful, and flexible. It is specific to a particular person with unique problems and allows for ongoing changes in the person's life. It should also include a mech-

anism for dealing with changes if the original plan no longer fits the person's needs so that certain outcomes will not be perceived as failures.

A person who doubts whether anything can be done to help should be assured, "If this doesn't work, we'll examine why and try something else." This feature of a plan is particularly important for people who distrust service agencies or who have experienced repeated disappointment in their efforts to obtain help.

8. *Inclusive of follow-up.* Finally, a good plan includes an agreement for follow-up contact after the apparent resolution of the crisis. This feature is too often neglected by crisis and mental health workers. If it is not initially placed in the plan and the service contract, it probably will not be done. In life-threatening crisis situations, a follow-up plan literally can mean the difference between life and death.

CASE EXAMPLE: MARY

Mary calls a crisis hotline at 11 P.M. She is very upset over the news of her husband's threat of divorce. After forty-five minutes, she and the telephone counselor agree that she will call a local counseling center the next day for an appointment. She is given the name and telephone number to help her make the contact. The plan includes an agreement that Mary will call back to the hotline for renegotiation if for any reason she is unable to keep the appointment.

Working Through a Crisis: Intervention Strategies

Effective crisis management fosters growth and avoids negative, destructive outcomes of traumatic events. Helping a person through healthy crisis resolution means carrying out the plan that was developed after assessment. The worker's crisis intervention techniques should follow from the way the person in crisis is thinking, feeling, and acting and should be tailored to the distinct origins of the crisis (see Figure 4.1, Boxes 1 and 3).

The manifestations of ineffective crisis coping in the case of George Sloan are spelled out on the assessment form illustrated in Chapter Three. The seventeen life areas and signals of distress represent a detailed picture of biophysical, emotional, cognitive, and behavioral functioning. Ineffective coping in any of these realms can be thought of as a red flag signaling possible negative crisis outcomes. The signals indicate that help is needed and that natural and formal crisis management strategies should be mobilized. Using any psychosocial techniques of intervention requires assessing the need for emergency medical services and establishing access to them if necessary. Common instances of such intervention are in the event of self-inflicted injury, victimization by crime, or injury by accident, as discussed in Chapters Seven, Eight, and Eleven. Having assessed the person's coping ability in each of the functional areas, the crisis worker helps the person avoid negative outcomes and move toward growth and development while resolving the crisis. The following crisis intervention strategies are suggested as ways to achieve this goal.

Loss, Change, and Grief Work

No matter what the origin of distress, a common theme observed in people in crisis is that of loss, including loss of:

- Spouse, child, or other loved one
- Health, property, and physical security
- Job, home, and country
- A familiar social role
- Freedom, safety, and bodily integrity
- The opportunity to live beyond youth

From this it follows that a pivotal aspect of successful crisis resolution is grief work. Bereavement is the response to any acute loss. Our rational, social nature implies attachment to other human beings and a view of ourselves in relationship to the rest of the world: our family, friends, pets, and home. Death and the changes following any loss are as inevitable as the ocean tide, but because loss is so painful emotionally, our natural tendency is to avoid coming to terms with it immediately and directly.

Grief work, therefore, takes time. Grief is not a set of symptoms to be treated, but rather, a process of suffering that a bereaved person goes through on the way to a new life without the lost person, status, or object of love. It includes numbness and somatic distress (tightness in the throat, need to sigh, shortness of breath, lack of muscular power), pining and searching, anger and depression, and finally a turning toward recovery (Lindemann, 1944; Parkes, 1975). Care of the bereaved is a communal responsibility (Parkes, 1975, p. 210). Traditional societies, however, have assisted the bereaved much more effectively than have industrialized ones. Material prosperity and the high value placed on individual strength and accomplishment tend to dull awareness of personal mortality and the need for social support. This issue will be discussed more fully in Chapters Thirteen and Fourteen. Because reconciliation with loss is so important in avoiding destructive outcomes of crises, the main features of bereavement reactions are included here:

- A process of realization eventually replaces denial and the avoidance of memory of the lost person, status, or object.
- An alarm reaction sets in, including restlessness, anxiety, and various somatic reactions that leave a person unable to initiate and maintain normal patterns of activity.

- The bereaved has an urge to search for and find the lost person or object in some form. Painful pining, preoccupation with thoughts of the lost person or role and events leading to the loss, and general inattentiveness are common.
- Anger may develop toward the one who has died, or toward oneself, or others: "Oh John, why did you leave me?" or "Why didn't I insist that he go to the hospital?" are typical reactions.
- Guilt about perceived neglect is typical—neglect by self or others—as is guilt about having said something harsh to the person now dead, or guilt about one's own survival—Lifton and Olson's (1976) "death guilt." There may also be outbursts against the people who press the bereaved person to accept the loss before he or she is psychologically ready.
- Feelings of internal loss or mutilation are revealed in such remarks as, "He was a part of me" or "Something of me went when they tore down our homes and neighborhood." The "urban villagers" (Gans, 1962) in Boston's West End are still mourning the loss of their community to an urban renewal project several decades later.
- By adopting the traits and mannerisms of the lost person or by trying to build another home of the same kind, the bereaved person recreates a world that has been lost.
- A pathological variant of normal grief may emerge, that is, the above reactions may be excessive, prolonged, inhibited, or inclined to take a distorted form. This is most apt to happen in the absence of social support.

These reactions have been observed in widows, disaster survivors, persons who lost a body part or who lost their homes in urban relocation, and among people who have lost a loved one to AIDS (Ericsson, 1993; Lindemann, 1944; Marris, 1974; Moffatt, 1986; Parkes, 1975; and Silverman, 1969).

Both normal and pathological reactions are influenced by factors existing before, during, and after a loss. These are similar to the personal, material, demographic, cultural, and social influences affecting the outcome of any other crisis. Examples of factors affecting the response to loss include an inflexible approach to problem solving, poverty, the dependency of youth or old age, cultural inhibition of emotional expression, and the availability of social support. Assisting the bereaved in avoiding pathological outcomes of grief is an essential feature of a preventive and developmental approach to crisis work. Grief work, then, can be viewed as integral to any crisis resolution process in which loss figures as a major theme.

Normal grief work (Johnson-Soderberg, 1981; Lindemann, 1944; Parkes, 1975) consists of the following:

1. *Acceptance of the pain of loss.* This means dealing with memories of the deceased.
2. *Open expression of pain, sorrow, hostility, and guilt.* The person must feel free to mourn his or her loss openly, usually by weeping, and to express feelings of guilt and hostility.

3. *Understanding of intense feelings associated with loss.* For example, the fear of going crazy is a normal part of the grieving process. When these feelings of sorrow, fear, guilt, and hostility are worked through in the presence of a caring person, they gradually subside. The ritual expression of grief, as in funerals, greatly aids in this process.

4. *Resumption of normal activities and social relationships without the person lost.* Having worked through the memories and feelings associated with a loss, a person acquires new patterns of social interaction apart from the deceased.

When people do not do grief work following any profound loss, serious emotional, mental, and social problems can occur. All of us can help people grieve without shame over their losses. This is possible if we are sensitized to the importance of expressing feelings openly and to the various factors affecting the bereavement process.

Other Intervention Strategies

1. *Listen actively and with concern.* When a person is ashamed of his or her ability to cope with a problem or feels that the problem is too minor to be so upset about, a good listener can dispel some of these feelings. Listening helps a person feel important and deserving of help no matter how trivial the problem may appear. Effective listening demands attention to possible listening barriers such as internal and external noise and the other factors influencing communication discussed earlier. Comments such as "hmm," "I see," and "Go on," are useful in acknowledging what a person says; they also encourage more talking and build rapport and trust. The failure to listen forms a barrier to all other intervention strategies.

2. *Encourage the open expression of feelings.* Listening is a natural forerunner of this important crisis intervention technique. One reason some people are crisis-prone is that they habitually bottle up feelings such as anger, grief, frustration, helplessness, and hopelessness. Negative associations with expressing feelings during childhood seem to put a damper on such expression when traumatic events occur later in life. The crisis worker's acceptance of a distressed person's feelings often helps him or her feel better immediately. It also can be the beginning of a healthier coping style in the future. This is one of the rewarding growth possibilities for people in crisis who are fortunate enough to get the help they need.

A useful technique for fostering emotional expression is role playing or role modeling. For example, the worker could say, "If that happened to me I think I'd be very angry," thus giving permission for the person in crisis to express feelings that she or he may hesitate to share, perhaps out of misdirected shame.

For extreme anxiety and accompanying changes in biophysical function, relaxation techniques and exercise can be encouraged. The increase in energy that follows a crisis experience can be channeled into constructive activity and socially approved outlets such as assigning tasks to disaster victims or providing athletic facilities in hospitals. The current popular emphasis on self-help techniques, such as physical exercise and leisure for stress reduction, should be encouraged as a wholesome substitute for chemical tranquilizers during crisis.

As important as listening and emotional and physical expression are, they do not constitute crisis intervention in themselves. Without additional strategies, these techniques may not result in positive crisis resolution. Together, grief work, listening, and facilitating the expression of feelings address *emotional* responses to crisis; but *cognitive* and *behavioral* elements of the crisis are also important. The next several strategies focus on these facets of the crisis resolution process.

3. *Help the person gain an understanding of the crisis.* The individual may ask, "Why did this awful thing have to happen to me?" This perception of a traumatic event implies that the event occurred because the person in crisis was bad and deserving of punishment. The crisis worker can help the person see the many factors that contribute to a crisis situation and thereby curtail self-blaming. The individual is encouraged to examine the total problem, including his or her own behavior as it may be related to the crisis. Thoughtful reflection on oneself and one's behavior can lead to growth and change rather than self-deprecation and self-pity.

4. *Help the person gradually accept reality.* Respond to the person's tendency to blame his or her problems on others. An individual in crisis may adopt the role of victim, but the counselor can help him or her escape that role. It may be tempting to agree with the person who is blaming others, especially when his or her story, as well as the reality, reveal especially cruel attacks, rejections, or other unfair treatment. Those whose crises stem primarily from social sources do not just *feel* victimized, they *are* in fact victimized. Such abused people, though, are also survivors (Hoff, 1990), and their survival skills can be tapped for constructive crisis resolution by encouraging them to channel their anger into action to change oppressive social arrangements and policies (see Figure 4.1, right circle, Box 3).

The tendency to blame and scapegoat is especially strong in family and marital crises. The crisis counselor should help such people understand that victim-persecutor relationships are not one-sided. This can be done effectively when the counselor has established an appropriate relationship with the person. If the counselor has genuine concern and is not engaging in rescue fantasies, the distressed person is more likely to accept the counselor's interpretation of his or her own role in the crisis event. The victim-rescuer-persecutor syndrome occurs frequently in human relationships of all kinds and is common in many helping relationships. People viewed as victims are not rescued easily, so counselors who try it are usually frustrated when their efforts fail. Their disappointment may move them to "persecute" their "victim" for failure to respond. At this point, the victim turns persecutor and punishes the counselor for a well-intended but inappropriate effort to help (Haley, 1969; James & Jongeward, 1971).

In such "meta-complementary" relationships (Haley, 1963), the egalitarian aspects of the service contract are sabotaged. That is, one person allows or pressures another to define a relationship in a certain way. For example, if person A acts helpless and provokes person B to take care of him or her, A is actually in control while being manifestly dependent. Translated to the helping relationship, a counselor may not wish to be controlled any more than a client would, hence the initiation of the troublesome victim-rescuer-persecutor cycle that is so difficult to disrupt once started. (See "Social Network Strategies" in Chapter Five for an effective means of interrupting the cycle and Chapter Six for rescue implications with self-destructive persons.)

5. *Help the person explore new ways of coping with problems.* Instead of responding to crises as helpless victims or with suicide and homicide attempts, people can learn new responses. Sometimes, people have given up on problem-solving devices that used to work for them.

CASE EXAMPLE: JANE

Jane, age thirty-eight, was able to weather many storms until her best friend died. Somehow after her friend's death, she could not find the energy to establish new friend-ships. Exploration revealed that Jane had never worked through the grief she experienced over the death of her friend. The lack of healthy resolution of this crisis made Jane more vulnerable than she might otherwise have been when her daughter, age eighteen, left home and married. Jane had temporarily given up and stopped using her effective problem-solving devices.

In Jane's case, a crisis worker might ask about previous successful coping devices and find out whether she thinks any of these might work for her now. Jane could also be assisted with delayed grief work and with exploring avenues for developing new friendships.

6. *Link the person to a social network.* The technique of exploring new coping devices leads naturally to this function. Just as disruption of social ties is an important precursor of crisis, so the restoration of those ties—or, if permanently lost, the formation of new ones—is one of the most powerful means of resolving a crisis. The crisis counselor takes an active role in reestablishing a person with his or her social network. This aspect of crisis management is also known as social network intervention—or the ecological approach to crisis intervention—and is discussed in detail in the next chapter.

Another way to enhance social network linkage is through "contemporary rites of passage" (see Figure 4.1, lower circle, Box 3). Such ritual support mechanisms are important in dealing with the common theme of loss during crisis, whether through unanticipated events or role changes. Chapter Thirteen discusses this strategy in detail.

7. *Reinforce the newly learned coping devices, and follow up after crisis resolution.* The person is given time to try the proposed solutions to the problem. Successful problem-solving mechanisms are reinforced; unsuccessful solutions are discarded, and new ones are sought. In any case, the person is not cut off abruptly.

A follow-up contact is carried out as agreed to in the initial plan. Some workers argue that follow-up contact maintains people in an unnecessary state of dependency. Others think that contacting a person later constitutes an invasion of privacy and an imposition of therapy on an unwilling client. Rarely does this argument hold when the person being helped has *initiated* the helping process, and follow-up is included in a mutually negotiated service contract. Unquestionably, imposing therapy or other services on people who do not want them would be unethical. Yet we need to consider whether the "invasion of privacy" and similar arguments may be covering a dearth of sensitively designed follow-up programs (Hoff, 1983).

Follow-up is more likely to be successful and less likely to be interpreted as an unwanted intrusion if:

- It is incorporated into the total service plan rather than added as an afterthought or an unexpected telephone call.
- It is based on the principle of self-determination (even if a person is in crisis) and on the avoidance of savior tactics as well as any denigration of others' values and abilities by counselors.

When carefully designed, then, follow-up work can often be the occasion for reaching people who are unable to initiate help for themselves *before* a crisis occurs. This is especially true for suicidal and very depressed people, those threatened with violence, and those especially vulnerable because of severe psychiatric illness. In such life-threatening situations, a person often feels worthless and is unable to reach out for help (see Chapters Six, Seven, Eight, and Eleven).

These crisis management techniques can be mastered by any helping person who chooses to learn them. Human service workers and community caretakers, volunteer counselors, social workers, nurses, physicians, police officers, teachers, and clergy increasingly incorporate crisis intervention as a part of their professional training in caring for distressed people. Whether in offices, institutions, homes, or mobile outreach programs, effective helping techniques save time and effort spent on problems that can develop from ineffectively resolved crises (Haley, 1987; Hoff & Miller, 1987; Zealberg, Santos, & Fisher, 1993). Primary prevention is much less costly in both human and economic terms. These basic strategies can be applied in a variety of settings and circumstances to be discussed in the remaining chapters. In highly charged and potentially violent crisis situations (both individual and group), additional techniques are indicated (see Part Two).

Tranquilizers: What Place in Crisis Intervention?

Advertisements bombard us constantly with the idea that drugs are a solution for many problems. We hear: Do you feel down or upset? Can't sleep? Can't control your kids? Take pills. Valium (diazepam), a mild tranquilizer that was once the most-prescribed mood-altering drug on the U.S. market may be supplanted by the antidepressant, Prozac (fluoxetine). The media suggest that this controversial drug, while not yet tested for long-term side effects, is already firmly established in popular culture as the psychoactive drug of choice (Barney, 1993; Breggin & Breggin, 1994; Cobb, 1994; Cohen, 1990). Of particular concern is the claim that Prozac precipitates suicidal impulses and violence (Ray & Ksir, 1993, p. 166). Statistics compiled by the National Institute on Drug Abuse (NIDA) show that 120 million prescriptions for tranquilizers—an estimated 4 billion doses—are prescribed annually in the United States. Only a small percentage of these prescriptions are authorized by psychiatrists. Considering that the total U.S. population is around 260 million, these figures are staggering. Women receive more than twice the amount of prescription drugs as men for the same psychological symptoms (Boston Women's Health Book Collective, 1992). On the other hand, poor, African-American women tend to be undermedicated, having been advised that their problems stem from a "character flaw" (Gubin, 1993; p. 5H).

The press, television, and major newspapers are repeatedly drawing attention to the drug dependency problem. It is noteworthy that health and human service practitioners and institutions are quieter about prescription drug abuse (Rogers, 1971). When confronted with the problem, it is not uncommon to hear practitioners say, "But they want the pills . . . They don't want to talk about or deal with what's troubling them . . . What am I supposed to do?" Admittedly, when a person seeks a tranquilizer and refuses to talk, it may be futile to refuse a prescription. Practitioners have reason to assume that someone else will provide drugs if they do not (Nellis, 1980). Yet, a more sophisticated example could hardly be found to illustrate what it means to blame the victim (Ryan, 1971) and reveal the limitation of an individual approach to a problem with social, political, and economic origins. This is not to say that crisis practitioners should avoid alerting people to the dangers and limitations of psychoactive drugs. Rather, it suggests the need to broaden our horizons, educate people about drugs (Doweiko, 1993; Ray & Ksir, 1993), look "upstream" to the origins of this problem, and ask ourselves:

- What is the deeper significance of the fact that someone else will, indeed, give a prescription on request?
- Despite people's use of mind-altering substances over many centuries, how did so many people, both professionals and the general public, come to believe that chemical tranquilization is a preferred way to deal with life's stresses and crises?
- What does the profit motive have to do with the overuse of these drugs? (See McKinlay, 1990, "A Case for Refocusing Upstream.")

These questions suggest that we should be cautious about placing the blame for this serious problem on the victims. Certainly, individuals cannot evade *personal* responsibility because of the *social* roots of a problem. Also, helpers must acknowledge defeat in certain situations. But sensitivity to the complexity of the personal and social dimensions of the widespread overdependence on drugs will be valuable in our crisis practice with individuals. With this overview of the problem, let us consider the criteria for use of tranquilizers for people in crisis.

Tranquilizers taken during crisis temporarily relieve tension but do nothing about the problem causing the tension. At best, they are a crutch. At worst, they are addictive and can displace effective problem solving at the psychosocial level. For the person in crisis, psychotropic drugs should *never* be used as a substitute for crisis counseling and problem solving. However, there are times when a tranquilizer can be used in addition to the crisis intervention techniques outlined above. These instances are: (1) when a person is experiencing extreme anxiety and fears losing control; (2) when a person is so distraught that it is impossible to engage him or her in the problem-solving process; (3) when extreme anxiety prevents sleep for a significant period of time. Sleeping pills should always be avoided. Exercise and nonchemical means of relaxation should be encouraged (see Chapter Seven).

Apart from these special circumstances, psychotropic drugs should be avoided whenever possible. By relieving anxiety on a temporary basis, tranquilizers can have the effect of reducing the person's motivation to effectively resolve a crisis. With chemical tranquilization, the person loses the advantages of his or her increased energy during a crisis state. The *opportunity* for psychosocial growth is often lost due to the temporary tranquility of a drugged psyche, while the *danger* is increased.

Caution is also suggested to crisis workers who have physicians or psychiatrist consultants available to them. Sometimes crisis workers ask for psychiatric consultation simply because of their own lack of clinical experience, not because the distinct service of a psychiatrist is needed. As long as the psychiatrist shares the worker's values regarding crisis work and has additional crisis intervention skills, there is no problem. However, this is not true of all psychiatrists (Hoff & Wells, 1989); some have little or no training or experience in crisis intervention but have the legal right to prescribe drugs.

While the traditional psychiatric management of behavioral emergencies has some features in common with crisis intervention, it should not be equated with the crisis model if a strictly medical approach is used. The nonmedical crisis worker should remember that a consultation request may result in a distressed person's receiving a drug prescription when actually what is needed is the experience of highly skilled crisis specialists. Such specialists include, but are not limited to, psychiatrists. On the other hand, a comprehensive plan for certain individuals in crisis may include measures available only through the professions of medicine and psychiatry. A psychiatrist has a medical degree and has skills and legal powers unique to his or her training and position in the field of medicine. Unlike the nonmedical counselor or psychiatric practitioner—a social worker for example—a psychiatrist can prescribe medications, admit people to hospitals, and make distinctions between psychological, psychiatric, and neurological disturbances. Psychiatrists also diagnose and treat the symptoms of drug overdose. In the United States, advanced practice nurses and psychologists can also prescribe medication in some jurisdictions. Ideally, psychiatric stabilization programs, such as those in emergency departments with holding beds, should include the services of skilled crisis counselors.

The appropriate use of a psychiatrist's special skills may be aided by reflection on the following opinion of psychiatrist Halleck in his book, *The Politics of Therapy* (1971). The book may be even more relevant today with the current emphasis on biological determinants of mental illness (Barney, 1994; Breggin, 1991; Parry, 1991):

> The focus of almost all psychiatric practice tends to be on the patient's internal system, that is, upon misery that the patient creates for himself. As a rule, the psychiatrist does not begin working with emotionally disturbed people until he has had considerable experience working with the physically ill. Physical illness, for the most part, implies a defect in the individual, not in society. The psychiatrist's medical training and his constant work with individuals who seem handicapped subtly encourage him to view human unhappiness as a product of individual disorder. Even if he is exceptionally aware of social forces that contribute to his patient's unhappiness, the psychiatrist's orientation as a physician tends to distract him from dealing with such forces. . . . This concept of unhappiness ignores the factors in the patient's immediate environment that make him behave peculiarly; rather it directs the physician to search for the causes of emotional suffering in the anomalies of his patient's biological and psychological past.

In short, all steps taken by the crisis intervention movement to reduce the large-scale dependence on drugs for problem solving during crisis and at other times will be steps forward.

Crisis Intervention Interview Example

Some of the recommended planning characteristics and techniques of intervention are illustrated by George Sloan's case (see Table 4.1), which is continued from Chapters Two and Three.

Summary

Without communication and rapport—the immediate context for crisis work—success will probably elude us. Resolution of crisis should occur in a person's or family's natural setting whenever possible. Planning well and using good crisis

TABLE 4.1. CRISIS INTERVENTION INTERVIEW EXAMPLE.

Intervention Techniques	Interview Between Mr. Sloan and Emergency Department Nurse
Exploring resources	**Nurse:** You said you really can't talk to your wife about your problems. Is there anyone else you've ever thought about talking with?
	George: Well, I tried talking to my doctor once, but he didn't really have time. Then a few months ago, my minister could see I was pretty down and he stopped by a couple of times, but that didn't help.
Facilitating client decision making	**Nurse:** Is there anyone else you think you could talk to?
	George: No, not really—nobody, anyway, that would understand.
Suggestion about new resources	**Nurse:** What about seeing a regular counselor, George? We have connections here in the emergency room with the psychiatric department of our hospital, where a program could be set up to help you work out some of your problems.
	George: What do you mean? You think I'm crazy or something? (defensively) I don't need to see a shrink.
Listening, accepting client's feelings	**Nurse:** No, George, of course I don't think you're crazy. But when you're down and out enough to see no other way to turn but suicide—well, I know things look pretty bleak now, but talking to a counselor usually leads to some other ways of dealing with problems if you're willing to give it a chance.
	George: Well, I could consider it. What would it cost? I sure can't afford any more medical bills.
Involving client in the plan *Facilitating client decision making* *Plan is concrete and specific* *Involvement of significant other*	**Nurse:** Here at our hospital clinic, if you can't pay the regular fee you can apply for medical assistance. How would you like to arrange it? I could call someone now to come over and talk with you and set up a program, or you can call them yourself tomorrow and make the arrangements.
	George: Well, I feel better now, so I think I'd just as soon wait until tomorrow and call them—besides, I guess I should really tell my wife; I don't know how she'd feel about me seeing a counselor. But then I guess suicide is kind of a coward's way out.
Reinforcing coping mechanism *Active encouragement* *Expression of empathy*	**Nurse:** George, you sound hesitant and I can understand what you must be feeling. Talking again with your wife sounds like a good idea. Or you and your wife might want to see the counselor together sometime. But I hope you do follow through on this, as I really believe you and your family could benefit from some help like this—after all, you've had a lot of things hit you at one time.
	George: Well, it's hard for me to imagine what anyone could do—but maybe at least my wife and I could get along better and keep our kid out of trouble. I just wish she'd quit insisting on things I can't afford.

TABLE 4.1, CONT.

Conveying realistic hope that things might get better	*Nurse:*	That's certainly a possibility, and that alone might improve things. How about this, George: I'll call you tomorrow afternoon to see how you are and whether you're having any trouble getting through to the counseling service?
Follow-up plan	*George:*	That sounds fine. I guess I really should give it another chance. Thanks for everything.
	Nurse:	I'm glad we were able to talk, George. I'll be in touch tomorrow.

management skills are the best ways to avoid extreme measures such as hospitalization and lengthy rehabilitation programs. Active involvement of a distressed person in a plan for crisis resolution is essential if crisis intervention is to succeed as a way of helping people. The service contract symbolizes this active involvement. The use of tranquilizers decreases such involvement and sabotages the growth potential of the crisis experience.

References

Bard, M. (1972). *Police family crisis intervention: An action research analysis.* Washington, DC: U.S. Department of Justice.

Barney, K. (1993). Psychiatry's swoon for the 'wonder' capsule. *New York Newsday,* October 31, p. 44.

Bateson, G. (1958). *NAVEN* (2nd ed.). Palo Alto, CA: Stanford University Press.

Boston Women's Health Book Collective. (1992). *The new our bodies, ourselves.* New York: Simon & Schuster.

Breggin, P., & Breggin, G. R. (1994). *Talking back to Prozac: What doctors won't tell you about today's most controversial drug.* New York: St. Martin's Press.

Breggin, P. (1991). *Toxic psychiatry.* New York: St. Martin's Press.

Campbell-Heider, N., & Pollock, D. (1987). Barriers to physician-nurse collegiality: An anthropological perspective. *Social Science and Medicine, 25*(5), 421–425.

Caplan, G., & Grunebaum, H. (1967). Perspectives on primary prevention: A review. *Archives of General Psychiatry, 17,* 331–346.

Cobb, N. (1994). The many faces of Prozac. *Boston Globe,* April 14, p. 55.

Cohen, D. (Ed.). (1990). Challenging the therapeutic state: Critical perspectives on psychiatry and the mental health system. *Journal of Mind and Behavior: Special Issue, 11*(3,4).

Capponi, P. (1992). *Upstairs in the crazy house.* Toronto: Penguin.

Dahnke, G. L., & Clatterbuck, G. W. (1990). *Human communication: Theory and research.* Belmont, CA: Wadsworth.

Doweiko, H. E. (1993). *Concepts of chemical dependency* (2nd ed.). Belmont, CA: Brooks/Cole.

Ericsson, S. (1993). *Companion through the darkness: Inner dialogues on grief.* New York: Harper Perennial.

Gans, H. (1962). *The urban villagers.* New York: Free Press.

Gerhardt, U. (1979). Coping and social action: Theoretical reconstruction of the life-event approach. *Sociology of Health and Illness, 1,* 195–225.

Gubin, S. (1993). Prozac: The miracle drug? *Sojourner: The Women's Forum,* March, pp. 5–6H.

Haley, J. (1963). *Strategies of psychotherapy.* New York: Grune & Stratton.

Haley, J. (1987). *Problem-solving therapy.* San Francisco: Jossey-Bass.

Haley, J. (1969). *Strategies of psychotherapy.* New York: Grune & Stratton.

Haley, J. (1969). The art of being a failure as a therapist. *American Journal of Orthopsychiatry, 39*(4), 691–695.

Hall, E. T. (1969). *The hidden dimension.* New York: Anchor Books.

Halleck, S. (1971). *The politics of therapy.* New York: Science House, Inc.

Haney, W. (1991). *Communication and interpersonal relations: Text and cases* (6th ed.). Baldwinsville, New York: Irwin.

Hansell, N. (1970). Decision counseling. *Archives of General Psychiatry, 22,* 462–467.

Hoff, L. A. (1990). *Battered women as survivors.* New York: Routledge.

Hoff, L. A. (1983). Interagency coordination for people in crisis. *Information and Referral, 5*(1), 79–89.

Hoff, L. A., & Miller, N. (1987). *Programs for people in crisis: A guide for educators, administrators, and clinical trainers.* Boston: Northeastern University Custom Book Program.

Hoff, L. A., & Wells, J. O. (1989). *Certification standards manual* (4th ed.). Denver: American Association of Suicidology.

James, M., & Jongeward, D. (1971). *Born to win.* Reading, MA: Addison-Wesley.

Johnson, A. B. (1990). *Out of bedlam: The truth about deinstitutionalization.* New York: Basic Books.

Johnson-Soderberg, S. (1981). Grief themes. *Advances in Nursing Science, 3*(4), 15–26.

Jourard, S. (1970). Suicide: An invitation to die. *American Journal of Nursing, 70,* 49–55.

Kelly, V. R., & Weston, H. B. (1974). Civil liberties in mental health facilities. *Social Work, 19,* 48–54.

King, J. M. (1971). The initial interview: Basis of assessment in crisis. *Perspectives in Psychiatric Care, 9,* 247–256.

Kottler, J. A. (1994). *Beyond blame: A new way of resolving conflicts in relationships.* San Francisco: Jossey-Bass.

Lifton, R. J., & Olson, E. (1976). The human meaning of total disaster: The Buffalo Creek experience. *Psychiatry, 39,* 1–18.

Lindemann, E. (1944). Symptomatology and management of acute grief. *American Journal of Psychiatry, 101,* 101–148. Also reprinted in H. J. Parad (Ed.) (1965). *Crisis intervention: Selected readings.* New York: Family Service Association of America.

Marks, I., & Scott, R. (Eds.). (1990). *Mental health care delivery: Innovations, impediments, and implementation.* Cambridge: Cambridge University Press.

Marris, P. (1974). *Loss and change.* London: Routledge & Kegan Paul.

McGee, R. K. (1974). *Crisis intervention in the community.* Baltimore: University Press.

McKinlay, J. B. (1990). A case for refocusing upstream: The political economy of illness. In P. Conrad & R. Kern (Eds), *The sociology of health and illness: Critical perspectives* (3rd ed., pp. 502–516). New York: St. Martin's Press.

Moffat, B. (1986). *When someone you love has AIDS: A book of hope for family and friends.* Santa Monica, CA: IBS Press, in association with Love Heals.

Nellis, M. (1980). *The female fix.* Boston: Houghton Mifflin.

Parkes, C. M. (1975). *Bereavement: Studies of grief in adult life.* Middlesex, England: Penguin.

Parry, J. W. (1991). Book reviews: Psychiatric treatment and justice at odds. *Mental and Physical Disability Law Reporter, 15,* 119–122.

Pennebaker, J. W. (1993). Putting stress into words: Health, linguistic, and therapeutic implications. *Behavior Research & Therapy, 31*(6), 539–548.

Pluckhan, M. L. (1978). *Human communication.* New York: McGraw-Hill.

Polak, P. (1967). The crisis of admission. *Social Psychiatry, 2,* 150–157.

Ray, O. S., & Ksir, C. (1993). *Drugs, society, & human behavior.* St. Louis, MO: Mosby.

Rogers, M. J. (1971). Drug abuse: Just what the doctor ordered. *Psychology Today, 5,* 16–24.

Ryan, W. (1971). *Blaming the victim.* New York: Vintage Books.

Silverman, P. (1969). The widow-to-widow program: An experiment in preventive intervention. *Mental Hygiene, 53,* 333–337.

Szasz, T. S. (1970). *The manufacture of madness.* New York: Harper & Row.

Thompson, T. L. (1988). *Communication for health professionals.* Lanham, MD: University Press of America.

Truax, C. B., & Carkhuff, R. R. (1967). *Toward effective counseling and psychotherapy.* Chicago: Aldine.

Vetterling-Braggin, M., Elliston, F. A., & English, J. (Eds.). (1977). *Feminism and philosophy, Part 3: Sexism in ordinary language* (pp. 105–170). Totowa, NJ: Littlefield, Adams & Co.

Zealberg, J. J., Santos, A. B., & Fisher, R. K. (1993). Benefits of mobile crisis programs. *Hospital and Community Psychiatry, 44*(1), 16–17.

CHAPTER FIVE

FAMILY AND SOCIAL NETWORK STRATEGIES DURING CRISIS

We are conceived and born into a social context. We grow and develop among other people. We experience crises around events in our social milieu. People near us—friends, family, the community—help or hinder us through crises. And finally, death, even for those who die alone and abandoned, demands some response from the society left behind.

Social Aspects of Human Growth

The results of multidisciplinary research increasingly support a shifting empha-sis from individual to social approaches to helping distressed people (e.g., Antonovsky, 1980, 1987; Berkman & Syme, 1979; Boissevain, 1979; Hoff, 1990; Mitchell, 1969). Despite the prevalence of individual intervention techniques, overwhelming evidence now shows that social networks and support are primary factors in a person's susceptibility to disease, the process of becoming ill and seek-ing help, the treatment process, and the outcome of illness, whether that be re-habilitation and recovery or death (e.g., Kaplan, Cassel, & Gore, 1977; Robinson, 1971; Sarason & Sarason, 1985). The prolific social science literature supporting social approaches is complemented by the clinical impressions of practitioners (see Garrison, 1974; Langsley & Kaplan, 1968; Polak, 1971). After using family and social network approaches, clinicians seldom return to predominantly indi-vidual practice (e.g., Satir, 1972; Satir, Stackowiak, & Taschman, 1975; Speck & Attneave, 1973). Hansell (1976) casts his entire description of persons in crisis in a social framework. Caplan (1964) laid the foundation for much of this work. The

Crisis Paradigm (see Figure 5.1) in this book similarly stresses the pivotal role of sociocultural factors in the development, manifestation, and resolution of crises. This chapter presents an overview of social approaches to crisis intervention and suggests strategies for family and social network practice.

An interrelated assumption underlies this discussion: people often avoid social approaches because they have not been trained to use them; their usefulness is still questioned. In addition, individual approaches are not evaluated for either their effectiveness or their underlying assumptions. Social strategies contrast strongly with approaches in which upsets are seen primarily as the result of personality dynamics and internal conflicts. Advocates of the latter view do not entirely disregard social factors nor do advocates of social-interactional approaches ignore individual factors. Rather, their differences are in emphasis and in their conviction of what constitutes an appropriate helping process.

A social network may consist of a person's family, friends, neighbors, relatives, bartender, employer, hairdresser, teacher, welfare worker, physician, lawyer—any-

FIGURE 5.1. CRISIS PARADIGM.

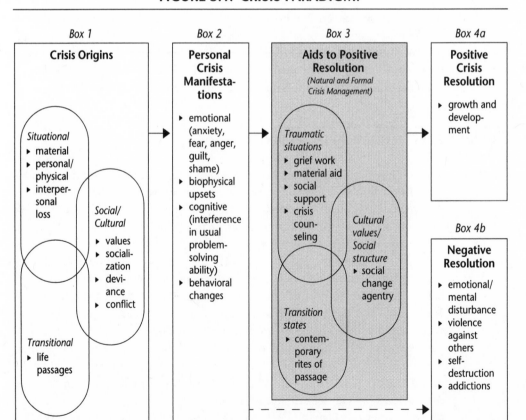

one with whom a person has regular social intercourse. Different individuals have different networks. The following interview with a cocktail waitress illustrates the diversity of social network support and how the *natural* crisis management process works.

CASE EXAMPLE: THE COCKTAIL WAITRESS

This is the dumpiest bar I've ever worked in, but I really enjoy it. I like the people. When I quit my last job and came here, a lot of old men followed me. There are all kinds of bars, but if it weren't for bars like this, a lot of old people and "down and outers" wouldn't have any place to go. Our regulars don't have anything or anyone, and they admit it. I feel like a counselor a lot of times. One of my customers, a pretty young woman, has had several children taken away. When her caseworker called me to ask if I thought she was ready to have her child back, I said no— and I told the woman so.

I think the people I feel closest to are the old men who are lonesome or widowed. One guy who shouldn't drink at all stayed on the wagon for quite a while, then went on a three-week binge. His girlfriend told him that she didn't want him anymore if he didn't stop drinking. So he came in here and got sick after two drinks. He fell on the floor and hurt himself. I called the police and asked them to take him to the hospital. I called the girlfriend, and she and I both convinced him to stay in the hospital for awhile. When he got out, he came in and thanked me. This is really rewarding.

I work hard at helping people get on the right track, and I'm really tough on people who don't do anything with their lives, like these old guys. I know just how much they can drink. Take Ben, he can drink only three and I tell him, "OK . . . you can have them either all at once or you can stick around for awhile." I was brought up to respect my elders, and I don't want to see these guys go out and fall on their faces . . . I have a good friend who's a priest. We argued for years about my work in the bar. Finally he agreed that it wasn't a bad thing to do. Someone has to do it.

The next case example highlights the individual, as opposed to the social, approach to *formal* crisis management.

CASE EXAMPLE: ELLEN

Ellen, age sixteen, ran away from home. Shortly after police found her and took her back, she attempted suicide with about ten aspirin tablets and five of her mother's tranquilizers. Ellen had exhibited many signs of depression. She was counseled individually at a mental health clinic for twelve sessions. Ellen's parents were counseled initially for one session as part of the assessment process. The counselor learned that Ellen was always somewhat depressed and withdrawn at home and that she was getting poor grades in school.

Counseling focused on Ellen's feelings of guilt, worthlessness, and anger toward her parents. She complained that her father was aloof and seldom available when there was a problem. She felt closer to her mother but said her mother was unreasonably strict about her friends and hours out. At the conclusion of the individual counseling sessions, Ellen was less depressed and felt less worthless, although things were essentially the same at home and school. Two months after termination of counseling, Ellen made another suicide attempt, this time with double the amount of aspirin and tranquilizers.

This case reveals that the involvement of Ellen's family and the school counselor—primary people in her social network—was not an integral part of the helping process. In contrast, a social network approach to Ellen's problem would have attended to her feelings of depression and worthlessness, but these feelings would have been viewed in the context of her interactions with those closest to her, not as the result of her withdrawn personality. In other words, in crisis intervention, people and their problems are seen in a psychosocial rather than a psychoanalytic context.

Within the psychosocial framework, Ellen's counselor would have included at least her family and the school counselor in the original assessment and counseling plan. This initial move might have revealed still other people who were important to Ellen and able to help. For example, when Ellen ran away, she went to her Aunt Dorothy's house; she felt closer to Dorothy than to her parents.

The social network is central to the process of human growth, development, and crisis intervention. Ellen is in a normal transition stage of development. The way she handles the natural stress of adolescence depends on the people in her social network: her parents, brothers and sisters, friends, teachers, and relatives. Her relationship with these people sets the tone for the successful completion of developmental tasks. A counselor with a social view of the situation would say that necessary social supports were lacking at a time in Ellen's life when stress was already high. So instead of normal growth, Ellen experienced a degree of stress that resulted in a destructive outcome: a suicide attempt. This was a clear message that support from members of her social network was weak.

Even when stress becomes so great that suicide seems the only alternative, it is not too late to mobilize a shaky social network on behalf of a person in crisis. Failure to do so can result in the kind of outcome that occurred for Ellen, that is, another crisis within two months. Individual crisis counseling was not necessarily bad for Ellen, it simply was not enough.

Before considering the specifics of how a person's social network is engaged or developed in crisis resolution, let us examine two important facets of the social network: the family and the community in crisis.

Families in Crisis

While social relations are important for an individual in crisis, often the members of a person's social network are themselves in crisis. The family unit can experience crises just as individuals can. Researchers consider family troubles in terms of sources, effect on family structure, and type of event affecting the family (Hill, 1965; Parad & Caplan, 1965). If the source of trouble is within the family, an event is usually more distressing than if the source is external, such as from a flood or from racial prejudice. Often, an individual in crisis may precipitate a family crisis. For example, if family members make suicide attempts or abuse alcohol, the family usually lacks basic harmony and internal adequacy—as suggested in the case of Ellen, discussed in the previous section.

Family troubles must be assessed according to their effect on the family configuration. Families experience stress from dismemberment (loss of family member), accession (an unexpected addition of a member), demoralization (loss of morale and family unity), or a combination of all three (Hill, 1965). This classification of stressor events casts in a family context the numerous traumatic life events associated with crises. Death and hospitalization—crisis-precipitating events for individuals— are examples of dismemberment for families. Unwanted pregnancy, a source of crisis for the girl or woman, is also an example of accession to the family and, therefore, a possible precipitant of family crisis as well. A person in crisis because of trouble with the law for delinquency or drug addiction may trigger family demoralization and crisis (Bishop & McNally, 1993; Seelig, Goldman-Hall & Jerrell, 1992). Divorce and acquisition by children of stepparents and stepfamilies (Stanton, 1986) also constitutes dismemberment and accession. The Stepfamily Association of America estimates from remarriage rates that 35 percent of children born today will live in a stepfamily (sometimes called blended or combined families) before their eighteenth birthday. Ahrons (1982) found in her study of families after divorce that role and relationship loss were the sources of greatest stress. Suicide, homicide, illegitimacy, imprisonment, or institutionalization for mental illness are examples of demoralization and dismemberment or accession.

The nuclear family (father, mother, and children) is the norm in most Western societies, whereas the extended family (including relatives) is the norm in most non-Western societies. According to U.S. census figures, only half of American children live in a nuclear family, that is, a married couple and their biological children.

Communal or "New Age" families may provide more avenues of support for some people than do traditional nuclear families. A current variation on these themes is the Cohousing approach, which is designed to address some of the "family" issues faced by all. Cohousing was initiated by a Danish divorced mother seeking greater support for rearing her children. Developed from the utopian ideal put forth by Thomas More in the fifteenth century (1965), the concept encompasses several features intended to:

• Provide privacy through separate, self-contained units for individuals and families
• Relieve isolation and alienation and promote community by an arrangement of clustered homes, a shared common house, a shared garden, play and work space, community dinners, and perhaps a computer center

- Encourage diversity by welcoming a broad range of residents and lifestyles
- Promote a sense of ownership and empowerment by participatory planning and design from the start

Pioneered primarily in Denmark during the 1970s and 1980s, the Cohousing movement "reestablishes many of the advantages of traditional villages within the context of late twentieth-century life" (McCamant & Durrett, 1988, p. 7). While hundreds of Cohousing communities exist in Western Europe, only a few are established in North America, although hundreds of groups are in start-up stages.[1]

In a similar vein, Lindsey (1981) writes in her *Friends as Family* of a time when she, a single woman, became ill and called on her friends for essential material and social support. Masnick and Bane's (1980) work on the "peer network" supports the increasingly common practice of finding substitutes for traditional family support. However, these new family forms can also be the source of unanticipated conflict when lines of authority are unclear, when opinions differ about privacy and intimacy, and when the group cannot reach consensus about how to get necessary domestic work done.

Whether or not stressful events lead to crisis depends on a family's resources for handling such events. Hill (1965, p. 33) gives a vivid description of the nuclear family and its burden as a social unit:

> Compared with other associations in society, the family is badly handicapped organizationally. Its age composition is heavily weighted with dependents, and it cannot freely reject its weak members and recruit more competent teammates. Its members receive an unearned acceptance; there is no price for belonging. Because of its unusual age composition and its uncertain gender composition, it is intrinsically a puny work group and an awkward decision-making group. This group is not ideally manned to withstand stress, yet society has assigned to it the heaviest of responsibilities: the socialization and orientation of the young, and the meeting of the major emotional needs of all citizens, young and old.

The family holds a unique position in society. It is the most natural source of support and understanding, which many of us rely on when in trouble, but it is also the arena in which we may experience our most acute distress or even abuse and violence. All families have problems, and all families have ways of dealing with them. Some are very successful in problem solving; others are less so. Much depends on the resources available in the normal course of family life. Despite the

---

[1]For further information about Regional Cohousing developments in North America and the network's journal, *Cohousing: Contemporary Approaches to Housing Ourselves,* contact: The Cohousing Network, P.O. Box 2584, Berkeley, CA 94702; Telephone (303) 494–8458 (editor); (510) 526–6124 (business).

burdens many face that can be traced to family stress, discord, or abuse, crisis workers can enhance individuals' prospects of moving beyond their family troubles. The labeling of so many families as "dysfunctional" can be just as damaging as the psychiatric labeling of individuals (Hillman & Ventura, 1992; Wolin, 1993).

Besides the ordinary stressors affecting families, in recent years, U.S. families have faced extraordinary stress stemming from a laissez-faire approach to public policy affecting families. Note the following:

- Approximately 40 million Americans have no health insurance coverage, and many lack money for the most basic health care.
- Because affordable, high-quality child care is unavailable, millions of children are left alone. Even though 70 percent of adults in a national survey want employers to provide on-site child care, only 9 percent do so (Rubin, 1987, p. 44).
- A total of 58 percent of caretakers in the few day-care centers that exist earn poverty-level wages or less, while 90 percent of women caring for children in their homes earn at that level (Trotter, 1987, p.38).
- Millions of families cannot afford to buy a home, and thousands of others are homeless due primarily to cuts in federal housing programs since 1981 (see Chapter Thirteen).
- Of the 72 percent of mothers in the labor force, most are there not only for personal fulfillment but because they need the money (Trotter, 1987, p. 34), yet North American women earn only about 70 percent of what similarly qualified men earn in spite of civil rights legislation decades ago.

Traditional caretaking patterns in the home are additional sources of stress for families, particularly for women (Goodrich, et al., 1988; Hoff, 1995; Reverby, 1987; Sommers & Shields, 1987). The disproportionate burden of caretaking placed on women is even more stark in less-industrialized societies. This source of stress on families will only increase with the AIDS crisis and with increasing numbers of old people needing care, unless the prevailing attitude and practice regarding the caretaking role shifts radically (see Chapters Thirteen and Fourteen).

A family's vulnerability to crisis is also determined by how it defines a traumatic event. For some families, a divorce or a pregnancy without marriage is regarded as nearly catastrophic; for others these are simply new situations to cope with. Much depends on religious and other values. Similarly, financial loss for an upper-middle-class family may not be a source of crisis if there are other reserves to draw upon. On the other hand, financial loss for a family with very limited material resources can be the last straw; such families are generally more vulnerable. If the loss includes a loss of status, however, the middle-class family that values external respectability will be more vulnerable to crisis than the family with little to lose in prestige.

As important as a family perspective is, one also needs to look beyond the family for influences on family disharmony and crisis. A well-known example of the failure to look further is Senator Daniel Patrick Moynihan's report, *The Negro Family, the Case for National Action* (1965). Moynihan concluded that causal relationships existed between juvenile delinquency and black households headed by women, and between black women wage earners and "emasculated" black men. When these factors were examined in relation to poverty, however, there was no significant difference between black and white female-headed households. This study is now largely discredited for its race, class, and sex bias, but it still represents a sophisticated example of blaming the victim (Ryan, 1971) and using scientific "evidence" that masks economic injustice.

Current debates about welfare reform take an either/or configuration: welfare dependency is due *either* to economic disparities *or* to illegitimacy. This argument fails to recognize the interrelatedness of poverty, race and gender bias, and widespread urban decay—the roots of problems instead of obvious symptoms (Allen & Baber, 1994; Medoff & Sklar, 1994; Wilson, 1987). These policy failures and the continuing rise in numbers of children born to single mothers is particularly revealing in light of the correlation between falling birth rates and the improvement in women's educational and economic status, regardless of race or ethnicity. This correlation has been established over five generations of women. It is easier, of course, to supply an individual woman with a welfare check and then blame her for dependency than to address the socioeconomic and cultural origins of welfare dependency.

Such blaming of families that are in crisis due to deeply rooted social problems becomes more significant when considering that the United States is the only industrialized country without a national family policy to deal with issues such as maternity and paternity leaves, child care, and flexible work schedules, even though the two-income family is the norm rather than the exception (see Chapter Thirteen). Although the U.S. Congress recently passed a bill permitting unpaid family leave without threat of job loss, few wage-earning parents can afford the loss of a regular paycheck. In contrast, most Western European parents can take such leave *with* pay.

The question of whether day care is harmful or helpful for infants and toddlers is frequently debated in the popular press. However, in spite of passionate arguments about abortion, the impending collapse of the family (according to some people), and traditional, as opposed to, alternative family structures, everyone agrees that human beings need other human beings for development and survival. In short, support from social network members—or the lack of it—influences the outcome of everyday stress, crisis, and illness whether the resolution of crisis is human growth or death (Hoff, 1990; Kaplan, Cassel, & Gore, 1977; McCubbin & Figley, 1983; Pearlin, et al., 1981). The probability, then, of people receiving support during crisis *includes* family issues but is not limited to them. Community stability and resources as well as public policies that affect individuals and families must also be considered (see Chapter Thirteen).

Communities in Crisis

Just as individuals in crisis are entwined with their families, so are families bound up with their community. An entire neighborhood may feel the impact of an individual in crisis. In one small community, a man shot himself in his front yard. The entire community, to say nothing of his wife and small children, was affected by this man's crisis. Also, the murder or abduction of a child in a small community invariably incites community-wide fear on behalf of other children. A crisis response to the entire community, including special sessions for school children, is indicated in these situations (NOVA, 1987). Increasingly in the United States, the school and its children and teachers are primary targets of violence, a situation calling for planning similar to disaster preparedness as discussed in Chapter Ten. Watson and colleagues (1990) offer detailed suggestions for preventing and containing crises in schools.

Clearly then, communities ranging from small villages to sprawling metropolitan areas can go into crisis. In small communal or religious groups, the deprivation of individual needs or rebellion against group norms can mushroom into a crisis for the entire membership. Some modern communal groups have dissolved because of such problems. Social and economic inequities among racial and ethnic groups can trigger a large-scale community crisis. For example, the Los Angeles race riots were sparked by the police beating of Rodney King, and violence in the South African township of Soweto reflects the legacy of apartheid (Holland, 1994; West, 1993). The risk of crisis for these groups is influenced by:

- Social and economic stability of individual family units within a neighborhood
- Level at which individual and family needs are met within the group or neighborhood
- Adequacy of neighborhood resources to meet social, housing, economic, and recreational needs of individuals and families
- Personality characteristics and personal strengths of the individuals within the group

Psychosocial needs must be met if individuals are to survive and grow. In the context of Maslow's (1970) hierarchy of needs: as a person meets basic survival needs of hunger, thirst, and protection from the elements, other needs emerge such as the need for social interaction and pleasant surroundings. We cannot actualize our potential for growth if we are barely surviving and using all our energy just to keep alive. To the extent that people's basic needs are unmet, they are increasingly crisis-prone.

This is true, for example, of millions of people worldwide who suffer from hunger, war, and other disasters, and of those living in large, inner-city housing projects. Poverty is rampant. Slum landlords take advantage of people who are already disadvantaged; there is a constant threat of essential utilities being cut off for persons with inadequate resources to meet skyrocketing rates. An elderly couple in an eastern state, unable to pay their bills, died of exposure after a utility company cut off their heat. Emergency medical and social services are often lacking or inaccessible through the bureaucratic structure.

The social and economic problems of the urban poor have been complicated further by the recent trend toward gentrification—the upgrading of inner-city property so that it is only affordable by the well-to-do. In a partial reversal of an earlier "white flight" from inner-city neighborhoods, middle- and upper-middle-class professionals (mostly white) are returning to the city. Housing crises or homelessness are the unfortunate outcome for many who are displaced (see Chapter Twelve).

Similar deprivations exist on North American Indian reservations, among migrant farm groups, and in sprawling cities with shanty towns (especially in the southern hemisphere) where millions of the world's poorest people eke out a way to survive. As a result of the personal, social, and economic deprivations in these communities, crime becomes widespread, adding another threat to basic survival. Another crisis-prone setting is the subculture of the average jail or prison. Physical survival is threatened by poor health service, and there is danger of suicide. Prisoners fear rape and physical attack by fellow prisoners. Social needs of prisoners go unmet to the extent that the term "rehabilitation" does not apply to what happens in prisons. This situation, combined with community attitudes, unemployment, and poverty, makes ex-offenders highly crisis-prone after release from prison (see Chapter Nine).

Natural disasters such as floods, hurricanes, and severe snowstorms are other sources of community crisis (see Chapter Ten). A community crisis can also be triggered by real or threatened acts of terrorism. This is true not only in internationally publicized cases but also in small communities. In one small town, families and children were threatened and virtually immobilized by an eighteen-year-old youth suspected of being a child molester. Another small community feared for everyone's safety when three teenagers threatened to bomb the local schools and police station in response to their own crises: the teenagers had been expelled from school and were unemployed.

Communities in crisis have several characteristics in common with those observed in individuals in crisis. First, within the group, an atmosphere of tension and fear is widespread. In riot-torn U.S. cities in the 1960s, for example, an atmosphere of suspicion prevailed. It was not uncommon for restaurant patrons to be questioned by police who were making routine rounds. Second, rumor runs rampant during a community crisis. Individuals in large groups color and distort facts out of fear and lack of knowledge. Third, as with individuals in crisis, normal functioning is inhibited or at a standstill. Schools and businesses are often closed; health and emergency resources may be in short supply.

However, as is the case with families, traumatic events can also mobilize and strengthen a group or nation (Holland, 1994; Medoff & Sklar, 1994). Examples include class-based prejudice, bombing by an enemy country, Nazi persecution of the Jews in Europe, and survivors of South Africa's apartheid policies.

Individual, Family, and Community Interaction

Individuals, families, and communities in crisis must be considered in relation to each other. Basic human needs and the prevention of destructive outcomes of crises form an interdependent network.

Privacy, Intimacy, Community

Human needs in regard to the self and the social network are threefold:

1. The need for privacy
2. The need for intimacy
3. The need for community

To lead a reasonably happy life free of excessive strain, people should have a balanced fulfillment of needs in each of these three areas. Many people support the Cohousing concept because it addresses the problem of meeting those needs. With a suitable measure of privacy, intimate attachments, and a sense of belonging to a community, people can avoid the potentially destructive effects of the life crises they encounter. Figure 5.2 illustrates these needs concentrically.

In the center of the interactional circle is the individual, with his or her personality, attributes and liabilities, view of self, view of the world, and goals, ambitions, and values. The centered person who is self-accepting has a need and a capacity for privacy. Well-adjusted people can retreat to their private world as a means of rejuvenating themselves and coming to terms with self and with the external world.

We all have differing needs and capacities for privacy. However, equally vital needs for intimacy and community affiliation should not be sacrificed to an excess of privacy. The need for privacy can be violated by the consistent deprivation of normal privacy and the retreat into an excess of privacy, that is, isolation. Privacy deprivation can occur, for example, when families are crowded into inadequate housing, or when one or both marriage partners are extremely clingy.

The excessively dependent and clinging person is too insecure to ever be alone in his or her private world. Such an individual usually assumes that there can be no happiness alone; the person's full psychosocial development has been stunted and the capacity for privacy is therefore unawakened. The person does not see how unfulfilling an overly dependent relationship can be. For example, a man involved in this kind of relationship is a prime candidate for a suicide attempt when, for example, his wife threatens to divorce him; the wife is also deprived of

FIGURE 5.2. PRIVACY, INTIMACY, COMMUNITY.

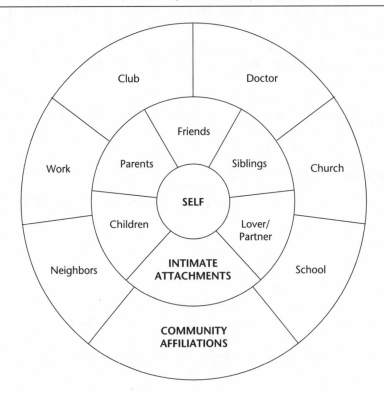

essential privacy and feels exhausted by the demand to relate continually to another person.

The problem of too much privacy leads to a consideration of the needs for intimacy and community. A person can seldom have too much privacy if his or her social needs are met. An example of social-need deprivation is the isolated person who eventually commits suicide because of extreme loneliness and feelings of rejection by others. The concentric circle of needs illustrates the continuous interaction between privacy, intimacy, and community.

The Individual's Extension Beyond Self

Individuals who feel in charge of themselves and capable of living in their private world are at a great advantage as they reach out and establish intimate attachments. They may have a mature marital relationship or a small circle of intimate friends to rely upon (see Figure 5.2). Need fulfillment in this second circle enables the individual to establish and enjoy additional relationships in the work world and in the larger community. The development of this interactional system can be halted in many situations: (1) if a person feels too insecure to establish intimate or communal attachments; (2) if a couple establishes an intimate attachment that is essentially closed and turned inward, thus limiting need fulfillment from the larger community (Dowrick, 1994); (3) if a small communal group turns in on itself and fails to relate to society outside of its confines. In all of these situations, healthy interaction is halted.

Social Network Influences on the Individual

The capacity of individuals to live comfortably with themselves and to move with ease in the world is influenced by families and communities. A child born into a chaotic, socially unstable family may find it difficult to settle into a hostile world. Such a child is more crisis-prone at developmental turning points such as entering school or beginning puberty. The child's family, in turn, is affected by the surrounding community. Both the child and the family are influenced by factors such as economic and employment opportunities, racial, ethnic, or other types of prejudice, the quality of available schools, family and social services, and recreational opportunities for youth. When a sufficient number of individuals and families are adversely affected by these factors, the whole community is more prone to crisis.

This concept of individuals, families, and communities interacting underscores the importance of assessing and managing human crises in a social framework. Certainly a person in crisis needs individual help. But this should always be offered in the context of the person's affectional and community needs. Halleck (1971) goes even further in urging a social approach to human problems and crises. He suggests that it may be unethical for a therapist to spend professional time focusing on a single individual in prison who has made a suicide attempt. Rather than tending only to the individual in crisis, a more responsible approach would be to use professional skills to influence the prison system that contributes to suicidal crises. As violence escalates and the subcultures of U.S. prisons explode with overcrowding and more violence, the crises in these communities will only increase as long as the socioeconomic and cultural roots of aggression are ignored (see Chapter Nine).

Gil (1987), discussing the social roots of violence, extends this argument. He suggests that emergency treatment of abused children and others must be combined with attention to social institutions such as schools and beliefs about parenting that perpetuate violent behavior. Research with battered women (Hoff, 1990) and rape victims (Holmstrom & Burgess, 1978) supports similar conclusions: these individuals' crises originate from society's values about women, marriage, the family, and violence (see Figure 5.1, the Crisis Paradigm).

Social and Group Process in Crisis Intervention

The foundations have been laid for a crisis paradigm that stresses the dynamic relationship between individual, family, and sociocultural factors. The task now is to consider the application of this perspective in actual work with people in crisis.

A Social Network Framework

Social approaches to crisis intervention never lose sight of the interactional network between individuals, families, and other social elements. Helping people resolve crises constructively involves helping them reestablish themselves in harmony with intimate associates and with the larger community. In practice, this might mean:

- Relieving the extreme isolation that led to a suicide attempt
- Developing a satisfying relationship to replace the loss of a close friend or spouse
- Reestablishing ties in the work world and resolving job conflicts
- Returning to normal school tasks after expulsion for truancy, drug abuse, or violence
- Establishing stability and a means of family support after desertion by an alcoholic parent
- Allaying community anxiety concerning bomb threats or child safety
- Identifying why an individual feels "no one is helping me" when, in fact, five agencies (or more) are officially involved

In each of these instances, an individual, psychotherapeutic approach is often used. However, a social strategy in these examples seems so appropriate and evidence supporting it seems so extensive that one wonders why so many practitioners rely primarily on individual approaches—including drug use—to crisis resolution. The reasons are complex, of course, and related to issues such as the medicalization of life problems and to the political and economic factors influencing illness (see Chapters One and Four).

Increasing numbers of practitioners, however, are choosing social strategies for helping distressed people. The experience of social psychiatrists (e.g., Halleck, 1971; Hansell, 1976; and Polak, 1971) and nonmedical practitioners (e.g., Garrison, 1974) suggests that social network techniques are among the most practical and effective available to crisis workers. Hansell (1976) refers to such network strategies as the Screening-Linking-Planning Conference Method. This method was developed and used extensively in community mental health systems in Chicago and Buffalo on behalf of high-risk former mental patients and others. Polak (1971) called this method "Social Systems Intervention" in his community mental health work in Colorado. The use of network strategies in resolving highly complex crisis situations is unparalleled in mental health practice. Their effectiveness is based on recognition and acceptance of the person's basic social nature. Social network techniques, therefore, are essential crisis worker skills.

An effective crisis worker has faith in members of a person's social network and in the techniques for mobilizing these people on behalf of a distressed person. A worker's lack of conviction translates into a negative self-fulfilling prophecy, that is, the response of social network members is highly dependent on what the worker *expects* will happen. A counselor skilled in social network techniques approaches people with a positive attitude and conveys an expectation that the person will respond positively and will have something valuable or essential to offer the individual in crisis. Such an attitude eliminates the need to be excessively demanding, an approach that could alienate the prospective social resource. Workers confident in themselves and in the use of social network techniques can successfully use an assertive approach that yields voluntary participation by those whose help is needed.

Social Network Strategies

Besides confidence in the usefulness of social approaches, the crisis worker also needs practice skills. Social network strategies can be used at any time during the course of service: at the beginning of intervention; when an impasse has been reached and evaluation suggests the need for a new strategy; or at the termination of service (Hansell, 1976; Garrison, 1974; Polak, 1971). The social network approach is particularly effective when chronic and crisis episodes intersect (see Figure 5.3). Its relevance is underscored by the world-wide trend toward community-based primary care as discussed in Chapter One. Putting social network strategies into operation involves several steps:

1. *Clarify with the client and others the purpose of a network strategy and their active participation in it.* Because a person who seeks help usually expects an individual approach, he or she may be surprised at the social emphasis. Tradition, after all, dies hard. Therefore, educating clients, based on our own convictions, is an essential aspect of success with social network strategies. Similarly, clients may be surprised to learn that they not only have an *opportunity* but are *expected* to participate actively in the crisis management process. This is especially true for people who may have developed unhealthy dependencies on agencies: the "agency shopper," the "revolving door client," the multiproblem family (Lynch & Tiedje, 1991), the repeat caller, or the person with "chronic stress" (Worthington, 1992).

The purpose of a network conference can be clarified with a statement such as the following: "John, you've been coming here for some months now, each time with a new crisis around an old problem, it seems. . . . We don't seem to be helping you with what you need. And you say other agencies aren't helping you either. I think we should all get together and try to figure out what's going wrong. Whatever it is we're doing now doesn't seem to be working." A positive presentation like this usually elicits a positive response.

2. *Identify all members of the social network,* including everyone involved with the person either before or because of the individual's crisis. This step will be accomplished by the comprehensive assessment suggested in Chapter Three.

Identification includes brainstorming and creative thinking with the client about possible substitutes for missing elements of a support network. This includes

FIGURE 5.3. COMPARISON OF CHRONIC PROBLEMS AND CRISES AND INTERVENTION STRATEGIES.

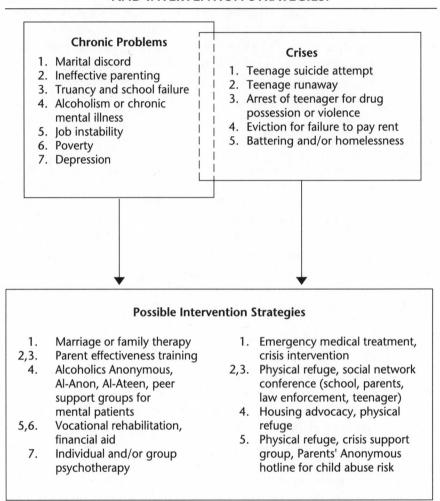

Chronic Problems

1. Marital discord
2. Ineffective parenting
3. Truancy and school failure
4. Alcoholism or chronic mental illness
5. Job instability
6. Poverty
7. Depression

Crises

1. Teenage suicide attempt
2. Teenage runaway
3. Arrest of teenager for drug possession or violence
4. Eviction for failure to pay rent
5. Battering and/or homelessness

Possible Intervention Strategies

1. Marriage or family therapy
2,3. Parent effectiveness training
4. Alcoholics Anonymous, Al-Anon, Al-Ateen, peer support groups for mental patients
5,6. Vocational rehabilitation, financial aid
7. Individual and/or group psychotherapy

1. Emergency medical treatment, crisis intervention
2,3. Physical refuge, social network conference (school, parents, law enforcement, teenager)
4. Housing advocacy, physical refuge
5. Physical refuge, crisis support group, Parents' Anonymous hotline for child abuse risk

The permeable boundaries between the two types of distress suggest the mutual influence these situations have on each other.

social resources that are currently unused but that could lead to successful crisis resolution. People who lack a *natural* support network (such as discharged mental patients who have been institutionalized for many years) may rely extensively on institutional network support. When such support is suddenly withdrawn, they are particularly vulnerable to recurring crises and need substitute sources of support (Hoff, 1993; Johnson, 1990). This problem has been particularly acute in communities where adequate community-based services were not developed in concert with the virtual emptying of state mental institutions (see "Homelessness" in Chapter Twelve). A network conference about such problems may also yield the necessary evidence for community political action to alleviate these problems.

3. *Identify the "symptom bearer" for a family or social network.* This is the person whose crisis state is most obvious. Sometimes this individual is called "crazy." Mental health workers often refer to this person as the "identified client"—recognizing that the entire family or community is, in fact, the client, but their role in the individual's crisis is unclear. The symptom bearer is also commonly called the scapegoat for a disturbed social system.

4. *Establish contact with the resource people identified and explain to them the purpose of the conference.* Elicit the cooperation of these people in helping the person in crisis. Explain how you perceive the crisis situation and how you think someone can be of help to the person in crisis. Finally, arrange the conference at a mutually satisfactory time and place.

If our approach is positive, others involved with a multiagency client will usually express relief that someone is taking the initiative to coordinate services. Families of people with repeated crisis episodes often respond similarly. Problems at

EXAMPLE: NETWORKING SESSION—ALICE

Mr. Rothman: (by telephone): "Mrs. Barrett, this is Mr. Rothman at the crisis clinic. Your daughter Alice is here and refuses to go home. . . . Alice and I would like to have you join us in a planning conference."

Mrs. Barrett: "So that's where she is. . . . I've done everything I know of to help that girl. There's nothing more I can do."

Mr. Rothman: "I know you must feel very frustrated, Mrs. Barrett, but it's important that you join us even if it's agreed that Alice doesn't go back home."

After a few more minutes, Mrs. Barrett agrees to come to the clinic with her husband. (Alice is thirty-four years old, has been in and out of mental hospitals, and cannot hold a job. She and her mother had a verbal battle about household chores. Mrs. Barrett threatened to call the police when Alice started throwing things. Alice left and went to the crisis clinic. . .)

Conference leader to Alice: "Alice, will you review for everyone here how you see your problem?"

To Mr. Higgins, counselor from emergency hostel: "Will you explain your emergency housing service, eligibility requirements, and other arrangements to Alice and her parents?"

To Alice: "How does this housing arrangement sound to you, Alice?"

To Alice's parents: "What do you think about this proposal?"

this stage may occur because the crisis worker is not convinced that there is a need for the conference, or people from other agencies may raise the issue of confidentiality. This is actually not an issue, since the client has been actively involved in the process of planning the conference: "Why, of course John consents. . . . He's right here with me now." Consent forms should not be a problem if the client participates actively. A straightforward approach is the most successful in using this method.

People may be concerned that conference participants will work together against the client. This is another nonissue, since the purpose of the conference is problem solving for the client's benefit, not punishment. If intentions are sincere, if the purposes of the conference are adhered to, and if the leader is competent, the group process should yield constructive, not destructive results. People tend to surpass their own expectations in situations like this—even the worker who is frustrated by dependent self-destructive persons. Often, the conference represents hope of success. This hope in turn is conveyed to the client. Another recommended strategy for diffusing fears about a client being harmed is to appoint a client advocate— someone who will ensure that the client's interests are not sacrificed in any way during the conference. Staff should thus work in teams of two in conducting these conferences.

5. *Convene the client and network members.* The network conference should be held in a place that is conducive to achieving the conference objectives. A conference might be held in the home, office, or hospital emergency department.

6. *Conduct the network conference with the person in crisis and with his or her social network.* During this time, starting with the client's view, the problem is explored as it pertains to everyone involved. The complaints of all parties are aired, and possible solutions are proposed and considered in relation to available resources.

7. *Conclude the conference with a plan of action for resolving the crisis.* For example, link the person in crisis to a social resource such as welfare, emergency or transitional housing, emergency hospitalization, or job training.

The details of the action plan are clearly defined: everyone knows *who* is to do *what* within a designated *time frame.* A contingency plan specifies what is to be done if the plan fails (see "Planning with a Person or Family in Crisis" in Chapter Four).

8. *Establish a follow-up plan,* that is, determine the time, place, circumstances, membership, and purpose of the next meeting.

9. *Record the results of the conference and distribute copies to all participants.* This step is based on the principles of contracting discussed in Chapter Four. It also provides the basis for evaluating progress or for finding out what went wrong if the plan fails.

Workers who have tried social network techniques seem very confident in them; the strategy usually yields highly positive results. Its success can be traced to the effective implementation of *group process* techniques combined with *active client involvement.* For example, a client can scarcely continue to protest that no one is helping when confronted with six to eight people whose purpose is to brainstorm together about ways to help more effectively. Nor can agency representatives continue to blame the victim for repeated suicide attempts or lack of cooperation when confronted with evidence that part of the problem may be:

- Lack of interagency coordination
- Cracks and deficits in the system that leave the clients' needs unmet
- Lack of financial resources to pay rent and utility bills
- Previous failure to confront the client (individuals and family) in a united, constructive manner

   As increasing numbers of discharged mental patients call crisis hotlines for routine support, the social networking technique suggested here is more relevant than ever. Social network strategies are also effective in avoiding unnecessary hospitalization. Certainly individual help and sometimes hospital treatment are indicated for a person in crisis. But once the person enters the subculture of a hospital, the functions of the natural family unit are disrupted. In the busy, bureaucratic atmosphere of institutions, it is all too easy to forget the family and community from which the individual came, although some hospital staffs do excellent work with families. Even when social network members (natural and institutional) contribute to the problem rather than offer support, they should be included in crisis resolution to help the person in crisis clarify the positive and negative aspects of social life. Steps of the social network intervention process are illustrated in Figure 5.4.

   A final observation is offered for readers who are new to this approach or feel intimidated by it. Social network principles—if not all the steps outlined here—can be applied in varying degrees. In noninstitutional crisis settings, for example, some of the steps may be unnecessary. A very simple example of network intervention in a highly charged situation was described in Chapter One (Ramona, the suicidal woman in a shelter). Years of special training are not required for success in network techniques. On the other hand, professionals and others trained in group process should be comfortable in applying this method even in complex situations.

Crisis Groups

The idea of helping people in groups developed during and after World War II. Because so many people needed help and resources were limited, it was impossible to serve everyone individually; group therapies were instituted. This experience, along with the success of the method, established the group mode of helping as often the method of choice rather than expediency. Whether or not workers use group modes in crisis intervention is influenced by their training and

FIGURE 5.4. STEPS IN IMPLEMENTING
SOCIAL NETWORK STRATEGIES.

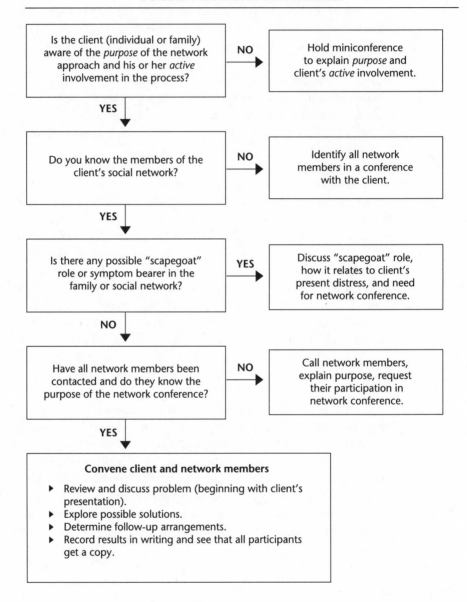

experience. Attitudes have been strongly influenced by psychiatric practice models that emphasize individual rather than social factors.

The traditional emphasis on individual rather than group approaches has contributed to the relative lack of study of group methods in crisis intervention (Allgeyer, 1970; Strickler & Allgeyer, 1967; Morley & Brown, 1968; Walsh & Phelau,

1974). As is true of social network techniques, success in working with groups depends on workers' conviction that the method is appropriate in the crisis intervention process. Group work is indicated in several instances:

1. *As a means of assessing a person's coping mechanisms,* as revealed through interaction with a group. Direct observation of a person in a group setting can uncover behaviors that may have contributed to the crisis situation. Examination of how a crisis developed is part of the process of crisis resolution. The individual is helped to grasp the reality and impact of his or her behavior in relation to others (Walsh & Phelau, 1974). Such understanding of the crisis situation can lead to discovery of more constructive coping mechanisms in interaction with others. The group is an ideal medium for such a process.

2. *As a means of crisis resolution* through the helping process inherent in a well-defined and appropriately led group. For the group members in crisis, the number of helpers is extended from one counselor to the whole group. The process of helping others resolve crises restores a person's confidence. It can also relieve a member's fear of going crazy or losing control.

3. *As a means of relieving the extreme isolation* of some individuals in crisis. For persons almost completely lacking in social resources or the ability to relate to others, the crisis group can be a first step in reestablishing a vital social network.

4. *As a means of immediate screening and assessment* in settings where large numbers of people come for help and the number of counselors is limited. This is the case in some metropolitan areas where the population is more crisis-prone due to housing, financial, employment, violence, and physical health problems.

Crisis Assessment in Groups

A crisis assessment group should be used only when counseling resources are so limited that the people asking for help would otherwise not be seen at all or would be placed on a waiting list. The chief value of a crisis assessment group is to screen out and assist people in most serious need of help before helping those in less critical need. This kind of screening is often necessary in busy emergency mental health clinics. Not all the people who come to such clinics are in crisis. The crisis assessment group is a means of quickly identifying those persons in need of immediate help. This method of assessment should not be used as a substitute for a comprehensive evaluation of individuals, including active involvement of the person's social network members.

Suggested Procedure for Group Crisis Assessment

Ideally, crisis assessment group work proceeds as in the following example:

1. Several people appear for service in an emergency mental health clinic within one hour: Joe, age twenty-eight; Jenny, age thirty-six; Charles, age thirty-

nine; Louise, age nineteen. Only two counselors are available for assessment, one of whom is involved in an assessment interview.

2. Each person is asked whether he or she is willing to be seen for initial assessment with a group of people who also desire crisis counseling. During this initial presentation, each person is also told that: (a) the reason for the group assessment is to give some immediate assistance and prevent a long period of waiting due to staff shortages; (b) the group assessment is not a substitute for individual assessment and counseling needs that are revealed in the group. If the person refuses, he or she is reassured of being seen individually as soon as a counselor is available.

3. The crisis counselor explores with each group member the nature of his or her problem. Each is asked to share the reason for coming to the emergency mental health service. Members are specifically asked why they came *today* rather than on another day. This line of questioning usually reveals the precipitating event as well as the person's current coping ability. Some responses might be:

Joe: "I had another argument with my wife last night and I felt like killing her—I couldn't control myself and got scared. Today I couldn't face going to work, so I thought I'd come in."

Jenny: "I've been feeling so depressed lately. . . . The only reason I happened to come in today is that I was talking with my best friend and she convinced me I should get some help."

Charles: "I've been so nervous at work—I just can't concentrate. Today I finally walked off and didn't tell anyone—I'm afraid to face my wife when I get home because we really need the money, so I decided to come here instead."

Louise: "I took an overdose of pills last night and they told me at the hospital emergency room to come in here today for some counseling."

4. Coping ability and resources are explored in detail. The counselor ascertains in each case the degree of danger to self or others. Members are asked how they have resolved problems in the past. Group members are invited to share and compare problem areas and ways of solving them:

Joe: "Usually I go out drinking or something just to keep away from my wife. Maybe if I'd have done that last night, too, I wouldn't have felt like killing her. . . . No, I've never hit her, but I came pretty close to it last night."

Jenny: "Usually it helps a lot to talk to my friend. We both think I should get a job so I can get out of the house, but my husband doesn't want me to. . . . No, I've never planned anything in particular to kill myself."

Charles: "I find, too, that it helps to talk to someone. . . . My wife has been really great since I've had this trouble on the job. She convinced me to talk with the company doctor. Maybe I could do that tomorrow and get medical leave or something for a while."

Louise: "My mother said I had to come in here. . . . They think I'm crazy for taking those pills last night. I feel like you, Joe. I can't stand going back home but I don't know where else to go. . . . Maybe if someone else could just talk to my folks."

5. Action plans are developed with the members. Again, members are invited to share ideas:

Joe's plan: An individual assessment is scheduled for later in the afternoon. A call to Joe's wife asking her to participate in the assessment is also planned. Joe is extremely tense and uses alcohol to calm his nerves. This, in turn, upsets his wife, so a referral to Alcoholics Anonymous will be considered after the full assessment.

Jenny's plan: An individual assessment interview is planned for Jenny three days later, as Jenny is depressed but not in crisis or in immediate danger of harming herself. She is also given the agency's emergency number should she become upset between now and her scheduled appointment (see "Assessment of the Suicidal Person" in Chapter Six). Jenny is also given the names and telephone numbers of private psychotherapists accepting referrals.

Charles's plan: He agrees to talk with the company doctor the next day and request medical leave. He will call in the results and return for a detailed assessment and exploration of his problem soon thereafter.

Louise's plan: A telephone call is planned to Louise's parents to solicit their participation in working with the counselor on Louise's behalf. If they refuse to come in, a home visit will be planned within twenty-four hours.

This example illustrates the function of the crisis assessment group as a useful way to focus helping resources intensely on people whose problems are most critical without neglecting others. The crisis assessment group rapidly reveals the degree of stress that people are feeling and their ability to cope with problems. It is apparent, for example, that Jenny has a problem with which she needs help, although she is not in crisis.

Mental health agencies with limited counseling resources need to develop techniques to assure that those in crisis or in life and death emergencies receive immediate attention (Hoff & Miller, 1987). The assessment worker who uses social resources and network techniques also facilitates the use of resources outside the agency and the individual. Charles, for example, is supported in his self-preservation plan to see the company doctor for medical leave; he intends to resolve his problem through counseling.

As is true with crisis groups generally, crisis assessment groups develop rapid cohesion. Members receive immediate help in a busy agency. Sharing their problems voluntarily with others and assisting fellow group members with similar or more difficult problems gives people a sense of self-mastery. It also strengthens their sense of community. An appropriately conducted crisis assessment group can lay the foundation for: (1) network techniques in each individual's own social milieu; (2) later participation in a crisis counseling group that may be recommended as part of the total plan for crisis resolution; (3) participation in self-help groups such as Alcoholics Anonymous (AA), widows' clubs, Parents-in-Crisis, and others.

Crisis Counseling in Groups

An important facet of crisis intervention is determining when group work is indicated. Counselors should guard against unnecessarily protecting people in crisis from groups. This attitude is often revealed in workers' statements such as: "I'll see her individually just for a few sessions"; or, "She's not ready for a group yet." These statements can be interpreted in several ways:

1. A person actually needs individual crisis counseling.
2. A person is so terrified of the prospect of a group experience that he or she is, in fact, not ready.
3. The counselor believes that counseling people individually is always better and that a group approach is indicated only when there is not enough time for individual work.

Consider the following responses to these interpretations:

1. The need for individual crisis counseling does not negate the need for group crisis counseling. If both are indicated, both should be offered simultaneously.
2. If a person is indeed terrified of a group experience, this may suggest an even greater need for it. In the individual sessions preparatory to the group experience, the counselor should convey the expectation that group work will be a helpful process. An overprotective attitude will confirm the person's fear that groups are basically destructive, and this can limit the person's learning of coping skills to individual encounters.
3. If the counselor believes in group work only as an expedient measure to be taken in certain instances rather than as the intervention of choice, he or she will not use this effective method of crisis counseling even when its use is indicated.

Group Structure

Another facet of crisis counseling in groups is the structure, content, and conduct of the group itself. Some crisis workers recommend structuring the group to a strict limit of six sessions. A more flexible approach takes into consideration the different coping abilities and external resources available to individuals. Therefore, while group members should be asked to attend sessions once or twice a week (average session length of one and one-half to two hours) for a minimum of six sessions, they might be permitted a maximum of ten sessions if a particular crisis situation warrants it. Group crisis counseling that extends beyond ten sessions indicates that: (1) the counselor does not recognize the difference between crisis counseling and longer-term therapy; (2) the person in crisis has an underlying, chronic mental health problem that should be dealt with in a traditional group-therapy setting; (3) the person in crisis may be substituting the group meetings for other, more regular social contacts, and the counselor is inadvertently fostering such restricted social engagement by not limiting the number of group sessions.

The content and conduct of the crisis counseling group are determined by its purpose: resolution of crisis by means of a group process. Therefore, the sessions focus on the crises identified by group members. Individual histories and feelings not associated with the crisis are restricted from group discussion. There is a continued focus on resolving the crisis that brought the person to the group. All techniques employed in crisis management for individuals should be used: encouraging expression of feelings appropriate to the traumatic event, gaining an understanding of the crisis situation, exploring resources and possible solutions to the problem, and examining social change strategies that might reduce crisis risk in the future (see Chapter Four).

A major difference between group and individual work is that in group work, the counselor facilitates the process of group members helping one another in the resolution of crises. Another difference is that individuals in crisis feel less isolated socially as a result of the bonds created in the group problem-solving process. The relief people feel at no longer being isolated, along with an accompanying sense of group solidarity, can be an important forerunner of other social action they can take to prevent future crises. For example, peer support groups are strongly recommended for people with cancer, parents who have lost a child, battered women, or widowed people.

We also need to consider whether a crisis group should be open or closed. The size of the agency and the potential number of clients can partially determine this. In an agency where many in crisis are seen daily, closed groups are indicated. That is, six or eight people are assigned to a crisis counseling group with the understanding of the contracted six- to ten-session limit, and no new members are admitted to the group once it is formed.

In an agency with fewer clients, where it is difficult to form an initial group of even five people, the group might be structured in an open fashion. This means that new members can be admitted up to a maximum of eight or ten. To avoid constantly dealing with the initiation of new members, admissions are best limited to every second or third session. Even though the group is open to new members, each individual is expected to abide by the six- to ten-session contract. The nature and structure of the group are explained to prospective members in orientation sessions conducted by the group crisis counselor.

Admission to and termination of the group can serve as a medium for discussion about the events that are often an integral part of life crises: loss, admission of a new family member by birth of a baby, revelation of minority sexual orientation, a divorce, an unwanted pregnancy, a rape, death, or absence of a family member through illness. As individuals come and go in the group, members are provided an opportunity to work through possible feelings associated with familiar personal losses. Crisis groups can also be viewed as contemporary substitutes for traditional rites of passage, an idea explored more fully in Chapter Thirteen.

Group counseling is a valuable means of facilitating individual and social growth from a crisis experience. More counselors are now availing themselves of this method of helping people in crisis.

Counseling Families in Crisis

Social network techniques generally apply to the family. Group crisis work resembles family crisis work, but scapegoating and established family patterns and roles make helping families in crisis more complex.

Determining who the scapegoat, or identified symptom bearer, is, along with his or her social network, will reveal the purpose of a person's symptoms in maintaining a family's function—unhealthy and maladjusted as the family may appear at times. For example, Julie, age fifteen, is identified by the school as a "behavior problem." She violates all the family rules at home. John, age seventeen, is seen as a "good boy." Through this convenient labeling process, the mother and father can overlook the chronic discord in their marital relationship and childrearing practices. Julie's mother and father always seem to be fighting about disciplining Julie. It is, therefore, easy for them to conclude that they would not be fighting if it weren't for Julie's behavior problems. Julie becomes very withdrawn, threatens to kill herself, and finally runs away from home to her friend's house. A naive counselor could simply focus on Julie as the chief source of difficulty in the family. If, however, the counselor were attuned to the principles of human growth, development, and life crises in a social context, the analysis would be different. Julie would be viewed as the symptom bearer for a disturbed family. The entire family would be identified as the client.

Crisis intervention for a family such as Julie's includes the following elements:

1. Julie's mother brings her to the crisis clinic as recommended by the school guidance counselor.
2. Julie and her mother are seen in individual assessment interviews.
3. A brief joint interview is held in which the counselor points out the importance and necessity of a family approach if Julie is to get any real help with her problem. The mother is directed to talk with her husband and son about

this recommendation with the understanding that the counselor will assist in this process as necessary.

4. Individual assessment interviews are arranged with the husband and son.

5. The entire family is seen together and a six- to eight-session family counseling contract is arranged.

6. Crisis counseling sessions are conducted with all family members participating. Julie does indeed have a problem, but the family is part of it. For example, Julie's mother and father give conflicting messages regarding their expectations: John is an "ideal boy," and Julie "never does anything right." Julie feels her father ignores her. The guidance counselor had asked Julie's parents to come to the school for a conference, but they "never had time."

   The sessions will focus on helping Julie and her parents reach compromise solutions regarding discipline and expected task performance. Parents are helped to recognize and change their inconsistent patterns of discipline. All members are helped to discover ways to give and receive affection in needed doses. Parents and John are helped to see how John's favored position in the family has isolated Julie and contributed to her withdrawing and running away.

7. A conference is held after the second or third session with the entire family, school guidance counselor, and Julie's friend. This conference will assure proper linkage to and involvement of the important people in Julie's social network.

8. During the course of the family sessions, basic marital discord between Julie's mother and father becomes apparent. They are referred to a marital counselor from a family service agency.

9. Family sessions are terminated with satisfactory resolution of the crisis as manifested by the family symptom bearer, Julie.

10. A follow-up contact is agreed on by the family and the counselor.

In some families, the underlying disturbance is so deep that the symptom bearer is forced to remain in his or her scapegoat position. For example, if Julie's father and mother refused to seek help for their marital problems, Julie would continue her role in the basic family disturbance. Unfortunately, these situations often get worse before they improve. For example, if in her desperation Julie becomes pregnant or carries out her suicide threat, the family might be jolted into doing something about the underlying problems that lead to such extreme behavior.

For children and adolescents in crisis, family crisis counseling is the *preferred* helping mode in nearly all instances. Bypassing this intervention method for young people does a grave disservice and ignores the concepts of human growth and development as well as the key role of family in this process. Langsley and Kaplan (1968) have demonstrated the effectiveness of family crisis intervention in other instances as well (see Getty & Humphreys, 1981; McKenry & Price, 1994; Minuchin, 1993; Satir, 1972).

When dealing with suicidal persons, family approaches may be lifesaving (see Chapter Seven; Hoff, 1981; Hoff & Resing, 1982). Figure 5.3 highlights the relationship between crises and chronic problems. It also illustrates:

- The interface between crisis and longer-term help for families such as Julie's and Ellen's
- The greater crisis vulnerability of people with chronic problems
- The inherent limitations of applying only a crisis approach to chronic problems
- The possible threat to life when crisis assistance is unavailable to people with chronic problems
- The consequent need to use a tandem approach to situations that contain elements of both a chronic and a crisis nature

Self-Help Groups

While social network and family groups are typically led by trained mental health professionals, self-help groups emphasize the strengths of the group members themselves. With roots in the consumer movement, self-help groups play an important part in all phases of crisis management: the acute phases, in prevention, and in follow-up support. Key factors in the success of such groups are the climate of empowerment that is created and the bonding among members that so often occurs. Among self-help groups, Alcoholics Anonymous (AA) and Al-Anon are the most familiar. Many self-help groups have adopted the AA twelve-step model and should be considered valuable sources of support by professionals working with people in crisis.

Grieving people who share with others an acute loss such as the death of a child from sudden infant death syndrome (SIDS) or the stress of having a child with AIDS may feel less isolated. The group is also a source of affirmation and information and a potential protection against suicide. Survivors of abuse, for example, can encourage one another to externalize their misfortunes rather than blaming themselves (Perloff, 1983, p. 57). Self-help groups exist in most communities for practically every kind of problem or health issue (e.g., parents of murdered children, incest survivors, families of people with AIDS, mastectomy patients). While professionals do not usually lead or facilitate such groups, they can help as catalysts and as resources for getting self-help groups started. They can also be a source of referrals. As a resource for people in crisis and with chronic problems, self-help groups have assumed growing importance in an era of increased consumer awareness of responsibility for one's own health. However, such groups should never become a substitute—at least not because of fiscal constraints—for the comprehensive professional health services to which every citizen is entitled.

Summary

Individuals, families, and communities interact with one another in inseparable ways. Crises arise out of this interaction network and are resolved by restoring people to their natural place. Attention to these principles can be the key to success in crisis intervention; inattention to the social network is often a source of destructive resolution of crises. In spite of the heavy influence of individualistic philosophies in all helping professions, a social network approach is being used effectively by increasing numbers of human service workers.

References

Ahrons, D. (1982). Sources of stress in family reorganization after divorce. Paper presented at the National Conference on Social Stress at the University of New Hampshire, Durham, NH.

Allen, K. R., & Baber, K. M. (1994). Issues of gender: A feminist perspective. In P. C. McKenry & S. J. Price (Eds.), *Families and change: Coping with stressful events* (pp. 21–39). Thousand Oaks, CA: Sage.

Allgeyer, L. (1970). The crisis group: Its unique usefulness to the disadvantaged. *International Journal of Group Psychotherapy, 20,* 235–240.

Antonovsky, A. (1980). *Health, stress, and coping.* San Francisco: Jossey-Bass.

Berkman, L. F., & Syme, S. L. (1979). Social networks, host resistance, and mortality: A nine-year follow-up study of Alameda County residents. *American Journal of Epidemiology, 109,* 186–204.

Bishop, E. E., & McNally, G. (1993). An in-home crisis intervention program for children and their families. *Hospital and Community Psychiatry, 44*(2), 182–184.

Boissevain, J. (1979). Network analysis: A reappraisal. *Current Anthropology, 20*(2), 392–394.

Caplan, G. (1964). *Principles of preventive psychiatry.* New York: Basic Books.

Dowrick, S. (1994). *Intimacy & solitude.* New York: W.W. Norton.

Garrison, J. (1974). Network techniques: Case studies in the screening-linking-planning conference method. *Family Process, 13,* 337–353.

Getty, C., & Humphreys, W. (Eds.). (1981). *Understanding the family: Stress and change in American family life.* New York: Appleton-Century-Crofts.

Gil, D. (1987). Sociocultural aspects of domestic violence. In M. Lystad (Ed.), *Violence in the home: Interdisciplinary perspectives* (pp. 124–149). New York: Brunner/Mazel.

Goodrich, T. J., Rampage, C., Ellman, B., & Halstead, K. (1988). *Feminist family therapy.* New York: W.W. Norton.

Halleck, S. (1971). *The politics of therapy.* New York: Science House.

Hansell, N. (1976). *The person in distress.* New York: Human Sciences Press.

Hill, R. (1965). Generic features of families under stress. In H. Parad (Ed.), *Crisis intervention: Selected readings* (pp. 32–52). New York: Family Service Association of America.

Hillman, J., & Ventura, M. (1992). Is therapy turning us into children? *New Age,* May/June, 60–65, 136–141.

Hoff, L. A. (1981). Families in crisis. In C. Getty & W. Humphreys (Eds.), *Understanding the family: Stress and change in American family life* (pp. 418–434). New York: Appleton-Century-Crofts.

Hoff, L. A. (1990). *Battered women as survivors.* New York: Routledge.

Hoff, L. A., & Miller, N. (1987). *Programs for people in crisis: A guide for educators, administrators, and clinical trainers.* Boston: Northeastern University Custom Book Program.

Hoff, L. A. (1993). Review essay: Health policy and the plight of the mentally ill. *Psychiatry, 56*(4), 400–419.

Hoff, L. A., & Resing, M. (1982). Was this suicide preventable? *American Journal of Nursing, 82,* 1106–1111. Also reprinted in B. A. Backer, P. M. Dubbert, & E.J.P. Eisenman (Eds.), (1985). *Psychiatric/mental health nursing: Contemporary readings* (pp. 169–180). Monterey, CA: Wadsworth.

Hoff, L. A. (1995). *Violence issues: An interdisciplinary curriculum guide for health professionals.* Ottawa: Health Canada, Health Series Directorate.

Holland, H. (1994). *Born in Soweto.* London: Penguin.

Holmstrom, L. L., & Burgess, A. W. (1978). *The victim of rape: Institutional reactions.* New York: Wiley.

Johnson, A. B. (1990). *Out of bedlam: The truth about deinstitutionalization.* New York: Basic Books.

Kaplan, B. H., Cassel, J., & Gore, S. (1977). Social support. *Medical Care, 15,* 47–58.

Langsley, D., & Kaplan, D. (1968). *The treatment of families in crisis.* New York: Grune & Stratton.

Lindsey, K. (1981). *Friends as family.* Boston: Beacon Press.

Lynch, I. & Tiedje, L. B. (1991). Working with multiproblem families: An intervention model for community health nurses. *Public Health Nursing, 8,* 8(3), 147–153.

Maslow, A. (1970). *Motivation and personality.* (2nd ed.). New York: Harper & Row.

Masnick, G. S., & Bane, M. J. (1980). *The nation's families.* Boston: Auburn House.

McCamant, K., & Durrett, C. (1988). *Cohousing: A contemporary approach to housing ourselves.* Berkeley: Ten Speed Press.

McCubbin, H., & Figley, C. (1983). Stress and the family. Vol. 2: *Coping with catastrophic stress.* New York: Brunner/Mazel.

McKenry, P. C., & Price, S. J. (Eds.). (1994). *Families and change: Coping with stressful events.* Thousand Oaks, CA: Sage.

Medoff, P., & Sklar, H. (1994). *Streets of hope: The fall and rise of an urban neighborhood.* Boston: South End Press.

Minuchin, S. (1993). *Family healing: Strategies for hope and understanding.* New York: Simon & Schuster.

Mitchell, S. C. (Ed.). (1969). *Social networks in urban situations.* Manchester, England: Manchester University Press.

More, T. (1965). *Utopia.* London: Penguin Classics.

Morley, W. E., & Brown, V. B. (1968). The crisis intervention group: A natural meeting or a marriage of convenience? *Psychotherapy: Theory, Research, Practice, 6,* 30–36.

Moynihan, D. P. (1965). The Negro family, the case for national action. In L. Rainwater & W. Yancy (Eds.), *The Moynihan report and the politics of controversy.* Washington, DC: Office of Policy Planning and Research, U.S. Department of Labor.

NOVA. (1987). *Crisis response.* Washington, DC: National Organization for Victim Assistance.

Parad, H., & Caplan, G. (1965). A framework for studying families in crisis. In H. Parad (Ed.), *Crisis intervention: Selected readings* (pp. 53–74). New York: Family Service Association of America.

Pearlin, L. E., et al. (1981). The stress process. *Journal of Health and Social Behavior, 22*(4), 337–356.

Perloff, L. S. (1983). Perceptions of vulnerability to victimization. *Journal of Social Issues, 39*(2), 41–61.

Polak, P. (1971). Social systems intervention. *Archives of General Psychiatry, 25,* 110–117.

Reverby, S. (1987). *Ordered to care.* Cambridge: Cambridge University Press.

Robinson, D. (1971). *The process of becoming ill.* London: Routledge & Kegan Paul.

Rubin, K. (1987). Whose job is child care? *MS, 15*(8), 32–44.

Ryan, W. (1971). *Blaming the victim.* New York: Vintage Books.

Sarason, A. G., & Sarason, B. R. (Eds.). (1985). *Social support: Theory, research, and application.* The Hague: Martinus Nijhof.

Satir, V. (1972). *People making.* Palo Alto, CA: Science and Behavior Books.

Satir, V., Stackowiak, J., & Taschman, H. A. (1975). *Helping people to change.* New York: Jason Aronson.

Seelig, W. R., Goldman-Hall, B. J., & Jerrell, J. M. (1992). In-home treatment of families with seriously disturbed adolescents in crisis. *Family Process, 31*(2), 135–149.

Sommers, T., & Shields, L. (1987). *Women take care: The consequences of caregiving in today's society.* Gainsville, FL: Triad.

Speck, R., & Attneave, C. (1973). *Family networks.* New York: Pantheon.

Stanton, G. (1986). Preventive intervention with stepfamilies. *Social Work,* May-June, 201–206.

Strickler, M., & Allgeyer, J. (1967). The crisis group: A new application of crisis theory. *Social Work, 12,* 28–32.

Trotter, R. J. (1987). Project daycare. *Psychology Today, 21*(12), 32–38.

Walsh, J. A., & Phelau, T. W. (1974). People in crisis: An experimental group. *Community Mental Health Journal, 10,* 3–8.

Watson, R. S., Poda, J. H., Miller, C. T., Rice, E. S., & West, G. (1990). *Containing crisis: A guide to managing school emergencies.* Bloomington, IN: National Educational Service.

West, C. (1993). *Race matters.* Boston: Beacon Press.

Wilson, W. J. (1987). *The truly disadvantaged: The inner city, the underclass, and public policy.* Chicago & London: University of Chicago Press.

Wolin, S. (1993). *The resilient self: How survivors of troubled families rise above adversity.* New York: Random House.

Worthington, J. G. (1992). Managing a crisis in a rehabilitation facility. *Rehabilitation Nursing, 17*(4), 187–196.

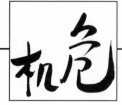

PART TWO

VIOLENCE AS ORIGIN OF AND RESPONSE TO CRISIS

The Crisis Paradigm presented in Part One links the origins of crisis with their possible outcomes. In Part Two, violence is discussed both as an origin of and a response to crisis. Violence toward oneself and others is a major, life-threatening factor for individuals, families, and whole communities in many crisis situations. Chapters Six and Seven focus on assessing and helping people who respond to crisis by suicide or other forms of self-destruc-tiveness. Chapters Eight and Nine deal with violence toward others, including the crises of both victims and perpetrators of violence. In Chapter Ten, violence affecting entire communities—disaster—is traced to natural and human sources. Because the effects of violence are destructive and often irreversible, the theme of prevention is reemphasized in discussing crisis and violence.

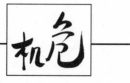

CHAPTER SIX

SUICIDE AND OTHER SELF-DESTRUCTIVE BEHAVIOR: UNDERSTANDING AND ASSESSMENT

S ome people respond to life crises with suicide or other self-destructive acts. George Sloan, whose case was noted in previous chapters, tried to kill himself in a car crash when he saw no other way out of his crisis (see Figure 6.1, Box 4b).

A Framework for Understanding Self-Destructive Behavior

Suicide is viewed as a major public health problem in many countries (McGinnis, 1987). In the United States, it is the eighth leading cause of death (McGinnis, 1987, p. 20). Suicide among adolescents and young adults has increased dramatically (Recklitis, Noam, & Borst, 1992); among young people ages fifteen to nineteen, it is the second leading cause of death (Holinger, 1990). Among adolescents ages fifteen to nineteen, the rate of suicide in 1990 was 11.1 per 100,000 (slightly lower than the overall rate), while among twenty- to twenty-four-year-olds the rate was 15.1 per 100,000 (Holinger, et al., 1994). The rate for women of all ages has remained stable—around 4.3 per 100,000 (McGinnis, 1987, pp. 23–24).

While white males constituted 70 percent of all suicides in the United States in 1980 (McGinnis, 1987, p. 21), Hendin (1987, pp. 152–153) found that in New York City the suicide rate among urban blacks of both sexes ages fifteen to thirty was consistently higher than for whites of the same age for the first seventy years of this century. This suggests black people's continuing struggle with devastating social and individual circumstances. Similar factors place many American

FIGURE 6.1. CRISIS PARADIGM.

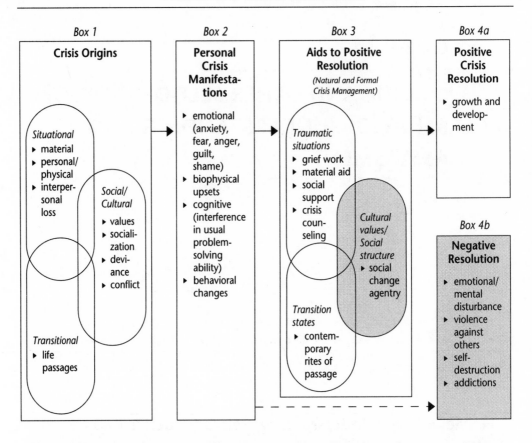

Crisis origins, manifestations, and outcomes, and the respective functions of crisis management have an interactional relationship. The intertwined circles represent the distinct yet interrelated origins of crisis and aids to positive resolution, even though personal manifestations are often similar. The arrows pointing from origins to positive resolution illustrate the opportunity for growth and development through crisis; the broken line at bottom depicts the potential danger of crisis in the absence of appropriate aids.

Indian adolescents at risk (Berlin, 1987). Although only recently commanding research attention, homosexuals are estimated to account for 30 percent of adolescent suicides, despite constituting only 5 to 10 percent of the general population (Remafedi, Farrow, & Deisher, 1991). On the other hand, Rich, et al. (1986) found little difference in suicide rates between adult homosexual and heterosexual men. The rate of suicide for all ages and groups in the United States is about 12 per 100,000 and has remained relatively constant over several decades (National Center for Health Statistics, 1986). Contrary to popular belief, suicide rates drop around the holidays, except for a slight fluctuation among white teenagers (Phillips & Wills, 1987).

In the United States, firearms are the method of choice for both men and women, while the second most common method used by men is hanging and by women is poisoning (Maris, 1991, p. 9). In spite of increased attention to adolescent suicide, the suicide rate among older white males is at least twice that of younger men (Maris, 1991; McGinnis, 1987, p. 21). White women's rates peak at around age fifty, while rates for nonwhite women remain low and fairly constant through old age (Canetto, 1992).

Suicide attempts occur at least ten times more frequently than suicides, with a total of approximately 300,000 annually. Among adolescents, particularly females, the attempt rate may be twenty to fifty times higher. Many of these adolescents have been physically or sexually abused. Stephens's (1985) research on suicidal women suggests strong links to conflict and abuse in intimate relationships. She suggests that women with histories of exaggerated passivity may be at greater risk of suicide than those who are rebellious. Women have higher rates of depression than men, which is commonly attributed to socioeconomic disparities (Brown & Harris, 1978). However, research remains to be done on why greater numbers of women who are abused or otherwise disadvantaged do not kill themselves.

Internationally, the wide range of suicide rates reveals further the complexity of the suicide problem. In Canada, the age-adjusted suicide rate is 13.6.[1] In England, France, Italy, Denmark, and Japan the rates for men are consistently higher than for women. England has the lowest rate for old people and Italy the lowest rate for the young. In most European countries, the rates are lowest among those of Catholic tradition (Kerkhof & Clark, 1993). In Japan, the rate for women between fifteen and twenty-four is half that for men (McGinnis, 1987, p. 25), while in India, for every 100 suicides, seventy are women (Menon, 1988). Because reporting systems differ widely, there are probably more suicides than are reported. Cultural taboos, insurance policies, and other factors strongly influence the reporting of suicide. Some coroners, for example, will not certify a death as suicide unless there is a suicide note. However, everyone who commits suicide does not leave a suicide note. Research supports the claim that the compilation of suicide statistics, like suicide itself, is a social—not strictly scientific—process affected by cultural, social, and economic considerations (Atkinson, 1978; Douglas, 1967). Because of all these factors, we lack accurate and comprehensive data. Statistics about suicide, therefore, should be used primarily as an indicator of trends, not as a substitute for sensitive interpersonal work with suicidal people. For

---

[1]For current comprehensive information on suicide, contact the Suicide Information and Education Centre (SIEC), 1615 10th Ave. SW., #201, Calgary, Alberta, Canada T3C 0J7. Telephone (403) 245–3900; fax (403) 245–0299. The SIEC, which is administered by the Canadian Mental Health Association of Alberta, contains a reference library that is kept current through international computer networking. Material is available to agency staff, educators, students, and researchers.

example, since suicide rates among adolescents and ethnic minority groups have increased the most dramatically in recent years, greater public attention is warranted than earlier, lower rates seemed to indicate.

Suicide as a response to crisis is used by all classes and kinds of people with social, mental, emotional, and physical problems—possibly including our relatives and neighbors. In short, people of every age, sex, religion, race, sexual identity, and social or economic class commit suicide. Perhaps most important of all, in the ethic of most world religions, suicide is generally considered the most stigmatizing sort of death.

In this and the following chapter, suicide and self-destructive behavior are discussed from the perspective of the Judeo-Christian value system and the development of social science and crisis intervention in industrialized societies. It assumes the psychosociocultural perspective presented in earlier chapters, with particular emphasis on themes of growth and empowerment despite the specter of death as a response to psychic pain during crisis. Suicide conveys universally the value, "death is preferred over life," making this discussion relevant in cross-cultural terms as well. However, particular belief systems will influence how and why suicide occurs and is interpreted in various non-Western societies. For a fuller cross-cultural discussion of suicide, see Counts (1987), Farberow (1975), and the journal, *Crisis*.

Perspectives, Myths, and Feelings About Self-Destructive People

Nearly everyone has had contact with self-destructive people. Some of us have relatives and friends who have committed suicide or made suicide attempts. We know others who slowly destroy themselves by excessive drinking or abuse of other drugs. Among the readers of this book, a certain percentage will have responded to a life crisis by some kind of self-destructive act. For example, the suicide rates among physicians and dentists are some of the highest among occupational groups. Also, narcotic addiction, as a way of coping with stress, is prevalent among physicians and nurses. It is a tragedy that those whose main work is service to others often find it difficult to ask for help for themselves when in crisis. All too often, physicians and nurses, particularly those who are in direct contact with people who have cut their wrists, attempted to kill themselves in a car crash, or overdosed on pills, will attempt to drown their own troubles in alcohol. These are only a few of the many consequences of self-destructive incidents with which emergency service personnel have to deal.

Volunteers and other workers in suicide and crisis centers are another group that has frequent contact with self-destructive people. About 20 percent of callers to these centers are in suicidal crisis. Counselors and psychotherapists also work with self-destructive people.

These workers, as well as other people, have varying degrees of knowledge about suicide and self-destructive people. Unfortunately, myths and false beliefs about suicidal people are widespread. The following are some of the most common myths and facts about suicide (Shneidman, 1981, pp. 213–214):

Myth: People who commit suicide are mentally ill. *Fact:* People who commit suicide are usually depressed or in emotional turmoil, but this is not the same as being "crazy" or mentally ill.

Myth: Good circumstances—a comfortable home or a good job—prevent suicide. *Fact:* Suicide cuts across class, race, age, and sex differences, although its frequency varies among different groups in society.

Myth: When gay, lesbian, and bisexual people recognize the "sinfulness" of their lives, most of them kill themselves. *Fact:* Although a significant number of this group commit suicide or make suicide attempts, they do so most often because of the prejudice, hatred, and sometimes violence they have endured from mainstream society.

Myth: People who talk about suicide will not commit suicide. *Fact:* People who die by suicide almost invariably talk about suicide or give clues and warnings about their intention through their behavior, even though the clues may not be recognized at the time.

Myth: People who threaten suicide, cut their wrists, or do not succeed with other attempts are not at risk for suicide. *Fact:* The majority of people who succeed in killing themselves have a history of previous suicide attempts. All threats and self-injury should be taken seriously. Not to do so may precipitate another attempt.

Myth: Talking about suicide to people who are upset will put the idea in their heads. *Fact:* Suicide is much too complex a process to occur as a result of a caring person asking a question about suicidal intent.

Myth: People who are deeply depressed do not have the energy to commit suicide. *Fact:* The energy level of another person is subjective and difficult to assess. People may kill themselves when depressed or following improvement; frequent and repeated assessment is therefore indicated.

Some of these myths can probably be recognized among ourselves, family, friends, and associates. Even among professional mental health workers, these ideas are more common than one would expect.

Professional suicidologists (those trained in the study of suicide and suicide prevention) believe that suicide prevention is everybody's business—a difficult order considering how many false beliefs about suicide still persist. But often, even nurses and physicians may resist dealing with self-destructive people by telling themselves, "That's somebody else's job." To be fair, people can hardly deal with something they know little about, and there are a number of difficulties in trying to learn more about self-destructive people:

- Cultural taboos against suicide
- Strong feelings about suicide and other self-destructive acts
- Limitations of doing research on human beings
- The intrinsic difficulty of examining the self-destructive process in those who commit suicide, since study is limited to determining the probable causes of suicide from survivors closely associated with the person

In spite of these limitations, research and direct work with self-destructive persons have yielded promising results. Suicidology—the study of suicide and suicide prevention—is still by no means an exact science. Yet the scientific knowledge and practices developed in the last few decades are a considerable advancement over responses based on myths and taboos. Knowledge alone, however, does not guarantee the use of that knowledge. Many false beliefs about self-destructive people and responses to them persist because of intense feelings about suicide, death, and dying. What are some of the most common feelings people have about a self-destructive person? And why are these feelings particularly intense in the helper-client interaction?

As we try to help self-destructive people, we may feel sadness, pity, helplessness, desire to rescue, anger, or frustration. Some of these feelings are mirrored in the following comments:

- *Curious bystander:* "Oh, the poor thing."
- *Friendly neighbor:* "What can I possibly do?"
- *Family:* "Why did she have to disgrace us this way?"
- *Nurse:* "I can't stand wasting my time on these people who are just looking for attention."

After a suicide, several feelings are common among survivors: *anxiety* that something we did or did not do caused the suicide; *relief*—which is not uncommon among family members or therapists who have exhausted themselves trying to help the suicidal person; or *guilt,* which often follows feelings of disgust or relief that the desperate person has died.

Understanding these feelings and their sources is crucial if we are to keep them from becoming impediments to helping distressed people find alternatives to suicide. Our feelings about suicide and responses to self-destructive persons can be clarified from three perspectives: social, psychological, and cultural.

Social Perspective

Physicians, nurses, and other helpers are often frustrated in working with self-destructive people. This can be traced, in part, to the socialization these professionals receive in their role of helping the sick person return to health. Success in this role depends partly on whether patients behave according to expectations of people in the "sick role." Parsons (1951, pp. 436–437) identified the following exemptions and responsibilities associated with the sick role:

1. Depending on the nature and severity of the illness, the person is exempt from normal social responsibility. This implies that the illness has been legitimized by a "mandated labeler," usually a physician (Becker, 1963; see also Chapter Three). Such legitimation gives moral approval to being sick and prevents people from using sickness inappropriately for secondary gains (Ehrenreich & Ehrenreich, 1978; Zola, 1978).
2. The sick person is expected to accept help and depend as necessary on the caregiver; it is understood that the person cannot improve merely by an act of will.
3. The person is obligated to want to get well as expeditiously as possible.
4. The person must seek technically competent help and cooperate with the helper.

   This concept of the sick role is unproblematic if applied to acute illness such as appendicitis or extreme pain caused by kidney stones. In fact, the study of persons with precisely such acute physical conditions resulted in Parsons's "sick role" formulation. However, the concept is inadequate if it is applied to chronic illnesses or to any condition with significant social, psychological, or cultural components—in short, any condition in which lifestyle or a willful act of the individual is directly related to the malady, such as smoking, drinking, or sexual contact (Levine & Kozloff, 1978).

   If so-called social illnesses do not fit the traditional sick role/helper model, think of the model's limitations when applied to a person who is self-destructive. Not only do suicidal people defeat the medical role of fostering and maintaining life, but self-injury appears to flout deliberately the natural instinct to live. The self-destructive person is requesting, directly or indirectly, a departure from the usual roles of patient and helper. If helpers deal with suicidal people according to rigid role expectations, the helper/patient relationship can lead to conflict. And if helping is limited to a medical approach when the problem is as philosophical, religious, and social as it is medical, the trouble that health professionals have when working with suicidal persons becomes more understandable.

Psychological Perspective

   Role conflicts are complicated further if helpers have an unrecognized or excessive need to be needed or to rescue the self-destructive person. Not only is the helper denied the fulfillment of traditional role expectations, but the suicidal person says, in effect, "I don't need you. How can you save me when I don't even want to save myself?" This is a very good question, considering what we know about the failure of therapy without the client's voluntary collaboration.

The most complex manifestation of the social-psychological roots of conflict with suicidal people is in the victim-rescuer-persecutor triangle discussed in Chapter Four. Of all the phases of crisis work, it is most important here that we be sensitive to a person's need for self-mastery, as well as to our own need to control our rescue fantasies. Not to do so could result in a vicious cycle of results that are exactly the opposite of our intentions:

- Our misguided rescue attempts are rejected.
- We feel frustrated in our helper role.
- We persecute the suicidal person for failing to cooperate.
- The suicidal person feels rejected.
- The suicidal person repeats the self-injury.
- The helper feels like a victim.

Preventing and interrupting the victim-rescuer-persecutor cycle is one of the most challenging tasks facing the crisis worker, especially in dealing with self-destructive people. The social network strategies discussed in Chapter Five are particularly helpful in this task.

Cultural Perspective

Self-destructive behavior takes on added meaning when placed in cultural-historical perspective. Suicide and self-destructive behavior have been part of the human condition from the beginning of time. Views about it—whether it is honorable or shameful—have always varied. In the Judeo-Christian tradition, neither the Hebrew Bible nor the New Testament prohibits suicide. Jews (defenders of Masada) and Christians (martyrs) alike justified suicide in the face of military defeat or personal attack by pagans. Later, however, suicide took on the character of a sinful act.

Over the centuries, we have seen suicide considered first from a religious standpoint and more recently from a legal and medical perspective as well. Today, these three major social institutions overlap in their interpretations of suicide. In spite of professionals' and civil libertarians' sophistication about the topic, suicide is still largely taboo. Now, however, it is seen less as a moral offense than as a socially disgraceful act.

When thus viewed in social, psychological, and cultural perspective, our beliefs and feelings about suicide are not surprising. We are, after all, members of a cultural community with distinct values about life, ourselves, and other people, as well as views about how people should behave. These cultural facts of life are even more complex when considering the multiethnicity of North American societies and the current emphasis on preserving one's unique cultural heritage. It is impossible for us to know in detail the beliefs and customs of cultures to which we have had little direct exposure. What we can do, however, is educate ourselves about ethnocentrism (see "Factors Influencing Communications" in Chapter Four) and to refrain from imposing our values on others. For example, in some belief systems the idea of an afterlife is meaningless, while for others suicide might be precisely the avenue toward a better life after reincarnation.

It is easier to accept and deal with our feelings if we remember that they have historical roots and are complicated by contemporary socialization to professional roles. Failing to recognize this can prevent us from being helpful to self-destructive people—which places an especially heavy burden on emergency and rescue personnel. Workers need an opportunity to express and work through their feelings about self-destructive behavior. Dealing with feelings and their origins, then, is a basic step in a worker's acquiring the knowledge and skills necessary to help people in suicidal crisis. Team relationships, peer support groups, and readily accessible consultation are some of the avenues that should be available to people working with suicidal persons.

Ethical Issues Regarding Suicide

Closely related to coping with feelings about self-destructive behavior are our positions on the right to die and on the degree of our responsibility for the lives of others. Within professional circles of suicidology, philosophy, and psychiatry, and in the general public the following are hotly debated topics (Battin & Mayo, 1980; Brandt, 1975; Humphrey, 1992; Richman, 1992):

- The right to die by suicide
- The right and/or responsibility to prevent suicide
- Related topics of euthanasia and abortion

Several ethical and legal questions have implications for the crisis worker:

- How do we respond to a person's declaration: "I have the right to commit suicide and you don't have the right to stop me"?
- If our own belief system forbids suicide, how might this belief influence our response to such a person?
- If a person commits suicide, whose responsibility is it?
- If we happen to believe the suicidal person alone is responsible, why do we often feel guilty?
- What is the ethical basis for depriving a person of normal, individual rights through commitment to a mental health facility to prevent suicide?

In considering these questions, the intent is not to persuade the reader to give up cherished beliefs or to impose a libertarian view about suicide. Rather, it is to provide an ethical and clinical basis for dealing with the issues without either abandoning our own beliefs or imposing them on others.

Some workers may confuse suicide prevention efforts with a distorted sense of obligation to prevent any and all suicides whenever physically possible and by whatever means possible. The term "distorted" is used to emphasize the fact that:

1. It is physically impossible to prevent suicide in some instances unless we place a person in a padded cell and strip him or her of all clothing. This does not mean that suicide is inevitable; it means that if social and psychological aid is lacking, physical protection alone is inadequate.
2. Forced physical protection attacks a person's basic need for mastery and self-determination and may result in the opposite of what is intended in the long run, even though suicide may be prevented in the short run. Such suicide prevention efforts may (a) impose on others the belief that people do not have the right to commit suicide, or (b) result in the worker's unresolved "savior complex."

These beliefs and unconscious conflicts often accompany a lack of scientific knowledge about self-destructive behavior and the inability to assess suicidal risk. The results may promote rather than prevent suicide through such practices as:

1. *Placing a hospitalized suicidal person in isolation.* This is done to allow closer observation, but it increases the person's sense of abandonment, which, for someone suicidal, is already acute.
2. *Committing a suicidal person involuntarily to a psychiatric facility* in the belief that others know what is best for a suicidal person. This can be an attack on the person's sense of dignity and self-worth, yet mental health laws in many states and provinces may encourage the practice among those working in public agencies or mental health professions. There is often little awareness that restricting individual freedom can give the suicidal person one more reason to choose death over life.
3. *Engaging in punitive practices* (though less common now), for example, using a larger tube than necessary to remove stomach contents if the person has taken an overdose of pills. Such a practice is based on the belief that physical discomfort will discourage future suicide attempts. In fact, the self-destructive person feels attacked and more worthless than ever.

The hidden function of these practices is probably the expression of anger against the self-destructive person for violating the suicide taboo and for frustrating the workers' helping role. The suicidal person has little or no ability to understand such messages. He or she already has an overdose of self-hatred. Rejection by helpers as they carry out their service responsibilities can only increase a person's self-destructiveness.

Opinions differ regarding the issue of responsibility to save others and the right to determine one's own death. The *ethical* and *legal* aspects of certain issues must be distinguished. For example, many people believe that suicide is ethically acceptable in certain circumstances, but regardless of personal beliefs, it is illegal in the United States and in most other countries to assist another in the act of suicide.[2] Conversely, while abortion is legal in the United States, people differ about whether it is ethically or morally acceptable. Crisis workers must consider the relevance of theoretical debates to their everyday interaction with suicidal people. The following case analyses illustrate some of the ethical questions.

CASE EXAMPLE: RACHEL'S "RIGHT" TO COMMIT SUICIDE

Rachel, age sixty-nine, lived with her daughter and son-in-law and was dying of cancer. The community health nurse learned that Rachel was considering suicide. In fact, Rachel spoke openly of her right to kill herself, although she had no immediate plan. After the nurse worked with the daughter and explored her feelings regarding her dying mother, the relationship between the daughter and mother improved. The daughter was put in touch with a respite service for families of cancer patients. Rachel was no longer suicidal and decided not to exercise her right.

This case demonstrates the philosophical dilemma posed by rational versus "manipulated" suicide (Battin, 1980). Among the rank and file of health and social service workers, the idea of manipulation is commonplace, especially with respect to suicidal people. But several things are noteworthy about this usage. When a person is unsuccessful in a suicide attempt, the assumption is that he or she is inappropriately trying to *manipulate* a staff person, family, or others. Thus, the term has a moral connotation. Yet crisis workers often do not acknowledge that manipulation is common in all social life. For example, the average person manipulates to get a larger salary, a different work shift, or better housing. When considering the right to commit suicide, we need to examine whether we, as members of a suicidal person's social world, have manipulated a person into "choosing" suicide. A person can be manipulated into suicide through material and social circumstances and through ideology.

Rachel's case illustrates (1) her social circumstances, highlighted by her relationship with her daughter and changed through home health care given to the daughter and (2) her ideology, that is, her belief about her value as an older person dying of cancer. As her view of herself changed from feeling nonproductive and worthless to feeling valuable in the eyes of her daughter and herself, she stopped arguing about her right to commit suicide. Thus, the argument about the right to die becomes moot if the reasons for choosing suicide are the failure to: (1) relieve intolerable pain (Fagerhaugh & Strauss, 1977); (2) provide relief to family

---

[2]Passage in Oregon of the recent ballot question on physician-assisted suicide is an exception to this general rule.

CASE EXAMPLE: DIANE AND ADOLESCENT SUICIDE

Diane, age eighteen and a high school senior, resisted all alternatives to suicide as proposed by a crisis counselor. She learned she
was pregnant; she was rejected by her lover
and could not share her distress with her
parents or friends. Abortion was not an acceptable alternative to her. She feared that
continuing the pregnancy would mean failing to graduate. The counselor agreed with

Diane's assertion of her basic right to commit suicide but expressed hope that she
would not follow through on that decision
during the peak of her crisis. This acknowl-
edgment seemed to give Diane a sense of
dignity and control over her life and a new
will to live, even though the only resource
she perceived at the moment was the
counselor.

caretakers[3] (Skorupka & Bohnet, 1982); and (3) examine critically a value system
that holds no place for the "nonproductive" old, ill, or disabled. Jourard (1970)
underscores this point in defining suicide as "an invitation [from social network
members] to die." Rachel's case suggests that the "right to commit suicide" argument can cloak hidden social processes and values at work. Ironically, acknowledging a person's right to commit suicide can have a curious suicide
prevention effect. Even if our own belief system disallows such a right, it is empowering (and therefore life-promoting) to respect and acknowledge others' beliefs.

At the other end of the age spectrum, let us consider the alarming increase
in adolescent suicides. We could profitably ask ourselves the following questions:

- What are our children telling us about the life and the world we have created
  for them if they choose death over life at a time when life has just begun?
- Have we perhaps "manipulated" our children into suicide by creating a material and social world and value system that they feel are not worth staying
  alive for?
- If we acknowledge the "right" of an adolescent to commit suicide, do we ignore a larger question about reasons for hope or despair among young people?

CASE EXAMPLE: JOHN AND MENTAL HEALTH COMMITMENT

John, age forty-eight, was placed in a public
mental health facility against his will when
he became highly suicidal after his wife divorced him. He also had a serious drinking
problem. John had two very close friends
and a small business of his own. The main

reason for hospitalizing John was to prevent
him from committing suicide. John found
the hospital worse than anything he had experienced. He had no contact with his
friends while in the hospital. After two
weeks, John begged to be discharged. He

---

[3]Current debates on voters' ballots about physician-assisted suicide and action intersect with
peoples' concerns about the adequacy of health and social services during terminal illness
and their dread of the prospect of "high technology" death in institutions. This issue is discussed more fully in Chapters Eleven and Thirteen.

Case Example, cont.

was no longer highly suicidal but was still depressed. John was discharged with antidepressant medicine and instructed to return for a follow-up appointment in one week. He killed himself with sleeping pills (obtained from a private physician) and alcohol two days after discharge. The staff of the mental hospital did not understand how they had failed John.

John's case represents the complexity of the debate between a commitment to protect against suicide and infringement on the right to self-determination. As the paralyzed hero of a movie by the same title put it, "Whose life is it, anyway?" He was speaking of his resistance to the treatment that kept him alive. Even though suicide can be seen as rational in certain circumstances, John's decision could also be seen as "not in his own best interest" (Brandt, 1975). Cases like John's reveal the ethical basis for depriving a person of personal freedom in the name of suicide prevention and treatment. That is, John had friends and by objective standards something to live for, even though he could not see that when he killed himself. It could be argued, therefore, that extreme rescue action by helpers is justified.

John's eventual suicide, though, illustrates the care that must be taken in implementing mental health laws on behalf of suicidal people. First of all, the decision to commit a person must be based on a thorough assessment. Second, even if he had been found to be a serious risk for suicide, involuntary hospitalization seemed to contribute to, rather than prevent, John's suicide. Hospitalization is indicated for suicidal people only when natural social network resources (such as John's friends) are not present. This case is analyzed further in "Team Analysis Following a Suicide" in the next chapter.

Some people choose suicide even after considering the alternatives with caring people. Public and controversial examples include the planned suicide of artist Jo Roman in the United States and the case of Sue Rodriguez in Canada. Ms. Roman's suicide plans and discussion with her family and friends were aired on national public television, followed by an interdisciplinary panel discussion of the

CASE EXAMPLE: PAUL—RATIONAL SUICIDE?

Paul, age sixty-four, had chronic heart disease. He had been depressed since his wife's death three months earlier. When he was laid off from his job, he became suicidal and talked with his doctor, who referred him to a community mental health center for therapy. He received individual and group psychotherapy and antidepressant drugs. After three months, Paul's depression lifted somewhat, but he was still unconvinced that there was anything left to live for. He had been very dependent on his wife and seemed unable to develop other satisfying relationships, even in the support group for widowed people that he had joined. Paul killed himself by carbon monoxide poisoning after terminating therapy at the mental health center.

Paul's situation does not imply that suicide is inevitable. Rather, it suggests the rationality of Paul's decision to commit suicide rather than live in circumstances to which he apparently could not adjust. However, Paul's case also shows us what can be done to help people find alternatives to suicide, even though these alternatives may be rejected. The people who tried to help Paul can take comfort in the fact that they acted humanely on his behalf, although they may still feel regret. But we must recognize our limitations in influencing the lives of other people (see "Survivors in Crisis" in the next chapter).

Currently, rational suicide is being discussed with respect to people with AIDS and those whose suicides were assisted by Dr. Jack Kevorkian.

CASE EXAMPLE: DENNIS—RATIONAL SUICIDE?

Dennis, age thirty-three, held a good job as a university professor at the time he was diagnosed with AIDS. Initially, Dennis was overwhelmed with shock, rage, and despair. He had been successful in his career, enjoyed a supportive circle of friends, and was comfortable with his gay identity. He had decided to kill himself but after surviving an antigay physical attack and helping two of his friends cope with a similar episode of violence, he became involved in a local activist group and no longer felt suicidal. Dennis reserves for himself, though, the possibility of suicide at a future time if AIDS progresses to the point of dementia for him.

Dennis's case illustrates the importance of control and self-determination for anyone in crisis. While we need to respect the decisions of people like Dennis, we must be particularly careful in reference to AIDS not to proffer rational suicide as a substitute for our humane response to this worldwide crisis (see Chapter Fourteen).

The following is offered as a practical guideline to helpers with respect to rights and responsibilities regarding suicide: each person has the final responsibility for his or her own life. This includes the right to live as one chooses or to end life. We have a communal responsibility to do what we reasonably can to help others live as happily as possible. This includes preventing suicide when it appears to be against a person's own best interests. It also involves examining values and social practices that inadvertently lead people to choose suicide only because they are socially disadvantaged and see no other way out. Choice in these instances is not truly free. Our social responsibility does not require that we prevent a suicide at all costs. We need to recognize that misguided "savior" tactics can result in suicide if overbearing help is interpreted as control. Workers in human service professions such as nursing, medicine, mental health, and law enforcement have an additional responsibility: they should learn as much as they can about self-destructive people and how to help them find alternatives to suicide.

Characteristics of Self-Destructive People

To be understood is basic to the feeling that someone cares, that life is worth living. When someone responds to stress with a deliberate suicide attempt, those around the person are usually dismayed and ask, "Why?" The wide range of self-destructive acts adds to the observer's confusion; there are many overlapping features of self-destructive behavior. For example, Mary, age fifty, has been destroying herself through alcohol abuse for fifteen years, but she also takes an overdose of sleeping pills during an acute crisis.

Volumes have been written about suicide—by philosophers, the clergy, psychiatrists and psychologists, nurses, and crisis specialists. Academics and researchers have profound discussions and varied opinions regarding the process, meanings, morality, and reasons involved in the act of self-destruction. While these debates continue, the focus in this book is on the *meaning* of self-destructive behavior and the importance of understanding and reaching out to those in pain (see O'Carroll, 1993; Shneidman, 1993). Precise definitions and a clear understanding of such behavior are complex and difficult to achieve. However, in spite of academic differences, most people agree that self-destructive behavior signals that a person is in turmoil or "perturbation" (Shneidman, 1976, p. 53). We can enhance our effectiveness in working with suicidal people by becoming familiar with several aspects of self-destructive behavior and intervention practices widely accepted by experts:

- The range and complexity of self-destructive behavior
- Communication and the meaning of self-destructive behavior
- Ambivalence and its relevance to suicide prevention
- The importance of assessing for suicidal risk
- Sensitivity to ethical issues as an aid to understanding, assessment, and appropriate intervention

Self-Destructiveness: What Does It Include?

Self-destructive behavior includes any action by which a person emotionally, socially, and physically damages or ends his or her life. Broadly, the spectrum of self-destructiveness includes biting nails, pulling hair, scratching, cutting one's wrist, swallowing toxic substances or harmful objects, smoking cigarettes, banging one's head, abusing alcohol and other drugs, driving recklessly, neglecting life-preserving measures such as taking insulin, attempting suicide, and committing suicide (Farberow, 1980; Menninger, 1938).

At one end of the spectrum of self-destructiveness is Jane, who smokes but is in essentially good emotional and physical health. She knows the long-range effects of smoking and chooses to live her life in such a way that may in fact shorten it. However, Jane would hardly be regarded as suicidal on a lethality assessment scale. Smoking by Arthur, who has severe emphysema, is another matter. His behavior could be considered a slow form of deliberate self-destruction. At the other end of the spectrum is James, who plans to hang himself. Unless saved accidentally, James will most certainly die by his own hand.

There are four broad groups of self-destructive people:

1. *Those who commit suicide.* Suicide is defined as a fatal act that is self-inflicted, consciously intended, and carried out with the knowledge that death is irreversible. This definition of suicide generally excludes young children, since a child's conception of death as final develops around age ten (Nagey, 1965; Pfeffer, 1986). Self-destructive deaths in young children are usually explained in terms of learning theory; the child learns—often by observing parents—that physical and emotional pain can be relieved by ingesting pills or banging one's head.

Classically defined, suicide is one of four modes of death; the others are natural, accidental, and homicidal. Shneidman (1973, p. 384) emphasizes the role of intention in an individual's death and proposes a reclassification of death as (1) intentioned, (2) subintentioned, (3) unintentioned. If full information is not available about the person's intentions, it is difficult to determine whether the act is suicidal or accidental. Suicide is not an illness or an inherited disease, as popular opinion and some professional practice seem to imply.

2. *Those who threaten suicide.* This group includes those who talk about suicide and whose suicidal plans may be either very vague or highly specific. Some in this group have made suicide attempts in the past; others have not. Note that only suicidal people threaten suicide; all suicide threats should be taken seriously and considered in relation to the person's intention and social circumstances.

3. *Those who make suicide attempts.* A suicide attempt is any nonfatal act of self-inflicted damage with self-destructive intention, however vague and ambiguous. Sometimes the individual's intention must be inferred from behavior. Technically, the term "suicide attempt" should be reserved for those actions in which a person *attempts* to carry out the *intention* to die but for unanticipated reasons, such as failure of the method or an unplanned rescue, the attempt *fails*. Other self-destructive behavior can more accurately be defined as "self-injury." The neutral term self-injury should be substituted for the term "suicide gesture," since the latter suggests that the behavior need not be taken seriously or that the person is "just seeking attention."

Some suicidal persons are in a state of acute crisis—in contrast to some who are chronically self-destructive—and therefore experience a high degree of emotional turmoil. As noted in Chapter Three, people in crisis may experience a temporary upset in cognitive functioning. This upset can make it difficult for a person to clarify his or her intentions or may interfere in making wise decisions. This feature of the crisis state is the basis for the general wisdom of delaying serious decisions such as getting married, selling one's house, or moving to a foreign country while in crisis. Certainly, then, it is similarly unwise to make an irrevocable decision such as suicide when in a state of emotional turmoil and crisis.

The ambiguity arising out of the crisis state should not be confused with a psychotic process, which may or may not be present. Nor should one subscribe to the prevalent myth that "only a crazy person could seriously consider, attempt, or commit suicide." Loss of impulse control influences some suicide attempts and completed suicides. In the large majority of instances, however, self-destructive behavior is something that people consciously and deliberately plan and execute.

4. *People who are chronically self-destructive.* People in this group may habitually abuse alcohol or other drugs and are often diagnosed with personality disorders. For many First Nations people, self-destructive behaviors are embedded in the abject poverty, unemployment, and other results of colonization and the near-destruction of Native cultures (Philp, 1993). A recent study of self-harm patients revealed that 65.8 percent had a previous history of self-harm (Barnes, 1986). The complex relationship between multiple self-harm episodes and suicide risk is discussed further in "Assessment of the Suicidal Person" later in this chapter. Other people may destroy themselves by the deliberate refusal to follow life-sustaining medical programs for such conditions as heart disease or diabetes. Still others engage in high-risk lifestyles or activities that bring them constantly into the face of potential death. Such individuals seem to need the stimulation of their risky lifestyles to make life seem worth living (Weisman, 1973). These behaviors are not, of course, explicitly suicidal. However, individuals who engage in them may, like others, become overtly suicidal. This complicates whatever problems already exist.

When considering chronic self-destructiveness, Maris's (1981, pp. 62–69) concept of *suicidal careers* is relevant. In this framework, suicide can be seen as "one product of a gradual loss of hope and the will and resources to live, a kind of running down and out of life energies, a bankruptcy of psychic defenses against death and decay" (p. 69). Or as Shneidman (1985, 1987) puts it: "People reach 'the point of no return' in response to unendurable psychological pain."

It is important to distinguish here between self-destructive persons and those who engage in self-mutilating activity (e.g., cutting, scraping, and bruising) that generally has no dire medical consequences, although some may end up killing themselves. Unlike suicidal behavior, self-mutilation is not characterized by an intent to die. Rather, it is a way of coping, usually employed by women. Many of these women are survivors of extreme childhood sexual abuse who have internalized their oppression (see Burstow, 1992, pp. 187–220).

The Path to Suicide

Suicidal behavior can be viewed on a continuum or as a "highway leading to suicide." The highway begins with the first suicide threat or attempt and ends in suicide. As in the case of any trip destined for a certain endpoint, one can always change one's mind, take a different road to another destination, or turn around and come back. The highway to suicide can be conceived either as a short trip—acute crisis—or a long trip—chronic self-destructiveness extending for years or over a lifetime. But in either case, it suggests that suicide is a *process* involving:

- One's perception of the meaning of life and death
- The availability of psychological and social resources
- Material and physical circumstances making self-destruction possible (for example, when a bedridden, helpless person is capable of self-destruction only through starvation)

The continuum concept is also useful in understanding suicides that appear to result from impulsive action, as sometimes happens with adolescents. Even with adolescent suicides, though, examination and hindsight usually reveal a process including, for example, alienation, family conflict, abuse, depression, self-doubt, and cynicism about life.

A destiny of suicide is not inevitable. Whether one continues down the highway to suicide depends on a variety of circumstances. People traveling this highway usually give clues to their distress, so the suicide continuum can be interrupted at any point: after a first attempt, fifth attempt, or as soon as clues are recognized. Much depends on the help available and the ability of the suicidal person to accept and use help. It is never too late to help a despairing person or to change one's mind about suicide.

Lacking help, some suicidal persons try to relieve their pain by repeated self-injury; each time, their gamble with death becomes more dangerous. As they move along the suicide highway repeating their cries for help, they are often labeled and written off as manipulators or attention seekers. This usually means that professional helpers and others regard them as devious and insincere in their "demands" for attention. Some conclude that if a person were serious about suicide, he or she would try something that "really did the job." Such a judgment implies a gross misunderstanding of the meaning of a suicidal person's behavior and ignores his or her real needs.

Individuals who are thus labeled and ignored will probably continue to injure themselves. The suicidal episodes typically become progressively more serious in the medical sense, signaling increasing desperation for someone to hear and understand their cries for help. They may also engage in the "no-lose game" as they plan the next suicide attempt (Baechler, 1979). The no-lose game goes something like this: "If they (spouse, friend, family) find me, they care enough and therefore life is worth living. (I win by living.) If they don't find me, life isn't worth living. (I win by dying.)"

The suicide method chosen is usually lethal but includes the possibility of rescue, such as swallowing sleeping pills. No-lose reasoning is ineffective in instances when one cannot reasonably expect rescue (for example, a family member rarely checks a person at 2 A.M.). It nevertheless indicates the person's extreme distress and illustrates the logic of the no-lose game.

The Messages of Self-Destructive People

Despite differing explanations for suicide, most people agree that self-destructive acts are a powerful means of communicating; suicidal people are trying to tell us something by their behavior. Interrupting the suicide continuum depends on understanding and responding appropriately to messages of pain, distress, or despair.

Most individuals get what they need or want by simply asking for it. Or friends and family are sensitive and caring enough to pick up the clues to distress before the person becomes desperate. Some people, however, spend a lifetime trying to obtain, without success, what they need for basic survival and happiness. This may be because they cannot express their needs directly, because their needs are insatiable and therefore unobtainable, or because others do not listen and try to meet their needs. Finally, these people give up and attempt suicide as a last effort to let someone know that they are hurting and desperate.

Typically, then, suicidal people have a history of unsuccessful communication. Their problems with communication follow two general patterns:

1. Some people habitually refrain from expressing feelings and sharing their concerns with significant others. People in this group use the "stiff upper lip" approach to life's problems. Men socialized to be cool and rational in the face of adversity and women socialized to be the social and emotional experts for everyone but themselves contribute to the withholding of feelings. This kind of failure in communication is typified by:
   a. A successful businessman who obtains a promotion, is threatened by his fear of not being able to handle his new responsibilities, and kills himself.
   b. A mother of five children who works devotedly and without complaint for her children and husband and is considered an ideal mother, one day kills two of her children and then herself.
   c. A boy, age seventeen, who is an honor student, plans to go to law school, and is the pride of his parents and the school, is found dead of carbon monoxide poisoning in the family car.

In each of these cases, the response is great shock and consternation: "He seemed to have everything . . . I wonder why? . . . There doesn't seem to be any

reason." Yet hindsight usually reveals that there were clues (Shneidman & Farberow, 1957). Subtle changes in behavior, along with a tendency to repress feelings, should be regarded as quiet cries for help. The messages of these suicidal
people are less explicit, and there often is no history of suicidal behavior. Caring
others, therefore, need great sensitivity; they need to encourage the suicidal person to share life's joys, troubles, and suicidal fantasies without feeling like an
"unmanly" man, a "failure" as a wife and mother, or a "sissy" as an adolescent.
Lacking invitations to share and live instead of to die, these people's despair
may be forever unexpressed in the eternity of death.

2. The second pattern of communication problems is less subtle than the first.
   People in this group typically include those who threaten suicide or have ac-
   tually injured themselves. Their suicidal messages are quite direct and are
   often preceded by other cries for help (Farberow & Shneidman, 1961). Con-
   sider, for example, an adolescent girl's signals that something is wrong:
   Age 11: Sullenness and truancy from school
   Age 12: Experimentation with drugs
   Age 13: Running away from home
   Age 14: Pregnancy and abortion
   Age 15: First suicide attempt

After a person's first suicide attempt, family members and other significant
people in the individual's life are usually shocked. They often are more disturbed
by a suicide attempt than by anything else the person might have done. Typically,
a parent, spouse, or friend will say, "I knew she was upset and not exactly happy,
but I didn't know she was that unhappy." In other words, the first suicide attempt is the most powerful of a series of behavioral messages or clues given over
a period of time.
    We should all be familiar with suicidal clues or cries for help such as:

- "You won't be seeing me around much anymore."
- "I've about had it with this job. . . . I can't take it anymore."
- "I'm angry at my mother. She'll really be sorry when I'm dead."
- "I can't take any more problems without some relief."
- "I can't live without my boyfriend. I don't really want to die, I just want him
  back or somebody in his place."
- "I can't take the pain and humiliation [from AIDS, for example] anymore."
- "There's nothing else left since my wife left me. I really want to die."

Behavioral clues may include making out a will, taking out a large life insurance policy, giving away precious belongings, being despondent after a financial
setback, or engaging in unusual behavior.
    Studies reveal that a majority of persons who commit suicide have made pre-

vious attempts. In the absence of attempts, 80 percent have given other significant clues of their suicidal intent (Barnes, 1986; Brown & Sheran, 1972). These behavioral, verbal, and affective clues can be interpreted in two general ways: (1) "I want to die," or (2) "I don't want to die, but I want something to change in order to go on living" or "If things don't change, life isn't worth living. . . . Help me find something to live for."

It is up to the interested helping person to determine the meaning of suicidal behavior and to identify clues in the distressed person's words and attitudes. This is done not by inferring the person's meaning but by asking, for example:

- "What do you mean when you say you can't take your problems anymore? Are you thinking of suicide?"
- "What did you hope would happen when you took the pills (or cut your wrists)? Did you intend to die?"

There is no substitute for *simple, direct communication* by a person who cares. Besides providing the information we need in order to help, it is helpful to the suicidal person. It tells the person we are interested and concerned about motives for the contemplated suicide. Often, self-destructive people have lacked the advantages of communicating directly about their feelings all of their lives.

Unfortunately, many people lack the knowledge or resources to respond helpfully to a suicidal person. The self-destructive person is often surrounded by others who potentially could help but whose own troubles prevent them from providing what the self-destructive person needs. Some families are so needy that the most they can do is obtain medical treatment for the suicidal person. This situation is not helped by the fact that twenty-four–hour crisis services are absent in some communities.

Some would-be helpers fail to communicate directly about suicide in the false belief that talking to the person about suicide intentions may trigger such ideas if he or she doesn't already have them. The process of deciding to commit suicide is much more complicated than such reasoning implies. A person who is not suicidal will not become so as a result of a question from someone intending to help. In fact, experience reveals that suicidal people are relieved when someone is sensitive enough to respond to their despair and thus help protect them from themselves.

For three reasons, then, communication is crucial in our work with people who respond to crisis by self-destructive behavior:

1. It is a key element in discerning the *process* of self-destruction (understanding).
2. It is the most effective means of ascertaining the person's intention regarding death (assessment of risk).
3. It is an essential avenue for helping the person feel reconnected to other human beings and finding a reason to live (crisis intervention).

Ambivalence: Weighing Life and Death

Suicidal people usually struggle with two irreconcilable wishes: the desire to live and the desire to die. They simultaneously consider the advantages of life and death—a state of mind known as ambivalence. As long as the person has ambivalent feelings about life and death, it is possible to help the individual consider choices on the side of life. Suicide is not inevitable. People can change their minds if they find realistic alternatives to suicide. The concept of ambivalence is basic to the purpose of suicide prevention and crisis work; those who are no longer ambivalent do not usually come to an emergency service or call police and suicide hotlines.

CASE EXAMPLE: SALLY

Sally, age sixteen, tried to commit suicide by swallowing six sleeping pills. In medical terms, this was not a serious attempt. Although she contemplated death, she also wanted to live. She hoped that the suicide attempt would bring about some change in her miserable family life so she could avoid the last resort of suicide. Before her suicide attempt, Sally was having trouble in school; she ran away from home once, experimented with drugs, and engaged in behavior that often brought disapproval from her parents.

All these behaviors were Sally's way of saying, "Listen to me! Can't you see that I'm miserable . . . that I can't control myself . . . that I can't go on like this anymore?" Sally had been upset for several years by her parents' constant fighting and playing favorites with the children. Her father drank heavily and frequently was away from home. When Sally's school counselor recommended family counseling, the family refused out of shame. Sally's acting out was really a cry for help. After her suicide attempt, her parents accepted counseling. Sally's behavior improved generally, and she made no further suicide attempts.

If Sally had not obtained the help she needed, it is probable that she would have continued down the highway to suicide. The usual pattern in such a case is that the attempts become medically more serious, the person becomes more desperate, and finally commits suicide. Helping the ambivalent person move in the direction of life is done by understanding and responding to the meaning of his or her behavior.

Assessment of the Suicidal Person

Communication leads to understanding, which is the foundation for decision and action. Helping suicidal people without understanding what their behavior means and without ascertaining the degree of suicide risk is difficult. *Suicide risk assessment* is the process of determining the likelihood of suicide for a particular person. *Lethality assessment* refers to the degree of physical injury incurred by a particular self-destructive act. Sometimes these terms are used interchangeably. *Suicide prediction,* in terms of current research, is "not very precise or useful" (Maris, 1991, p. 2) and, according to Motto (1991, p. 75) should probably be eliminated from scientific terminology. The main focus here is to provide clinicians with guidelines about the risk of suicide that are based on clinical experience and on empirical and epidemiological findings. Clinical assessment tries to answer the question: what is the risk of death by suicide for this individual at this time, considering the person's life as a whole?

Some workers use lethality assessment scales, which are primarily research tools, to assess suicidal risk. Most of these scales are not very effective (Brown & Sheran, 1972). Motto (1985, p. 139) states: "The use of a scale has never been intended to predict suicide, but simply to supplement clinical judgment at the time an evaluation is done." Nor can a rating scale ever substitute for a clinician's sensitive inquiry, for example, "Can you tell me what's happening to cause you so much pain?" (Motto, 1991). The problem with most scales is that they do not exclude the nonsuicidal population. For example, let us consider depression as a predictive sign. A large number of people who commit suicide (approximately 70 percent) have been diagnosed as depressed; however, the majority of depressed people do not commit suicide. Similarly, the majority of people who commit suicide have made previous suicide attempts; yet eight out of ten people who attempt suicide never go on to commit suicide. These statistics do not invite complacency; they simply indicate that something changed—a cry for help was heard. Standard psychological tests such as the Minnesota Multiphasic Personality Inventory (MMPI) are also not very helpful in assessing suicide risk.

The Importance of Assessing Suicide Risk

The importance of suicide risk assessment can be compared to the importance of diagnosing a cough before beginning treatment. Effective assessment of suicide risk should accomplish the following:

- Cut down on guesswork in working with self-destructive people
- Reduce the confusion and disagreement that often occur among those trying to help suicidal people
- Provide a scientific base for service plans for self-destructive people
- Assure that hospitalization of suicidal persons is used appropriately
- Decrease a worker's level of anxiety in working with suicidal persons

Failure to assess the degree of suicide risk results in unnecessary problems. For example, Linda, age twenty-two, who lives alone and feels alienated from her family, was treated medically for her cut wrist and discharged without follow-up counseling. The emergency department staff assumed that she was not serious about committing suicide; rather, she was just seeking attention. Since the message and long-range risk of Linda's suicide attempt were missed, she will very probably make another attempt in the future.

Another problem arising out of guesswork about suicide risk is unnecessary hospitalization. It is inappropriate to hospitalize a suicidal person when the degree of suicide risk is very low and other sources of protection are available. A person who hopes, by a suicide attempt, to relieve his or her isolation from family may feel even more isolated in a psychiatric hospital. This is especially true when community and family intervention are indicated instead.

Sometimes, community and hospital workers hospitalize suicidal people because of their own anxiety about suicide. Unresolved feelings of guilt and responsibility about suicide usually precipitate such action. On the other hand, hospitals can be places in which isolation can be relieved and suicide prevented when social supports in the community are lacking. As with personal factors, assumptions about the presence or absence of social supports should not be made without a systematic social assessment (see Chapters Three and Five).

Signs That Help Assess Suicide Risk

Risk assessment techniques are based on knowledge obtained from the study of completed suicides. Such research is among the most difficult of scientific studies (Maris, 1991; Smith & Maris, 1986), but the study of completed suicides has explained much about the problem of risk assessment. Maris, et al. (1992), Brown and Sheran (1972), and others have identified signs that help us assess the degree of risk for suicide. The most reliable indicators help us distinguish people who commit suicide from the population at large and also from those who only attempt suicide. These signs, however, have their limitations. For instance, there is not enough research on suicide to warrant general conclusions about suicide for different population groups (Smith & Maris, 1986). One should never be overconfident in applying signs to a suicidal person. It is impossible to predict suicide in any absolute sense; the focus for clinicians should be on assessing immediate and long-term risk. However, attention to the known signs of suicide risk is a considerable improvement over an approach based on myth, taboo, and unresearched guesswork. The chaos of a crisis situation and anxiety about suicide can be reduced by thoughtful attention to general principles based on research.

The following material regarding signs that help us assess suicide risk is summarized from the works of Alvarez (1971); Brown and Sheran (1972); Durkheim (1951); Farberow (1975); Furst & Huffine (1991); Hatton, Valente, and Rink (1984); Hendin (1982; 1987); Litman (1987); Maris (1981); Maris et al. (1992); Shneidman (1985); and Wandrei (1985). These principles for assessing suicide risk apply to *any* person in *any* setting contacted through *any* helping situation: telephone, office, hospital, home, jail, nursing home, school, or pastoral care. The discussion is based on research in Western societies; suicide signs and methods vary in other cultural settings (see Farberow, 1975). Sensitivity to these differences, however, is important in helping various immigrant and ethnic groups in distress in North America.

Suicide Plan. Studies reveal that the majority of persons who die by suicide deliberately planned to do so. This is in contrast to the myth that people who commit suicide do not know what they are doing or are "crazy." In respect to the plan, people suspected of being suicidal should be asked several direct questions concerning the following subjects:

1. *Suicidal ideas:* "Are you so upset that you're thinking of suicide?" or "Are you thinking about hurting yourself?"
2. *Lethality of method:* "What are you thinking of doing?"

High-lethal methods:

Gun

Barbiturate and prescribed sleeping pills

Jumping

Hanging

Drowning

Carbon monoxide poisoning

Aspirin (high dose) and acetaminophen (Tylenol)

Car crash

Exposure to extreme cold

Antidepressants (such as Elavil)

Low-lethal methods:

Wrist cutting

Nonprescription drugs (excluding aspirin and Tylenol)

Tranquilizers (such as Valium and Dalmane)

The helper should also determine the person's knowledge about the lethality of the chosen method. For example, a person who takes ten tranquilizers with the mistaken belief that the dose is fatal is alive more accidentally than by intent.

3. *Availability of means:* "Do you have a gun? Do you know how to use it? Do you have ammunition? Do you have pills?" Lives have often been saved by removing very lethal methods such as guns and sleeping pills. A highly suicidal person who calls a crisis center is often making a final effort to get help, even though

he or she may be sitting next to a loaded gun or bottle of pills. Such an individual will welcome a direct, protective gesture from a telephone counselor such as, "Why don't you put the gun away?" or, "Why don't you throw the pills out . . . and then let's talk about what's troubling you." When friends and family are involved, they too should be directed to get rid of the weapon or pills. In disposing of lethal weapons, it is important to engage the suicidal person actively in the process, keeping in mind that power ploys can trigger rather than prevent suicide. If trust and rapport have been established, engaging the suicidal person is generally not difficult to do.

4. *Specificity of plan:* "Do you have a plan worked out for killing yourself? How do you plan to get the pills? How do you plan to get the gun?" A person who has a plan that is well thought out—including time, place, and circumstances—with an available high-lethal method is an immediate and very high risk for suicide. We should also determine whether any rescue possibilities are included in the plan, for example, "What time of day do you plan to do this?" or "Is there anyone else around at that time?" We should also find out about the person's intent. Some people really intend to die; others intend to bring about some change that will help them avoid death and make life more liveable.

We can seldom discover a person's suicide plan except through *direct questioning.* An individual who believes in the myth that talking about suicide may suggest the idea will hesitate to ask direct questions. The suicide plan is a less important sign of risk in the case of people with a history of impulsive behavior. This is true for some adults and for adolescents in general, who are inclined to be impulsive as a characteristic of their stage of development.

History of Suicide Attempts. In the North American adult population, suicide attempts occur eight to ten times more often than actual suicide. Among adolescents, there are about fifty attempts to every completed suicide. Most people who attempt suicide do not go on to commit suicide. Usually some change occurs in their psychosocial world that makes life more desirable than death. On the other hand, the majority of people who kill themselves have made previous suicide attempts. A history of suicide attempts (65 percent of completed suicides) is especially prominent among suicidal people who find that self-destructive behavior is the most powerful means they have of communicating their distress to others. Those who have made previous high-lethal attempts are at greater risk for suicide than those who made low-lethal attempts. Another historical indicator is a change in method of suicide attempt. A person who makes a high-lethal attempt after several less lethal attempts that elicited increasingly indifferent responses from significant others is a higher risk for suicide than a person with a consistent pattern of low-lethal attempts. This is particularly true in the case of suicidal adolescents.

We should also determine the outcome of previous suicide attempts, for example, "What happened after your last attempt? Did you plan any possibility of rescue, or were you rescued accidentally?" A person living alone who overdoses with sleeping pills, then has unexpected company and is rescued, is alive more by accident than by intent. He or she falls into a high-risk category for future suicide if there are other high-risk indicators as well. Suicide risk is also increased if the person has a negative perception of a psychiatric hospital or counseling experience. This finding underscores the importance of extreme caution in employing mental health laws to hospitalize suicidal people against their will for self-protection.

Resources and Communication with Significant Others. Internal resources consist of strengths, problem-solving ability, and personality factors that help one cope with stress. External resources include a network of persons on whom one can rely routinely as well as during a crisis. Communication as a suicide sign includes: (1) the statement to others of intent to commit suicide, and (2) the quality of the bond that exists between the suicidal person and significant others. A large number of people who finally commit suicide feel ignored or cut off from significant people around them, some to the point of feeling there are no significant people in their lives. This is extremely important in the case of adolescents, especially regarding their attempts to communicate with their parents. Research suggests that most adolescents who kill themselves are at odds with their families and feel very misunderstood or have experienced various external stressors (Berman & Jobes, 1991; Brent, et al., 1993).

Institutionalized racism and the unequal distribution of material resources in the United States appear to contribute to the rapidly increasing rate of suicide among minority groups. This is especially true among young (under thirty) people who realize early in life that many doors are closed to them. Their rage and frustration eventually lead to despair, suicide, and other violent behavior. An example of violence that is closely linked to suicide is *victim-precipitated homicide.* In this form of homicide, the person killed is suicidal, but instead of committing suicide, the victim incites someone else to kill, thus precipitating the homicide.

Others may have apparent resources such as a supportive, caring spouse, but the conviction of their worthlessness prevents them from accepting and using such support. This is especially true for suicidal people who are also extremely depressed. Adequate personality resources include the ability to be flexible and to accept mistakes and imperfections in oneself. Some people who kill themselves seem to have happy families, good jobs, and good health. Observers therefore assume that these people have no reason to kill themselves. Research by Breed (1972) reveals that this kind of person perceives him- or herself in very rigid roles imposed by culture, sexual identity, or socioeconomic status. A typical example is the middle-aged male executive who rigidly commits himself to success by climbing up the career ladder in his company. A threatened or actual failure in this self-imposed and rigid role performance can precipitate suicide for such a person.

Such perceived failure is usually sex-specific: work failure for men (Morrell,

et al., 1993) and family or mate failure for women (Stephens, 1985). Other research, however, suggests that a woman might commit suicide in response to "su-
perwoman" demands that she be both the perfect, unpaid domestic worker and
the perfect paid public worker (Hoff, 1985; Neuringer, 1982). Investigation of completed suicides reveals that a person with rigid role perceptions commits suicide
after receiving, for example, a long-anticipated promotion, an event that leads the
person to doubt his or her ability to fulfill higher expectations (Perrah & Wichman, 1987). Such rigidity in personality type is also revealed in the person's approach to problem solving. The individual sees narrowly, perceiving only one
course of action or one solution to a problem: suicide. This has sometimes been
described as telescopic or "tunnel vision" (Hatton, Valente, & Rink, 1984, p. 29;
Shneidman, 1987, p. 57). Such people typically are candidates for psychotherapy
to help them develop more flexible approaches to problem solving. We should recognize this rigidity as a possible barrier in our efforts to help suicidal people consider alternatives. Thus, a person of this type whose personal and social resources
are exhausted and whose only remaining communication link is to a counselor or
helping agency is a high risk for suicide.

Research and clinical experience suggest that workers should look not only at
such signs of risk but also at the complex *patterning* of signs (Brown & Sheran 1972;
Farberow, 1975) in concert with clinical judgment (Motto, 1991). Let us apply this
evidence to the pattern of the signs considered above. If the person (1) has a history of high-lethal attempts; (2) has a specific, high-lethal plan for suicide with
available means; and (3) lacks both personality and social resources, his or her immediate and long-range risk for probable suicide is very high, regardless of other
factors. The risk increases, however, if factors such as those discussed next are also
present.

Sex, Age, Race, Marital Status, and Sexual Identity. The suicide ratio among
North American men and women is approximately three males to one female, although female suicides are increasing at a faster rate than male suicides. Among
children between the ages of ten and fourteen, the suicide rate is 0.3 to 0.6 per
100,000. Among children below the age of ten, suicide is almost nonexistent—
less than one annually in the United States. Suicide risk increases with age only
for white males. Among blacks, Chicanos, and First Nations people, the suicide
rate reaches its peak under the age of thirty.

The overall suicide rate among white persons is three times that among black
persons. However, among young, urban, African-American men between twenty
and thirty-five years of age, the rate is twice that of white men the same age. In
Native North American communities, the suicide rate varies from group to group.
In general, suicide rates are increasing among adolescents, racial minority groups,
and among youth experiencing sexual identity crisis.

If a person is separated from a spouse, widowed, or divorced, the risk of
suicide increases. Those who are married or who have never been married are

at less risk (Smith, Mercy, & Conn, 1988). This seems related to the loss factor among suicidal people but does not seem to apply to two specific groups: older, married, white men who are simply "tired of living," and married black people who have lost a love relationship. See Maltsberger (1986) and Motto (1991) regarding limitations of statistical data to predict suicide in particular individuals.

Recent Loss. Loss or the threat of loss of a spouse, parent, status, money, or job increases a person's suicide risk. Loss is a very significant suicide indicator among adolescents. Loss should also be kept in mind as a common theme in most people's experience of crisis (see "Loss, Change, and Grief Work" in Chapter Four).

Physical Illness. Studies reveal that many people who kill themselves are physically ill. Also, three out of four suicide victims have been under medical care or have visited their physician within four to six months of their death. The visit to a physician does not necessarily imply that the person is physically ill. However, it highlights the fact that a large number of people with any problem seek out either physicians or the clergy. In the case of suicidal people, the visit may be their last attempt to find relief from distress. Of twelve men with AIDS who committed suicide, five had seen a psychiatrist within four days of committing suicide, and two had seen psychiatric consultants within twenty-four hours of suicide (Marzuk, et al., 1988, p. 1336).

These facts suggest the influential role physicians can have in preventing suicide if they are attentive to clues. The physician's failure to ascertain the suicide plan or to examine the depression disguised by a complaint with no physical basis often leads to the common practice of prescribing a mild tranquilizer without listening to the person and making a referral for counseling. Such a response by a physician can be interpreted by the individual as an invitation to commit suicide.

The possibility of suicide is even greater if a person receives a diagnosis that affects his or her self-image and value system or demands a major switch in lifestyle, for example, AIDS, degenerative neurological conditions, heart disease, breast cancer, amputation of a limb, or cancer of the sex organs.

Drinking and Other Drug Abuse. Drinking increases impulsive behavior and loss of control and therefore increases suicide risk, especially if the person has a high-lethal means available. Alcohol also reduces the number of sleeping pills needed for a lethal overdose. Alcohol is involved in many deaths by suicide (Motto, 1980); often, adolescents who die by suicide were involved in drug or alcohol abuse before their death.

Physical Isolation. If a person is isolated both emotionally and physically, risk of suicide is greater than if he or she lives with close significant others. According to Durkheim (1951), "egoistic" suicide occurs when people feel they do not belong to society; "anomic" suicide occurs among people who cannot adjust to change and social demands. One of the basic human needs is approval by others of our performance in expected roles. The lack of such approval leads to social isolation.

Negative reactions from significant people are incorporated into the sense of self. Rejection from significant others can lead to a conviction of worthlessness. When this happens, the person believes that others also see him or her as worthless. People who suffer from discrimination are at risk for "egoistic" suicide. However, once minority groups and women achieve equality and better conditions, studies indicate that their risk for "anomic" suicide will increase. If white society or male dominance can no longer be blamed, the person may internalize failure. This process can lead to suicide. As one black person put it: "Being on the ground floor left no room to jump." Thus, upward mobility may increase suicide risk.

A person who is physically alone and socially isolated is often a candidate for hospitalization or other extraordinary means to relieve isolation. In such cases, hospitalization can be a life-saving measure.

Unexplained Change in Behavior. Changes in behavior, such as reckless driving and drinking by a previously careful and sober driver, can be an indicator of suicide risk. It is particularly important to observe behavior changes in adolescents, since these changes are often clues to inner turmoil. Again, direct communication about observed behavior changes can be a life-saving measure, signaling that someone cares and is sensitive to another's distress, even though talking about it initially may seem impossible.

Depression. Depressed people may experience sleeplessness, early wakening, slowed-down functioning, weight loss, menstrual irregularity, loss of appetite, inability to work normally, disinterest in sex, crying, and restlessness. Feelings of hopelessness are an even more important indicator of suicidal danger than depression (Beck, et al., 1993). Depressed adolescents are often overactive; they may fail in school or withdraw from usual social contacts. While not all people who kill themselves show signs of depression, enough suicide victims are depressed to make this an important indicator of risk. This is particularly true for the depressed person who is convinced of his or her worthlessness and is unable to reach out to others for help. Depression is a significant avenue for opening direct discussion of possible suicide plans: "You seem really down. . . . Are you so depressed that perhaps you've considered suicide?"

Social Factors. Social problems such as family disorganization, a broken home, and a record of delinquency, truancy, and violence against others increase a person's risk of suicide. Many adolescents who kill themselves had prior physical fights with their families. A person with a chaotic social background is also likely to follow the suicide attempt pattern of significant others. Suicide risk also increases for people who are unemployed or forced to retire or move, especially when these upsets occur during a developmental transition stage. Among women who attempt suicide, many have a history of sexual or other abuse (Egmond, et al., 1993; Hoff, 1992; Hoff & Rosenbaum, 1994; Stephens, 1985).

Mental Illness. Some people falsely believe that only a mentally ill person could commit suicide. If an individual hears voices directing him or her to commit suicide, the risk of suicide is obviously increased. However, the number of individuals who fall into this category is extremely small. People who are diagnosed as psychotic should also be assessed for suicide risk according to the criteria outlined in this section.

Table 6.1 illustrates how signs of suicide risk help distinguish people who kill themselves from those who injure themselves nonlethally and from the general population. In the next section, the pattern of these signs is described in a typology of suicide risk.

Typology of Suicidal Behavior: Assessing Immediate and Long-Range Risk

People tend to classify the seriousness of self-destructive behavior according to whether there is immediate danger of death. A person might engage in several kinds of self-destructive behavior at the same time. For example, an individual who chronically abuses alcohol may threaten, attempt, or commit suicide—all in one day. We should view these behaviors on the continuum noted earlier; *all are serious and important* in terms of life and death. The difference is that for some the danger of death is immediate, whereas for others it is long-range. Still others are at risk because of a high-risk lifestyle, chronic substance abuse, and neglect of medical care.

Distinguishing between immediate and long-range risk for suicide is not only a potential life-saving measure, it is also important for preventing or interrupting a vicious cycle of repeated self-injury. If immediate risk is high and we do not uncover it in assessment, a suicide can result (see Hoff & Resing, 1982). On the other hand, if immediate risk is low, as in medically nonserious cases of wrist slashing or swallowing a few sleeping pills, but we respond medically as though life were at stake while failing to address the *meaning* of this physical act, we run the risk of *reinforcing* self-destructive behavior. The person, in effect, is told by our behavior, "Do something more serious (medically) and I'll pay attention to you." In reality, medically nonserious self-injury is a life and death issue. That is, if the person's cries for help are repeatedly ignored, there is high probability that eventually the person will accept the invitation to do something more serious—actually commit suicide.

The following schema assists in assessing suicide risk by means of a structured guide (see Table 6.2). Examples illustrate the application of risk criteria to people at low risk, moderate risk, and high risk. This assessment guide highlights the

TABLE 6.1. SIGNS COMPARING PEOPLE WHO COMPLETE OR ATTEMPT SUICIDE WITH THE GENERAL POPULATION.

Signs	Suicide	Suicide Attempt	General Population
Suicide plan*	Specific, with available, high-lethal method; does not include rescue	Less lethal method, including plan for rescue; risk increases if lethality of method increases	None, or vague ideas only
History of suicide attempts*	65% have history of high-lethal attempts; if rescued, it was probably accidental	Previous attempts are usually low-lethal; rescue plan included; risk increases if there is a change from many low-lethal attempts to a high-lethal one	None, or low-lethal with definite rescue plan
Resources* • **psychological** • **social**	Very limited or nonexistent; or, person *perceives* self with no resources	Moderate, or in psychological and/or social turmoil	Either intact or able to restore them through nonsuicidal means
Communication*	Feels cut off from resources and unable to communicate effectively	Ambiguously attached to resources; may use self-injury as a method of communicating with significant others when other methods fail	Able to communicate directly and non-destructively for need fulfillment
Recent loss	Increases risk	May increase risk	Is widespread but is resolved nonsuicidally through grief work, etc.
Physical illness	Increases risk	May increase risk	Is common but responded to through effective crisis management (natural and/or formal)
Drinking and other drug abuse	Increases risk	May increase risk	Is widespread but does not in itself lead to suicide
Isolation	Increases risk	May increase risk	Many well-adjusted people live alone; they handle physical isolation through satisfactory social contacts

Unexplained change in behavior	A possible clue to suicidal intent, especially in teenagers	A cry for help and possible clue to suicidal ideas	Does not apply in absence of other predictive signs
Depression	65% have a history of depression	A large percentage are depressed	A large percentage are depressed
Social factors or problems	May be present	Often are present	Widespread but do not in themselves lead to suicide
Mental illness	May be present	May be present	May be present
Age, sex, race, marital status, sexual identity	These are statistical predictors that are most useful for identifying whether an individual belongs to a high-lethal risk group, not for clinical assessment of individuals	May be present	May be present

*If all four of these signs exist in a particular person, the risk for suicide is very high regardless of all other factors. If other signs also apply, the risk is increased further.

importance of the *patterns* of signs and the use of *clinical judgment* along with a database—not simply a mechanical rating—in evaluating suicidal risk (Motto, 1991).

Low-Risk Suicidal Behavior. This includes verbal threats of suicide with no specific plan or means of carrying out a plan. Also defined in this behavior is an attempt that, with knowledge of the effects of the method, involves no physical danger to life or clearly provides for rescue. Ambivalence in low-risk behavior tends more in the direction of life than death.

The immediate risk of suicide is low, but the risk of an attempt, a repeat attempt, and eventual suicide is high, depending on what happens after the threat or attempt. The risk is increased if the person abuses alcohol and other drugs. Social and personal resources are present but problematic for people in this behavior group.

CASE EXAMPLE: SARAH

Sarah, age forty-two, took five sleeping pills at 5:00 P.M., with full knowledge that the drug would not kill her, and obtained the temporary relief she wanted in sleep. When her husband found her sleeping at 6:00 P.M., he got at least some indication of her distress. Sarah is troubled by her marriage. She really wants a divorce but is afraid she cannot easily make it on her own. Sarah also takes Prozac every day. She has not made any other suicide attempts.

TABLE 6.2. LETHALITY ASSESSMENT SCALES: SELF.*

Key to Scale	Danger to Self	Typical Indicators
1	No predictable risk of suicide now	No suicidal ideation or history of attempt, has satisfactory social support system, and is in close contact with significant others
2	Low risk of suicide now	Person has suicidal ideation with low lethal methods, no history of attempts, or recent serious loss. Has satisfactory support network; no alcohol problems; basically wants to live
3	Moderate risk of suicide now	Has suicidal ideation with high lethal method but no specific plan or threats. Or has plan with low lethal method, history of low lethal attempts; e.g., employed female, age 35, divorced, with tumultuous family history and reliance on Valium or other drugs for stress relief; is weighing the odds between life and death
4	High risk of suicide now	Has current high lethal plan, obtainable means, history of previous attempts, is unable to communicate with a significant other; e.g., female, age 50, living alone, with drinking history; or black male, age 29, unemployed, and has lost his lover; depressed and wants to die
5	Very high risk of suicide now	Has current high lethal plan with available means, history of suicide attempts, is cut off from resources; e.g., white male, over 40, physically ill and depressed, wife threatening divorce, is unemployed, or has received promotion and fears failure

*Adapted from specifications for use of forms discussed in Chapter Three.

Suicide risk for Sarah: The immediate risk of suicide is low (rating scale: 2). The risk of repeat suicide attempts is moderate to high, depending on what Sarah is able to do about her problem.

Moderate-Risk Suicidal Behavior. This includes verbal threats with a plan and available means more specific and potentially more lethal than those involved in low-risk behavior. Also included are attempts in which the possibility of rescue is more precarious. The chosen method, although it may result in temporary physical disability, is not fatal, regardless of whether or not there is rescue. Ambivalence is strong; life and death are seen more and more in an equally favorable light. The immediate risk for suicide is moderate. The risk for a repeat suicide attempt and eventual suicide is higher than for low-risk behavior if no important life changes occur after the attempt or revelation of the suicide plan. The risk is significantly increased in the presence of chronic alcohol and drug abuse.

CASE EXAMPLE: SUSAN

Susan, age nineteen, came alone in a taxi to a local hospital emergency department. She had taken an overdose of Prozac a half hour earlier. Susan and her three-year-old child, Debbie, live with her parents. She has never gotten along well with her parents, especially her mother. Before the birth of her child, Susan had two short-lived jobs as a waitress. She dropped out of high school at age sixteen and has experimented off and on with drugs. Since the age of fifteen, Susan had made four suicide attempts. She took overdoses of nonprescription drugs three times and cut her wrists once. These attempts were assessed as being low-lethal.

At the emergency department, Susan had her stomach pumped and was kept for observation for a couple of hours. She was discharged without a referral for follow-up counseling. While in the emergency department, Susan could sense the impatience and disgust of the staff. A man having a heart attack had come in around the same time. Susan felt that no one had the time or interest to talk to her. She and the nurses knew each other from emergency service visits after her other suicide attempts. Twice before, Susan had refused referrals for counseling, so the nurses assumed that she was hopeless and did not really want help.

Suicide risk for Susan: Susan is not in immediate danger of suicide (rating scale: 3). She does not have a high-lethal plan and has no history of high-lethal attempts. Her personal coping ability is poor—she used drugs and failed in school—but she is not cut off from her family, despite their disturbed relationship. She has not suffered a serious personal loss. However, because there is no follow-up counseling or evidence of any changes in her troubled social situation, she is at risk of making more suicide attempts in the future. If such attempts increase in their medical seriousness, Susan's risk of eventual suicide also increases significantly. On the ambivalence scale, life and death may begin to look the same for Susan if her circumstances do not change.

High-Risk Suicidal Behavior. This includes a threat or a suicide attempt that would probably be fatal without accidental rescue. Such behavior also includes instances when a suicide attempt fails to end in death as expected, such as in a deliberate car crash. Another example is a threat that will be carried out unless a potential rescuer, such as a friend, family member, or crisis worker, can convince the person that there are good reasons to go on living. Ambivalence in high-risk behavior tends more in the direction of death than life.

The present and long-range risk of suicide is very high unless immediate help is available and accepted. Chronic self-destructive behavior increases the risk even further.

CASE EXAMPLE: EDWARD

Edward, age forty-one, had just learned that his wife Jane had decided to divorce him. He threatened to kill himself with a gun or carbon monoxide on the day she filed for the divorce. Jane's divorce lawyer proposed that their country home and the twenty adjoining acres be turned over completely to Jane. Edward told his wife, neighbors, and a crisis counselor that his family and home were all he had to live for. Indeed, all Edward could afford after the divorce was the rental of a single, shabby room. He and Jane have four children. Edward also has several concerned friends but does not feel he can turn to them, as he always kept his family matters private. Jane's decision to divorce Edward has left him feeling like a complete failure. He has several guns and is a skilled hunter. A major factor in Jane's decision to divorce Edward was his chronic drinking problem. He had threatened to shoot himself eight months earlier after a violent argument with Jane when he was drinking.

Several strong signs of high risk can be identified in Edward's case:

1. He has a specific plan with an available high-lethal means: the gun.
2. He threatened suicide with a high-lethal method eight months previously and is currently communicating his suicide plan.
3. He is threatened with a serious interpersonal loss and feels cut off from what he regards as his most important social resources—his family and home.
4. Edward has a rigid expectation of himself in his role as husband and provider for his family. He sees himself as a failure in that role and has a deep sense of shame about his perceived failure.
5. His coping ability is apparently poor, as he resorts to the use of alcohol and is reluctant to use his friends for support during a crisis.
6. Edward is also a high risk in terms of his age, sex, race, marital status, and history of alcohol abuse.

Suicide risk for Edward: Edward is in immediate danger of committing suicide (rating scale: 5). Even if he makes it through his present crisis, he is also a long-range risk for suicide because of his chronic self-destructive behavior—abuse of alcohol and threats of suicide by a readily available, high-lethal means.

CASE EXAMPLE: BARBARA

Barbara, age seventy-seven, is noted in the nursing care facility for her disagreeable personality and suspiciousness of staff and other residents. She has diabetes, heart disease, and asthma, the symptoms of which are exacerbated when she has an unpleasant encounter with others. Barbara has been moved to several different wings of the institution because the staff "can take only so much of her." After her last move, Barbara refused to eat or receive visits from other residents, resisted taking her medication, and said she just wanted to die. Barbara has a daughter and son-in-law who see her every few months. She also attends religious services routinely, the only activity she has continued.

Suicide risk for Barbara: Barbara is a high risk for suicide both immediately and in the future (rating scale: 4). The outcome of her self-destructive behavior will depend on how staff and her family understand and respond to her distress. On the ambivalence scale, unless her circumstances change, Barbara will probably continue to see death as more desirable than life.

CASE EXAMPLE: SHIRLEY

A woman went to visit her mother, Shirley, at a psychiatric facility, although she was advised on arrival not to see her mother at that time; Shirley was hearing voices telling her to kill herself and had therefore been placed in a special room with restraints. Her treatment consisted of psychotropic drugs and periodic checks by staff members. After the staff convinced the daughter that a visit would not benefit Shirley, the daughter asked to be allowed to see her mother through the peek hole, unobserved by her mother. The daughter had had a dream about her mother dying and told the psychiatrist she would not be able to forgive herself if her mother did die and she had not seen her. The psychiatrist refused, claiming then to be protecting the daughter.

Suicide risk for Shirley: Shirley is an immediate and long-range risk for suicide (rating scale: 5). Shirley's physical restraint decreased her immediate risk; however, it is now known that social isolation only promotes suicidal tendencies. Therefore, the long-range probability of suicide by Shirley is increased by the coercive measures used and by the psychiatrist's refusal to allow a caring daughter to visit. The immediate and long-range risks of these suicidal behaviors are summarized in Table 6.3.

Understanding and Assessing Risk in Special Populations

This chapter describes the wide range of people who are self-destructive and need help. The general principles of assessment apply to all people who are actually or potentially suicidal—the old, the young, different ethnic and sexual identity groups, institutionalized people, the unemployed, the educated, patients in medical/surgical wards, and psychotic and nonpsychotic persons in psychiatric settings. Still, trends and issues in the suicidology field suggest the need to highlight the special needs of adolescents, distinct ethnic groups, and suicidal people in hospitals and other institutions.

Young People

As we have seen, suicidal behavior is a cry for help, a way to stop the pain when nothing else works. Unnecessary death by suicide is a tragedy regardless of age,

TABLE 6.3. SUICIDE RISK DIFFERENTIATION.

Suicidal Behavior	Ambivalence Scale		Rescue Plan	Immediate Risk	Long-Range Risk	
Low-Risk	Life	Desires life more than death	Present	Low	High	
Moderate-Risk		Life and death seem equally desirable	Ambiguous	Moderate	High	Depending on immediate response, treatment, and follow-up
High-Risk	Death	Desires death more than life	Absent, or rescue after past attempts was accidental	Very high	High	

gender, class, race, or sexual identity, and regardless of variations in suicide rates among these different groups. But suicidal death by those who have barely begun life's journey is particularly poignant—for the victims themselves, their families, and all of society. The tragedy of youth suicide must not be missed in statistical comparisons to other at-risk groups. Young people who kill themselves not only prefer death over life, but they are telling us in powerful behavioral language that they do not even want to try out the society we have created for them. The question is, Why? What can we do to prevent these premature deaths? And how is youth suicide related to other problems such as substance abuse, violence against others, and entrenched social problems?

Increased public attention to these questions has resulted in a recent surge in literature on the topic (e.g., Berman & Jobes, 1991; Deykin & Buka, 1994; Goodman & Hoff, 1990; Leenaars & Wenckstern, 1991; Pfeffer, 1986). The general criteria for assessing risk of suicide, as already discussed, are similar for adolescents and adults, except for adolescents' greater tendency toward imitation and impulsivity as seen in cluster suicides (Coleman, 1987; Maris, 1985; Smith & Crawford, 1986). However, the issues are complex and the answers are not always clear. Recognition of the individual developmental, familial, and societal factors that interact in self-destructive youth will enhance the understanding and empathic communication necessary for risk assessment and suicide prevention among young people.

Teens in North America and other industrial societies today feel great pressure to avoid failure in a social milieu that is very achievement oriented, while facing employment uncertainties affected by global economic shifts and turmoil. As a distinct and increasingly prolonged phase in the life cycle, adolescence exaggerates the challenge of finding one's place in the world, while cultural messages emphasize that anything can be had in modern society if one only works hard and takes advantage of opportunities. This means, among other things, that traumatic life events such as failing an exam or the breakup of a relationship are perceived as disasters by at-risk teens. Furthermore, the brutal reality for many is that individual efforts are not enough to overcome obstacles such as race and class divisions that are deeply embedded in the social structure and cultural values. This is particularly true for black urban males in the United States, who face unemployment rates as high as 50 percent (Hendin, 1987; Maris, 1985, p. 100), and for Native youth on reservations, whose futures are even more bleak.

Complicating teenagers' lives today is the flux and change occurring throughout many societies, particularly in traditional roles for women and men. All adolescents face normal role confusion and sexual identity issues, but family instability and the frequency of divorce create additional stresses for children. Thousands of teens also encounter problems with alcoholism, violence, and incest. (Chapter Eight discusses in greater detail the relationship between victimization and self-destructiveness. See also Figure 2.2 in Chapter Two.) Many suicidal runaway teens are victims of these family problems. Considered together, these factors make a teenager's hopelessness and disillusionment with planning a career and entering adult life understandable (Goodman & Hoff, 1990; Joan, 1986).

This is not to suggest that living in an era of global change and unrest causes teen suicide. Rather, an attitude of cultural pessimism and financial uncertainties combine with individual stressors, family, and other social factors to create a climate from which many teens today will want to escape (see Chapters One and Two on crisis origins). These issues are elaborated further in Chapters Eight, Nine, and Thirteen.

Distinct Ethnic and Sexual Orientation Groups

The tragedy of suicide among ethnic minority and Native groups in U.S. society is often hidden behind the predominant presence of the white majority. Similarly, research about suicide among gay, lesbian, and bisexual people has been neglected in favor of the heterosexual majority. Social and cultural factors have been cited as the origin of many crises, especially among those disadvantaged by the economic, political, and related factors stemming from personal and institutionalized racism and homophobia (Hendin, 1987; Remafedi, 1994, 1991; Rofes, 1983) (see Chapters Thirteen and Fourteen). Understanding and assessing individual pain and suicide risk in these instances is incomplete without attention to the cultural context of this pain. It is ironic to speak of the right of disadvantaged people to commit suicide when the basic rights of life are enjoyed on an unequal basis. Our common humanity demands a renewed effort to combine understanding of individuals in crisis with keen sensitivity to the social and political origins and ramifications of these crises (see Boxes 1 and 3 in the right circle, Figure 6.1, the Crisis Paradigm).

People in Hospitals and Other Institutions

Finally, a number of people are in institutions because they are suicidal or for other reasons: illness, infirmity, crime, or behavioral problems. Admission to an institution is often a crisis in itself. Not infrequently, the culture shock experienced in this process is so extreme that suicide seems the only way out. Osgood's (1992) research supports the relationship between adverse environmental factors (e.g., frequent staff turnover) and suicidal behavior and death in long-term care facilities. Such factors also contribute to the greater frequency of suicide in temporary holding centers than in prisons. Often, a person already suicidal feels so disempowered by the experience of institutionalization that suicide is the single action that says, "I am in charge of my life (and death)."

Preventing suicide, self-injury, and indirect self-destruction in institutions demands that:

- We do not use hospitals as a "catch-all" to prevent suicide.
- We abandon the notion that when a patient is under a physician's care, responsibility for intelligent assessment and intervention by others ceases.
- We recognize that the general principles of suicidology and risk assessment apply equally to institutionalized and other people. If physical and social isolation and powerlessness increase suicidal risk, people in hospitals and other institutions who are isolated and powerless are at increased suicide risk (Farberow, 1981; Haycock, 1993).

This discussion of special population groups and the previous case examples is continued in the next chapter.

Two final points about the assessment of suicide risk must be noted:

1. *Suicide risk assessment is an ongoing process.* A person at risk should be reassessed continually. If important social and attitudinal changes occur as a result of a suicide attempt, the person who is suicidal today may not be suicidal tomorrow or ever again. The opposite is also true: a crucial life event or other circumstance can drastically affect a person's view of life and death. Someone who has never been suicidal may become so.
2. *Suicide risk assessment is an integral aspect of the crisis assessment process.* No assessment of a person who is upset or in crisis can be considered complete if evaluation of suicide risk is not included. See Chapter Three for interview

examples of how to incorporate these suicide risk assessment principles and techniques into routine crisis and mental health practice in emergency settings and elsewhere (see also Hoff & Resing, 1982).

Summary

Suicide and self-destructive behavior are extreme ways in which some people respond to crisis. The pain and turmoil felt by a self-destructive person can be compared to the confusion and mixed feelings of those trying to help. People destroy themselves for complex reasons. Understanding what a self-destructive person is trying to communicate is basic to helping that person find alternatives to suicide. Assessment of suicide risk is a difficult task, but it is made possible by recognition of signs that portend the likelihood of suicide for particular individuals. Assessment of suicide risk is an important basis for appropriate response to self-destructive people.

References

Alvarez, A. (1971). *The savage god*. London: Weidenfield & Nicolson.

Atkinson, J. M. (1978). *Discovering suicide: Studies in the social organization of death*. Pittsburg: University of Pittsburg Press.

Baechler, J. (1979). *Suicide*. New York: Basic Books.

Barnes, R. A. (1986). The recurrent self-harm patient. *Suicide & Life-Threatening Behavior, 16*(4), 399–408.

Battin, M. P. (1980). Manipulated suicide. In M. P. Battin & D. J. Mayo (Eds.), *Suicide: The philosophical issues* (pp. 169–182). New York: St. Martin's Press.

Battin, M. P., and Mayo, D. (Eds.). (1980). *Suicide: The philosophical issues*. New York: St. Martin's Press.

Beck, A. T., Steer, R. A., Beck, J. S., & Newman, C. F. (1993). Hopelessness, depression, suicidal ideation, and clinical diagnosis of depression. *Suicide & Life-Threatening Behavior, 23*(2), 120–129.

Becker, H. (1963). *Outsiders: Studies in the sociology of deviance*. New York: Free Press.

Berlin, I. N. (1987). Suicide among American Indian adolescents: An overview. *Suicide & Life-Threatening Behavior, 17*(3), 218–232.

Berman, A. L & Jobes, D. A. (1991). *Adolescent suicide: Assessment and intervention*. Washington: American Psychological Association.

Brandt, R. B. (1975). The morality and rationality of suicide. In S. Perlin (Ed.), *A handbook for the study of suicide* (pp. 61–76). New York: Oxford University Press.

Breed, W. (1972). Five components of a basic suicide syndrome. *Suicide & Life-Threatening Behavior, 2*, 3–18.

Brent, D. A., Perper, J. A., Moritz, G., Baugher, M., Roth, C., Balach, L., & Schweers, J. (1993). Stressful life events, psychopathology, and adolescent suicide: A case control study. *Suicide & Life-Threatening Behavior, 23*(3), 179–187.

Brown, G. W., & Harris, T. (1978). *The social origins of expression*. London: Tavistock.

Brown, T. R., & Sheran, T. J. (1972). Suicide prediction: A review. *Suicide and Life-Threatening Behavior, 2*, 67–97.

Burstow, B. (1992). *Radical feminist therapy: Working in the context of violence.* Newbury Park, CA: Sage.

Canetto, S. (1992). Gender and suicide in the elderly. *Suicide & Life-Threatening Behavior, 22*(1), 80–97.

Coleman, L. (1987). *Cluster suicides.* London: Faber & Faber.

Counts, D. A. (1987). Female suicide and wife abuse: A cross-cultural perspective. *Suicide & Life-Threatening Behavior, 17*(3), 194–204.

Deykin, E. Y., & Buka, S. L. (1994). Suicidal ideation and attempts among chemically dependent adolescents. *American Journal of Public Health, 84*(4), 634–639.

Douglas, J. (1967). *The social meanings of suicide.* Princeton, NJ: Princeton University Press.

Durkheim, E. (1951). *Suicide* (2nd ed.). New York: Free Press (Original work published 1897).

Egmond, M. V., Garnefski, N., Jonker, D., & Kerkhof, A. (1993). The relationship between sexual abuse and female suicidal behavior. *Crisis, 14*(3), 129–139.

Ehrenreich, B., & Ehrenreich, J. (1978). Medicine and social control. In J. Ehrenreich (Ed.), *The cultural crisis of modern medicine* (pp. 39–79). New York: Monthly Review Press.

Fagerhaugh, S. & Strauss, A. (1977). *The politics of pain management.* Menlo Park, CA: Addison-Wesley.

Farberow, N. L. (Ed.). (1975). *Suicide in different cultures.* Baltimore: University Park Press.

Farberow, N. L. (Ed.). (1980). *The many faces of death.* New York: McGraw-Hill.

Farberow, N. L. (1981). Suicide prevention in hospitals. *Hospital and Community Psychiatry, 32*(2), 99–104.

Farberow, N., Gallager-Thompson, D., Gilewski, M., & Thompson, L. (1992). The role of social support in the bereavement process of surviving spouses of suicide and natural deaths. *Suicide & Life-Threatening Behavior, 22*(1), 107–124.

Farberow, N. L., & Shneidman, E. S. (Eds.). (1961). *The cry for help.* New York: McGraw-Hill.

Furst, J., & Huffine, C. L. (1991). Assessing vulnerability to suicide. *Suicide & Life-Threatening Behavior, 21*(4), 329–344.

Goodman, L. M., & Hoff, L. A. (1990). *Omnicide.* New York: Praeger.

Hatton, C., Valente, S., & Rink, A. (1984). *Suicide: Assessment and intervention* (2nd ed.). New York: Appleton-Century-Crofts.

Haycock, J. (1993). Double jeopardy: Suicide rates in forensic hospitals. *Suicide & Life-Threatening Behavior, 23*(2), 130–138.

Hendin, H. (1982). *Suicide in America.* New York: W.W. Norton.

Hendin, H. (1987). Youth suicide: A psychosocial perspective. *Suicide & Life-Threatening Behavior, 17*(2), 151–165.

Hoff, L. A. (1985). Book review: C. Neuringer & D. Lettieri (1982). *Suicidal women: Their thinking and feeling patterns.* New York: Gardner Press. In *Suicide & Life-Threatening Behavior, 15*(1), 69–73.

Hoff, L. A. (1992). Battered women: Understanding, identification, and assessment—A psychosociocultural perspective, Part I. *Journal of American Academy of Nurse Practitioners, 4*(4), 148–154.

Hoff, L. A., & Resing, M. (1982). Was this suicide preventable? *American Journal of Nursing, 82*(7), 1106–1111.

Hoff, L. A., & Rosenbaum, L. (1994). A victimization assessment tool: Instrument development and clinical implications. *Journal of Advanced Nursing, 20*(4), 627–634.

Holinger, P. C. (1990). The causes, impact, and preventability of childhood injuries in the United States: Childhood suicides in the United States. *American Journal of Disease in Children, 144*, 670–676.

Holinger, P. C., Offer, D., Barter, J. C., & Bell, C. C. (1994). *Suicide and homicide among adolescents.* New York: Guilford.

Humphrey, D. (1992). Rational suicide among the elderly. *Suicide & Life-Threatening Behavior,* *22*(1), 125–129.

Joan, P. (1986). *Preventing teenage suicide: The living alternative handbook.* New York: Human Sciences Press.

Jourard, S. M. (1970). Suicide: An invitation to die. *American Journal of Nursing, 70,* 273–275.

Kerkhof, A.J.F.M., & Clark, D. C. (1993). Stability of suicide rates in Europe. *Crisis, 14*(2), 50–51.

Leenaars, A. A., & Wenckstern, S. (1991). *Suicide prevention in schools.* New York & Washington: Hemisphere.

Levine, S., & Kozloff, M. A. (1978). The sick role: Assessment and overview. *Annual Review of Sociology, 4,* 317–343.

Litman, R. E. (1987). Mental disorders and suicidal intention. *Suicide & Life-Threatening Behavior, 17*(2), 85–92.

Maltsberger, J. T. (1986). *Suicide risk: The formulation of clinical judgment.* New York: New York University Press.

Maris, R. W. (1985). The adolescent suicide problem. *Suicide & Life-Threatening Behavior, 15*(2), 91–109.

Maris, R. (1991). Assessment and prediction of suicide: Introduction. *Suicide & Life-Threatening Behavior* (Special Issue) *21*(1), 1–17.

Maris, R. (1981). *Pathways to suicide.* Baltimore: Johns Hopkins University Press.

Maris, R. W. (Ed.), Berman, A. L., Maltsberger, J. T., & Yufit, R. I. (1992). *Assessment and prediction of suicide.* New York: Guilford.

Marzuk, P. M., et al. (1988). Increased risk of suicide in persons with AIDS. *Journal of American Medical Association, 259*(9), 1333–1337.

McGinnis, J. M. (1987). Suicide in America—moving up the public health agenda. *Suicide & Life-Threatening Behavior, 17*(1), 18–32.

Menninger, K. (1938). *Man against himself.* New York: Harcourt Brace Jovanovich.

Menon, R. (1988, June 26). Personal communication. Publisher: Kali for Women. New Delhi, India.

Morrell, S., Taylor, R., Quine, S., & Kerr, C. (1993). Suicide and unemployment in Australia. *Social Science & Medicine, 36*(6) 749–756.

Motto, J. (1985). Preliminary field testing of a risk estimation for suicide. *Suicide & Life-Threatening Behavior, 15*(3), 139–150.

Motto, J. (1991). An integrated approach to estimating suicide prediction. *Suicide & Life-Threatening Behavior, 21*(1), 74–89.

Motto, J. (1980). Suicide risk factors in alcohol abuse. *Suicide & Life-Threatening Behavior, 10,* 230–238.

Nagey, M. I. (1965). The child's view of death. In H. Fiefel (Ed.), *The meaning of death* (pp. 79–98). New York: McGraw-Hill.

National Center for Health Statistics. Births, marriages, divorces, and deaths for January 1986. *Monthly Vital Statistics Report, 35,* 1–12.

Neuringer, C. (1982). Suicidal behavior in women. *Crisis, 3,* 41–49.

O'Carroll, P. (1993). Suicide causation: Pies, paths, and pointless polemics. *Suicide & Life-Threatening Behavior, 23*(1), 27–36.

Osgood, N. (1992). Environmental factors in suicide in long-term care facilities. *Suicide & Life-Threatening Behavior, 22*(1), 98–106.

Parsons, T. (1951). The case of modern medical practice. *The social system.* Glencoe, IL: Free Press.

Perrah, M., & Wichman, H. (1987). Cognitive rigidity in suicide attempters. *Suicide & Life-Threatening Behavior, 17*(3), 251–255.

Pfeffer, C. R. (1986). *The suicidal child*. New York: Guilford.

Phillips, D. P., & Wills, J. S. (1987). A drop in suicides around major holidays. *Suicide & Life-Threatening Behavior, 17*(1), 1–12.

Philp, M. (1993, September 20). Roots of solvent abuse run deep. *Globe and Mail*, pp. 1,4.

Remafedi, G. (Ed.). (1994). *Death by denial: Studies of gay and lesbian teenagers*. Boston: Alyson Publishers.

Remafedi, G., Farrow, J. A., & Deisher, R. W. (1991). Risk factors for attempted suicide in gay and bisexual youth. *Pediatrics, 87*(6), 869–875.

Recklitis, C. J., Noam, G. G., & Borst, S. R. (1992). Adolescent suicide and defensive style. *Suicide & Life-Threatening Behavior, 22*(3), 374–387.

Rich, C. L., Fowler, R. C., Young, D., & Blenkush, M. (1986). San Diego suicide study: Comparison of gay to straight males. *Suicide & Life-Threatening Behavior, 16*(40), 448–457.

Richman, J. (1992). A rational approach to rational suicide. *Suicide & Life-Threatening Behavior, 22*(1), 130–141.

Rofes, E. E. (1983). *"I thought people like that killed themselves": Lesbians, gay men and suicide*. San Francisco: Grey Fox Press.

Shneidman, E. S. (1981). Suicide. *Suicide & Life-Threatening Behavior, 11*, 198–220.

Shneidman, E. (1987). At the point of no return. *Psychology Today, 21*(3), 54–58.

Shneidman, E. (1985). *Definition of suicide*. New York: Wiley.

Shneidman, E. (1993). Some controversies in suicidology: Toward a mentalistic discipline. *Suicide & Life-Threatening Behavior, 23*(4), 292–298.

Shneidman, E. S. (1973). Suicide. *Encyclopedia Britannica*. Reprinted in *Suicide & Life-Threatening Behavior, 11*, 198–220.

Shneidman, E. S. (1976). *Suicidology: Contemporary developments*. New York: Grune and Stratton.

Shneidman, E. S., & Farberow, N. L. (Eds.). (1957). *Clues to suicide*. New York: McGraw-Hill.

Skorupka, P., & Bohnet, N. (1982). Primary caregivers' perceptions that met their needs in a home care hospice setting. *Cancer Nursing, 5*, 371–374.

Smith, K., & Crawford, S. (1986). Suicidal behavior among "normal" high school students. *Suicide & Life-Threatening Behavior, 16*(3), 313–325.

Smith, J. D., Mercy, J. A., & Conn, J. M. (1988). Marital status and the risk of suicide. *American Journal of Public Health, 78*(1), 78–80.

Smith, K., & Maris, R. (1986). Suggested recommendations for the study of suicide and other life-threatening behaviors. *Suicide & Life-Threatening Behavior, 16*(1), 67–69.

Stephens, B. J. (1987). Cheap thrills and humble pie: The adolescence of female suicide attempters. *Suicide & Life-Threatening Behavior, 17*(2), 107–118.

Stephens, B. J. (1985). Suicidal women and their relationships with husbands, boyfriends, and lovers. *Suicide & Life-Threatening Behavior, 15*(2), 77–90.

Wandrei, K. E. (1985). Identifying potential suicides among high-risk women. *Social Work*, Nov/Dec, 511–517.

Weisman, A. (1973). Death and self-destruction. In *Suicide prevention in the 1970s*. Washington, DC: U.S. Government Printing Office, Pub. no. (HSM) 72–9054.

Zola, I. K. (1978). Medicine as an institution of social control. In J. Ehrenreich (Ed.), *The cultural crisis of modern medicine* (pp. 80–100). New York: Monthly Review Press.

CHAPTER SEVEN

HELPING SELF-DESTRUCTIVE PEOPLE AND THOSE MOURNING SUICIDE

Several agencies or helpers are usually needed to provide distinct facets of service for suicidal people. All, however, should be aware of what constitutes comprehensive care for this at-risk population and establish linkages that actually work for clients.

Comprehensive Service for Self-Destructive People

Everyone who threatens or attempts suicide should have access to all the services the crisis calls for. Three kinds of service should be available for suicidal and self-destructive people:

1. Emergency medical treatment
2. Crisis intervention
3. Follow-up counseling or therapy

Emergency Medical Treatment

Emergency medical treatment is indicated for anyone who has already made a suicide attempt. Unfortunately, this is still all that is received by a large number of people who attempt suicide. Everyone—friend, neighbor, family member, passer-by—is obligated by simple humanity to help a suicidal person obtain medical treatment. First-aid can be performed by police, volunteers in fire departments, rescue squads, or anyone familiar with first-aid procedures.

Any time a person is in immediate danger of death, the police should be called because police and rescue squads have the greatest possibility of assuring rapid transportation to a hospital. If there is any question about the medical seriousness of the suicide attempt, a physician should be called. The best way to obtain a medical opinion in such cases is to call a local hospital emergency service. In large communities, a physician is always there; in small ones, a physician is on call.

Most communities also have poison control centers, usually attached to a hospital. In cases of drug overdose, when the lethality level of the drug is not certain, a poison control center should be called. The amount of a drug necessary to cause death depends on the kind of drug, the size of the person, and the person's tolerance for the drug in cases of addiction. Sleeping pills are the most dangerous.

In general, *a lethal dose is ten times the normal dose*. In combination with alcohol, only half that amount can cause death. Aspirin is also much more dangerous than is commonly believed. One hundred five-grain tablets can cause death; less is needed if other drugs are also taken. Tylenol (acetaminophen), an aspirin substitute, is even more dangerous, as it cannot be removed from body tissue by dialysis. Tranquilizers are less dangerous; antidepressant drugs, however, can be used as a suicide weapon.

Some suicidal people have gone through hospital emergency rooms, intensive care and surgical units, and on to discharge with no explicit attention paid to the primary problem that triggered the suicide attempt. The urgency of medical treatment for a suicidal person can be so engrossing that other aspects of crisis intervention are omitted. For example, if a person is in a coma from an overdose or is being treated for injuries from a car crash, a careful suicide risk assessment may be forgotten after the person is out of physical danger. Great care should be taken to ensure that this does not happen.

If a person whose suicide attempt is medically serious does not receive follow-up counseling, the risk of suicide within a few months is very high. Medical treatment, of course, is of primary importance when there is danger of death; still, we should remember that the person's physical injuries are a result of the suicide attempt; treating those injuries is only a first step. The attitude of hospital emergency department staff can be the forerunner of more serious suicide attempts or the foundation for crisis intervention and acceptance of a referral for follow-up counseling. Emergency personnel should also consider carefully the appropriate use of drugs for suicidal people in crisis, as discussed in Chapter Four, since prescribed drugs are one of the weapons used most frequently for suicide.

Crisis Intervention

People who threaten or attempt suicide as a way of coping with a crisis usually lack more constructive ways of handling stress. The crisis intervention principles outlined in Chapters Four and Five should be used on behalf of self-destructive persons. Several additional techniques are important for a person in suicidal crisis:

1. *Relieve isolation.* If the suicidal person is living alone, physical isolation must be relieved. If there is no friend or supportive relative with whom the person can stay temporarily and if the person is highly suicidal, he or she should probably be hospitalized until the active crisis is over.

2. *Remove lethal weapons.* Lethal weapons and pills should be removed either by the counselor, a relative, or friend, keeping in mind the active collaboration of the suicidal person in this process. If caring and concern are expressed and the person's sense of self-mastery and control are respected, he or she will usually surrender a weapon voluntarily so it is safe from easy or impulsive access during the acute crisis.

3. *Encourage alternate expression of anger.* If the person is planning suicide as a way of expressing anger at someone, we should actively explore with the individual other ways of expressing anger short of paying with his or her life. For example: "I can see that you're very angry with her for leaving you. Can you think of a way to express your anger that would not cost you your life?" Or, "Yes, of course she'll probably feel bad if you kill yourself after the divorce. . . . But she most likely would talk with someone about it and go on with her life. Meanwhile, you've had your revenge, but you can't get your life back."

4. *Avoid a final decision about suicide during crisis.* We should assure the suicidal person that the suicidal crisis, that is, seeing suicide as the only option, is a temporary state. Also, we should try to persuade the person to avoid a decision about suicide until he or she has considered all other alternatives during a noncrisis state of mind, just as other serious decisions should be postponed until the crisis is over.

A cautionary note about contracts is in order here. The "no-suicide contract" is a technique employed by some therapists and crisis workers in which the client promises not to harm him- or herself between sessions and to contact the therapist if contemplating such harm. Such contracts offer neither special protection against suicide nor legal protection for the therapist (Clark & Kerkhof, 1993). This is because any value the contract may have flows from the *quality of the therapeutic relationship*—ideally, one in which the therapist conveys caring and concern about the client. In no way should a contract serve as a convenient substitute for the time spent in empathetic listening and in planning alternatives to self-destruction with a suicidal person. If contracts are used, they should be situated within the context of the overall service plan as discussed here and in Chapter Four, including such specifics as relieving isolation, finding substitutes for losses, and planning to control impulsive behavior.

5. *Reestablish social ties.* We should make every effort to help the suicidal person reestablish broken social bonds. This can be done through family crisis counseling sessions or finding satisfying substitutes for lost relationships. Active links to self-help groups such as Widow-to-Widow or Parents-Without-Partners clubs can be life-saving (see Chapter Five).

6. *Relieve extreme anxiety and sleep loss.* If a suicidal person is extremely anxious and also has been unable to sleep for several days, he or she may become even

more suicidal as a result. To a suicidal person, the world looks more bleak and death seems more desirable at 4:00 A.M. after endless nights of sleeplessness. A good night's sleep can temporarily reduce suicide risk and put the person in a better frame of mind to consider other ways of solving life's problems.

In such cases, it is appropriate to consider medication on an emergency basis (Bonger, et al., 1992). This should never be done for a highly suicidal person, however, without daily crisis counseling sessions. Without effective counseling, the extremely suicidal person may interpret such an approach as an invitation to commit suicide. A tranquilizer will usually alleviate the anxiety and thus improve sleep, since anxiety is the major cause of sleeplessness. If medication is needed, the person should be given a *one-to-three-day supply at most*—*always* with a return appointment scheduled for crisis counseling.

Sometimes nonmedical crisis counselors need to seek medical consultation and emergency medicine for a suicidal person. In such cases, the counselor must clearly advise the consulting physician of the person's suicidal state and of the recommended limited dose of drugs. This is particularly important when dealing with physicians who lack training in suicide prevention or who seem hurried and disinterested. Some practitioners accustomed to using medication in treatment programs may recommend tranquilization during crisis; however, tranquilizers are indicated only if a person is so upset that he or she cannot be engaged in the process of problem solving (see Chapter Four). Nonchemical means of inducing sleep should be encouraged. This assumes a thorough assessment and an effort to apply various psychosocial strategies before prescribing drugs. Crisis workers should never forget that many suicide deaths in North America are caused by *prescribed* drugs.

Crisis assessment is never more important than when working with a self-destructive person. It determines our immediate and long-range response to the individual. A person who is threatening or has attempted suicide is either in active crisis or is already beyond the crisis and is at a loss to resolve it any other way.

Not everyone who engages in self-destructive acts is in a life-and-death emergency. Anyone distressed enough to be self-destructive to any degree should be listened to and helped; however, if the suicide attempt is medically nonserious, the counselor's response should not convey a sense of life-and-death urgency. This does not mean that the person's action is dismissed as nonserious. Rather, the underlying message of the behavior—its social-psychological dynamics—should receive the greatest part of our attention. To do otherwise may inadvertently lead to further suicide attempts. A helper reinforces self-destructive behavior by a dramatic and misplaced medical response while ignoring the problems signaled by the self-destructive act. For example, while suturing a slashed wrist, the physician and nurse should regard the physical injury neutrally, with a certain sense of detachment, while focusing on the *meaning* of self-injury: "You must have been pretty upset to do this to yourself. What did you hope would happen when you cut your wrists?"

Thus, persons at all levels of risk warrant a response. The helper must differentiate between the types of response. Emergency measures are used when there is immediate danger of death from a medically serious failed suicide attempt. If the risk of death is long-range, the therapeutic approach should be long-range as well. If the attempt is medically nonserious, we should avoid using only medical treatment or a life-and death approach. We should help the person bring about needed psychosocial changes through aids to constructive crisis management rather than self-destructive acts.

Follow-up Service for Suicidal People

Beyond crisis counseling, all self-destructive persons should have the opportunity to receive counseling or psychotherapy as an aid in solving the problems that led them to self-destructive behavior (Bongar, et al., 1992). People who respond to life crises with self-destructive behavior often have a long-standing pattern of inadequate psychological and social coping (McLeavey, et al., 1987; Snyder, Pitts, & Pokorny, 1986). Individual or group psychotherapy, therefore, is frequently indicated (Frederick & Farberow, 1970). Drug treatment for depression may also be indicated.

Counseling and Psychotherapy.   Psychotherapy is the proper work of specially trained people, usually clinical psychologists, psychiatric nurses, psychiatrists, and psychiatric social workers. Others qualified to do counseling may be clergy, laypersons who are volunteers, and counselors in community mental health settings. Of main concern is that the counselor or psychotherapist be properly trained and supervised (Hoff & Miller, 1987).

Counseling should focus on resolving situational problems and expressing feelings appropriately. The person is helped to change various behaviors that are causing discomfort and that he or she usually is conscious of. Psychotherapy involves uncovering feelings that have been denied expression for a long time. It may also involve changing aspects of one's personality and deep-rooted patterns of behavior, such as an inability to communicate feelings or inflexible approaches to problem solving. People usually engage in psychotherapy because they are troubled or unhappy about certain features of their personality or behavior.

In most instances, counseling or psychotherapy should be made available to the suicidal person. It is particularly recommended for crisis-prone people who approach everyday problems with drug and alcohol abuse and other self-destructive behaviors. Such people have difficulty expressing feelings verbally, and self-destructive acts become an easier way to communicate. People who are extremely dependent, or who have rigid expectations for themselves combined with inflexible behavior patterns, are also good candidates for psychotherapy (Barnes, 1986). A severely depressed, suicidal person should always have follow-up counseling or psychotherapy (Doweiko, 1993; Williams, 1984). When hospitalization also is indicated for seriously suicidal persons, practitioners should observe carefully the current standards of care for hospitalized people who are at risk of harming themselves (see Bongar, et al., 1993; Farberow, 1981).

Counseling and psychotherapy can take place on an individual or group basis, in outpatient and inpatient settings. A group experience is valuable for nearly everyone, but it is particularly recommended for the suicidal person who has underlying problems interacting socially and communicating feelings. For adolescents who have made suicide attempts, family therapy should frequently follow family crisis counseling (Richman, 1985). Marital counseling should be offered whenever a disturbed marriage has contributed to the person's suicidal crisis. These therapies can be used in various combinations, depending on the needs of the individual and family.

Whether conducted in a group or individually, counseling and psychotherapy goals should be directed toward

- Correcting psychological and social disturbances in the person's life
- Improving the person's self-image
- Finding satisfactory social resources
- Developing approaches to problems other than self-destructive behavior
- Discovering a satisfying life plan

Crisis counselors should keep in mind that a satisfying and constructive resolution of a crisis is an excellent foundation for persuading people to seek follow-up counseling or psychotherapy for the problems that made them crisis-prone in the first place. However, if people in crisis are placed on waiting lists, they will find other ways to resolve their crises. If such people are suicidal, the chances of a tragic outcome are greatly increased (Hoff & Resing, 1982). This is because, with or without our help, the pain of the crisis state compels one to move toward resolution—positive or negative. If waiting lists prevent people from getting help at the time they need it and later appointments are not kept, we should examine the adequacy of our service arrangements rather than conclude that the client was not motivated for therapy (Hoff & Miller, 1987).

Drug Treatment for Depression. Antidepressants are not emergency drugs. However, these drugs may be used successfully for some suicidal persons who experience severe, recurring depression. Classic drugs for treating depression include tricyclic antidepressants (TCA) and monoamine-oxidase inhibitors (MAOI). Successful response to antidepressant therapy is highly variable, and debate about the use of psychotropic drugs as a new "magic bullet" continues (Johnson, 1990, pp. 38–52). This may be due in part to the unclear demarcation between reactive depression and major depressive episodes, sometimes called endogenous depression. Thus, while some people respond favorably to antidepressant treatment, there are high rates of spontaneous remission as well as favorable response to placebos (Extein, Gold, & Pottash, 1984, pp. 504–507).

Antidepressants should be used sparingly or not at all for a person who is going through normal grief and mourning (Worden, 1991, p. 54). Nor should they be used when the person is suffering from a reactive depression; grief work and crisis counseling are indicated instead, except when the person does not respond to interpersonal interventions (Worden, 1991, p. 31). A reactive depression occurs when a person in crisis because of a loss does not express normal feelings of sadness and anger *during* the crisis and later reacts with depression—sometimes called a delayed grief reaction. Psychotherapy is indicated for such persons.

Classic symptoms of a major depressive episode (endogenous depression) include weight loss, early morning wakening, loss of appetite, slowed down body functions, sexual and menstrual abnormality, and extreme feelings of worthlessness. The symptoms usually cannot be related to a conscious loss, specific life event, or situation. The assumption, therefore, is that the depression arises from sources within the person, whereas in reactive depression one is aware of the loss or depressing situation (see "Loss, Change, and Grief Work" in Chapter Four). Even in cases of endogenous depression, however, research suggests that the sources are social rather than physiologic; repression of painful situations clouds them from current awareness (Brown & Harris, 1978; Cloward & Piven, 1979; Gordon & Ledray, 1985). For example, depression in the women studied by Brown and Harris was significantly associated with their economic circumstances and large numbers of children: less money and more children meant greater depression.

Antidepressant drugs are dangerous and should be prescribed with extreme caution for suicidal persons (Bongar, et al., 1992). When taken with alcohol, an overdose of drugs can easily cause death. People using these drugs can experience side effects such as feelings of confusion, restlessness, or loss of control. Persons with a past history of psychosis or with symptoms of "borderline psychosis" can have serious side effects from antidepressants.

Another problem with antidepressant drugs is that they take so long to work. Ten to fourteen days elapse before depression lifts noticeably, even though the person sleeps better as a result of the sedative side effect. This delayed action should be explained carefully, because most people expect to feel better immediately after taking a drug. And during the pretherapeutic phase, a suicide could occur as a result of confusion and agitation—other drug side effects. As discussed in Chapter Four, Prozac is currently at the center of debate about the benefits versus the side effects of psychotropic drugs.

Another danger of suicide occurs after the depression lifts during drug treatment. This is especially true for the person who is so depressed and physically slowed down that he or she did not previously have the energy to carry out a suicide plan. Because of all these factors, it is preferable to use antidepressant drugs in combination with psychiatric hospitalization for a depressed person who is highly suicidal, especially if he or she is also socially and physically isolated.

Crisis counselors should always remember that antidepressants are not emergency drugs. These drugs should usually not be prescribed for a highly suicidal

CASE EXAMPLE: JACK

Jack, age sixty-nine, had seen his physician about bowel problems. He was also quite depressed. Even after a complete examination and extensive tests, he was obsessed with the idea that he might have cancer and was afraid that he would die. Jack also had high blood pressure and emphysema. Months earlier, he had had prostate surgery. His family described him as a chronic complainer. Jack's doctor gave him a prescription for an antidepressant drug and referred him to a local mental health clinic for counseling. Jack admitted to the crisis counselor that he had ideas of suicide, but he had no specific plan or history of attempts. After two counseling sessions, Jack killed himself by carbon monoxide poisoning. This suicide might have been prevented if Jack had been hospitalized and if the delayed reaction of the drug had been properly explained. He lived alone and probably expected to feel better immediately after taking the antidepressant. An alternative might have been to prescribe a drug to relieve his acute anxiety in combination with a plan to live with relatives for a couple of weeks.

person during the acute crisis state unless the individual is hospitalized. The crisis counselor should routinely ask a person in crisis what drugs he or she is taking or possesses. The prescription of *any* drug as a substitute for effective counseling is irresponsible. Not only can drugs such as Prozac provoke suicidal ideation and subsequent litigation (Breggin, 1994; Bongar, et al., 1992), but the unwarranted prescription of drugs can also lead to serious drug abuse problems (Rogers, 1971).

Intervention with Self-Destructive People: Case Examples

The following cases are continued from Chapter Six. They illustrate the resolution of ethical dilemmas regarding suicide, as well as planning for emergency, crisis, and follow-up services for self-destructive people.

The Right to Die Dilemma

CASE EXAMPLE

Rachel (age sixty-nine, dying of cancer, and feeling suicidal; see p. 177)

Rachel: This cancer is killing me. I have nothing to live for.

Nurse: You sound really depressed, Rachel.

Rachel: I am. I'm a burden to my daughter. . . . I don't want to live like this anymore.

Nurse: You mean you're thinking of suicide, Rachel?

Rachel: Yes, I guess you could say that— at least I don't want to go on living like this. . . . Yes, I want to die, and no one can stop me. I'm old and I'm sick. If there is a God, I'm sure I wouldn't be punished. How could any God expect me to go on living with this? Yes, I want to die. It's my right.

Case Example, cont.

Nurse: I know you feel old and I know you're sick, and I agree, Rachel, that you have the right to determine your own life. But I'd feel bad if you acted on that now, Rachel, when you're feeling so depressed and like such a burden to your daughter. I'd really like to help you find some other way . . . (Rachel interrupts).

Rachel: There's no other way that I can see. I've thought about it a lot. I don't know

exactly what I'd do, but I'd figure something out. I just don't know how things could change for me . . . After all, my daughter's got her own life.

Nurse: Rachel, I'd like to go back to something you said earlier. You seem to feel you're a burden to your daughter. Can you tell me more about that? (Conversation continues.)

Other possible elements of service plan for Rachel include the following:

1. Continue problem exploration on a one-to-one basis.
2. Talk with daughter (with Rachel's consent) after exploring the "burden" issue further with Rachel.
3. Have a joint session with Rachel and her daughter (see Chapter Five).
4. Continue weekly visits.
5. Explore home health respite service for daughter (see Skorupka & Bohnet, 1982).

Low-Risk Suicidal Behavior

CASE EXAMPLE

Sarah (age forty-two, troubled by her marriage; see p. 199)

Emergency medical: Medical treatment for Sarah is not indicated because pills are absorbed from the stomach into the bloodstream within thirty minutes. The dose of five sleeping pills is not lethal or extremely toxic. Therefore, other medical measures such as dialysis are not indicated.

Crisis intervention: Crisis counseling should focus on the immediate situation re-

lated to Sarah's suicide attempt and decision-making about her marriage.

Follow-up service: In follow-up counseling, Sarah can examine her extreme dependency on her marriage, her personal insecurity, and her dependency on drugs as a means of problem solving. Sarah might also be linked to a women's support group that focuses on career counseling and the midlife transition faced by women (see Chapter Thirteen).

Moderate-Risk Suicidal Behavior

CASE EXAMPLE

Susan (age nineteen, with a history of repeat suicide attempts; see p. 201)

Emergency medical: Treatment for the

overdose is stomach lavage (washing out the stomach contents).

Crisis intervention: Crisis counseling for

Case Example: . . . Cont.

Susan should include contacts with her parents and should focus on situational problems she faces: unemployment, upsets with her parents, and dependence on her parents.

    Follow-up service: Since Susan has had a chaotic life for a number of years, she could benefit from ongoing counseling or psychotherapy if she so chooses. Family therapy may be indicated if she decides to remain in her parents' household. Group therapy is strongly recommended for Susan.

High-Risk Suicidal Behavior

CASE EXAMPLE

Edward (age forty-one, recently divorced, and threatening to shoot himself; see p. 201)

    Emergency medical: No treatment is indicated, since no suicide attempt has been made. Depending on the level of engagement in crisis counseling, an antianxiety agent may be indicated for temporary stabilization, as discussed in Chapter Four.

    Crisis intervention: Remove guns (and alcohol, if possible) or have wife or friend remove them with Edward's collaboration. Arrange to have Edward stay with a friend on the day his wife files for divorce. Try to get Edward to attend a self-help group, such as Alcoholics Anonymous, and to rely on an AA member for support during his crisis. Arrange daily crisis counseling sessions for Edward.

    Follow-up service: Edward should have on-going therapy—both individually and in a group—focusing on his alcohol dependency and his rigid expectations of himself; therapy should help Edward find other satisfying relationships after the loss of his wife by divorce.

CASE EXAMPLE

Barbara (age seventy-seven, in a nursing home, and refusing to eat; see p. 202)

    Emergency medical and crisis intervention: Barbara should be assigned to a nurse or other staff person she trusts who can persuade her noncoercively to take her medication. Her daughter and son-in-law should be called and urged to visit immediately so Barbara has some evidence that someone cares whether she lives or dies. A stable staffing arrangement should be instituted and any further moving of Barbara to different wings of the nursing facility should be avoided. Thus a trusting, caring relationship can be established with at least one or two staff members, which is necessary for understanding what makes Barbara upset and suspicious.

    Follow-up service: Organize problem-solving and service-planning meetings with Barbara, her daughter and son-in-law, the chaplain, and the nursing staff who have worked with Barbara the most closely—her social network (see Chapter Five). Examine the rotation practices and support system for staff, which provide temporary "relief" from troublesome residents like Barbara. Frequent rotations exacerbate the underlying insecurity of an older person who has decreased ability to adjust to environmental changes and disruptions in staff/resident relationships.

CASE EXAMPLE

Shirley (age fifty-five, acutely suicidal and psychotic in a psychiatric setting; see p. 203)

Emergency medical and crisis intervention: Institute routine precautions with regard to sharp objects, belts, and so on (see Farberow, 1981). Assign a staff member for one-to-one care of Shirley. Place Shirley in a bedroom arrangement with at least one other patient, close to the nurses' station. Engage patients or other volunteers to assist in offering support and protection to Shirley during her acute psychotic episodes. Contact relatives and encourage frequent visits.

Follow-up service: Family meetings are recommended to encourage on-going support and help prevent future psychotic and suicidal episodes; drug therapy can help alleviate thought disorder and depression. Institute daily ward meetings in which patients' acute suicidal episodes can be discussed openly and dealt with cooperatively among all residents. Develop staff in-service training programs on suicide prevention as a means of critically examining and eliminating destructive and inhumane measures such as isolation and physical restraint of suicidal people.

Suicide Prevention and Intervention with Special Populations

As noted in Chapter Six, certain groups in contemporary society are at special risk of suicide. These groups need particular service programs commensurate with their assessed needs.

Young People

The tragedy of youth suicide has commanded international attention at several levels recently. In the United States, the National Institute of Mental Health convened a Task Force on Youth Suicide in several locations to address the problem. Since the occurrence of cluster suicides in recent years, a National Committee on Youth Suicide has been formed, with a focus on suicide education in the schools. The American Association of Suicidology has information about model school suicide prevention programs. Current information about these activities is available from: AAS Central Office, 4201 Connecticut Ave. NW Suite 310, Washington, D.C. 20008; telephone (202) 237–2280; fax: (202) 237–2282.

In general, suicide prevention programs for young people focus on educational and support activities for the young themselves, their parents, and teachers (Leenaars & Wenckstern, 1991). Pastors, recreation workers, school nurses, physicians, and police officers should also receive such education. Intervention in community settings should include drop-in services, where troubled youth can receive individual help without being stigmatized and can be referred to peer support groups or family counseling services. School health programs, counseling agencies, and local suicide prevention centers usually collaborate on such programs.

If suicidal young people are referred to mental health and psychiatric agencies, the treatment of choice should include the family in an active way (Richman, 1986). This is particularly true for an adolescent still living with parents. The adolescent's cry for help might otherwise be misunderstood; often the problem is related to family issues, or the adolescent depends on the family for necessary support during this hazardous transition state (see Chapters Five and Thirteen). Suicide prevention programs that focus their activities primarily on depression may miss their target (Shaffer, 1993, p. 172). A study by Garrison, et al. (1993) reveals a powerful relationship between suicidal behavior, aggression, and alcohol use, especially by high school males.

Suicide prevention for young people is illustrated in a special program developed by the Tompkins County Suicide Prevention and Crisis Service in Ithaca, New York (Joan, 1986). Among the elements of this countywide service and similar programs are:

- A suicide prevention information program each semester for students in junior and senior high schools and colleges, including cards listing warning signs, myths and facts about suicide, and emergency telephone numbers
- Training of students in communication skills, including role playing and modeling of reaching out to others
- Developing suicide prevention curriculum packets to be used by faculty
- Conducting special information programs for parents
- Providing drop-in centers staffed by trained persons sensitive to the special needs of adolescents

Although many communities now have such programs (Leenaars & Wenckstern, 1991; Webb, 1986), denial of suicide by school authorities and failure to provide *prevention* and *postvention* programs still occurs despite the international efforts noted above (contact AAS Central Office for further information). In school-based programs, students are trained to become peer counselors for classmates who feel left out, lonely, and depressed. Such programs include role playing real-life crises and exploring dramatically how to avert tragedy.

Distinct Ethnic and Sexual Orientation Groups

Besides the general principles of helping suicidal people, some other points should be kept in mind with respect to individuals in these groups.

1. *In agencies routinely serving people with language, cultural, and other differences, staff should be recruited from the distinct communities served.* This does not mean that a distressed person can only be helped by someone from his or her own ethnic or sexual identity group. Rather, it provides a resource for special problems related to different belief systems and lifestyles. It also helps to avoid the appearance of

discriminatory practices, which can be a barrier to accepting help. In cases of immigrants who speak rare languages, International Institute staff can be called on to assist (see Chapter Twelve). Communication with respect to *process, intention,* and *helping* is pivotal during suicidal crises; thus, human bonds formed through language, culture, lifestyle, and sexual identity are crucial (Blumenfeld & Lindop, 1994).

2. *The suicidal crises of people in these groups may be strongly linked to their disadvantaged social position.* When this appears to be the case, the social change strategies discussed in Chapter Two are a particularly important aspect of follow-up after crisis intervention. For example, a poor, immigrant woman with three small children became suicidal each time she was threatened with cutting off the heat because she could not pay the bill. To offer this woman only crisis counseling without linking her to social support or social action groups would not approach the social roots of the problem. In Boston, for example, there is an organization called the Coalition for Basic Human Needs, a welfare rights group. Gay rights organizations are also becoming increasingly visible in their advocacy work for civil rights. People in crisis because of discriminatory treatment should be linked to such groups or at least be informed that they exist on their behalf (see Figure 6.1, right circle, Box 3).

People in Hospitals and Other Institutions

People in crisis, like other human beings, have a need for self-mastery and control of their lives. Sensitivity to this need is an important element of positive crisis resolution. People in crisis who are suicidal not only do not lose their need for self-determination, but also frequently feel powerless to solve their problems except by the ultimate act of self-determination: suicide. As noted earlier in Shirley's case, staff members in institutions should examine various approaches to suicidal people; many approaches to protecting people from suicide may result in exactly the opposite of what is intended. While physical restraint and isolation may prevent immediate self-injury, these methods may actually increase the long-term suicide risk. Such results are especially probable if the physical measures are carried out with authoritarian attitudes and an absence of communication, warmth, and genuine concern. People who already feel powerless may interpret such harsh, outmoded practices as another attack on their self-esteem and ability to control their lives. As Farberow (1981, p. 101) states, people in hospitals (and other institutions) "are continually impressed with a sense of powerlessness; their lives must conform to a schedule designed essentially for the convenience of the staff. Most things happen *to* them, not because of or *for* them; other people continually make the most important decisions about their lives" (see also Berman, et al., 1993; Berman & Cohen-Sandler, 1982; Osgood, 1992).

Many people expect institutionalized people to conform to the sick role, but it is unrealistic to conduct our practice within this framework for suicidal people.

The problem of expecting suicidal people to fit the traditional sick role is exacerbated if there is no systematic effort to include family or other social contacts in hospital treatment programs. Once institutionalization has taken place, a person's natural social community is often forgotten (Polak, 1967). Or, if the person is suicidal because such community support is lacking, it takes a special effort by hospital staffs to help develop substitute support systems, such as transitional housing services, prior to discharge. Also, admission to institutions is frequently the occasion of suicidal impulses based on culture shock for people not acculturated to institutions through routine work or residence.

Attention to these points can help prevent self-injury and suicides in hospitals and other institutions as well as reduce the high rate of suicide after discharge from mental hospitals. See Farberow's work (1981) and Bongar, et al. (1993) for additional recommendations and standards for suicide prevention in hospitals.

Suicide prevention in holding centers and correctional institutions presents similar but even more complex problems (Haycock, 1993). A study in the Netherlands (cited in Kerkhof & Clark, 1993) revealed four types of stressors faced by prisoners: problems with relatives or the problems of relatives; legal process issues; conflicts with staff or other inmates; and issues of drug abuse. In one sense, the isolation cell is like an instrument of death. Yet relieving the physical isolation of a suicidal inmate may expose the person to possible abuse or attack by fellow inmates.

The crisis of suicide behind bars is gaining attention (Danto, 1981). A unique program—Lifeline—is operated by staff of The Samaritans in Boston. Similar to the Prisoner Befriender program in several prisons in the United Kingdom, Lifeline is conducted in the county jail. Inmates—including murderers, arsonists, and rapists—receive special training to work as befrienders of the lonely and depressed. Besides reducing the number of suicides in this jail, the program is noted for its benefits to the befriending inmates: they have the satisfaction of saving others' lives and of feeling useful and appreciated for their caring (McGinnis, 1993).

Halleck (1971) addresses chronic self-destructiveness among inmates. He suggests that prisoners' repeated suicide attempts are a symptom of conditions in the institution that bear examination and probable reform. Halleck questions whether it is ethical for a psychotherapist to use professional time in such institutions primarily for treating individual suicide attempters without also consulting with prison authorities about the meaning of these attempts in relation to prison conditions (see Chapter Nine). As crime and prison populations in the United States soar, suicide attempts are probable as long as real prison reform lags and primary prevention of crime takes a back burner in policy circles.

Helping Survivors in Crisis

When a suicide occurs, it is almost always the occasion of a crisis for survivors: children, spouse, parents, other relatives, friends, crisis counselor, therapist—anyone closely associated with the person. The term "survivor" in the suicidology literature properly refers to *completed suicides,* not to those who survive a suicide attempt. The usual feelings associated with any serious loss are felt by most survivors of a suicide: sadness that the person ended life so tragically and anger that the person is no longer a part of one's life.

In addition, however, survivors often feel enormous guilt, primarily from two sources:

1. The sense of responsibility for not having prevented the suicide. This is especially true when the survivors were very close to the person who has died.
2. The sense of relief that some survivors feel after a suicide. This happens when relationships were very strained or when the person attempted suicide many times and either could not or would not accept the help available.

A common tendency among survivors of suicide is to blame or "scapegoat" someone for the suicide. This reaction often arises from a survivor's sense of helplessness and guilt about not preventing the suicide. Deeply held beliefs about suicide also contribute to this response. Some survivors deny that the suicide ever took place because they have no other way to handle the crisis. Often, this takes the form of insisting that the death was an accident.

CASE EXAMPLE: DENIAL OF SUICIDE

One couple instructed their nine-year-old daughter, who was a patient in the pediatric ward, to tell the hospital supervisor that her older brother had died in an accident. (The supervisor knew the family through the hospital psychiatric unit.) The parents had insisted that the brother be discharged from psychiatric care, even though he was highly suicidal and the physician advised against it. A few days later, the boy shot himself at home with a hunting rifle. The parents were apparently very guilt-ridden and went to great lengths to deny the suicide.

Various authors (Dunne, et al., 1987; Cain, 1972) have documented problems that can occur throughout survivors' lives if they do not have help at the time of the crisis of suicide. A study by Farberow, et al. (1992) revealed that suicide survivors among bereaved elderly people received significantly less support than those whose spouses died by natural death; men received less support than women. Reed & Greenwald (1991) found that survivor-victim *attachment* and the quality of the relationship is more important in explaining grief reactions than the survivor's status. Problems for survivors include depression, serious personality disturbances, and obsession with suicide as the predestined fate for oneself, especially on the anniversary of the suicide or when the person reaches the same age.

The tragic effect of suicide is particularly striking in the case of children after a parent's suicide. In studies of child survivors, some of the symptoms found were learning disabilities, sleep-walking, delinquency, and setting fires (Cain & Fast, 1972). Crisis counseling should therefore be available for all survivors of suicide. Shneidman (1972) calls this "postvention," an effort to reduce some of the possible harmful effects of suicide on the survivors. Making such support available, however, presents a special challenge, particularly in settings such as schools (Wenckstern & Leenaars, 1991).

Team Analysis Following a Suicide

Some people commit suicide while receiving therapy or counseling through a crisis center, mental health agency, or private practitioner, or while receiving hospital or medical care. In these cases, the counselor, nurse, or physician is in a strategic position to help survivors. Unfortunately, workers often miss the opportunity for postvention because they may be struggling with the same feelings that beset the family. It is more effective to deal with the family immediately than to wait for an impasse to develop, but if staff have not dealt with their own feelings, they may avoid approaching family survivors.

The most useful preventive measure is for helpers to learn as much as they can about suicide and about constructive ways of handling the feelings that often accompany working with self-destructive people. There will always be strong feelings following a suicide. However, a worker with a realistic concept of the limits of responsibility for another's suicide can help other survivors work through their feelings and reduce the scapegoating that often occurs.

In counseling and health care settings, a counselor or nurse should immediately seek consultation with a supervisor after a suicide occurs. Team meetings are also important, as they provide staff with an opportunity to air feelings and evaluate the total situation. For example, team analysis of John's case (Chapter Six) illustrates how easy it is to forget a person's natural place in the world and to fail to draw on social resources once the patient is in an institutional subculture. John's friends were never contacted, nor was a peer support source like Alcoholics Anonymous considered. Involuntary commitment for self-protection, although well-intentioned, was not enough. Analysis of this case sharpened the staff's awareness that the sense of isolation and powerlessness often experienced in mental health facilities may increase rather than decrease suicide risk. Through open discussion, staff members were able to acknowledge that John's suicide might have been prevented with a different approach to intervention, including helping him to reestablish himself socially after a serious interpersonal loss (see Chapter Five). If suicide prevention efforts are based on current standards in suicidology, the staff is less likely to feel guilty, and malpractice suits are less likely (Bongar, et al., 1993). In addition, self-examination and hindsight after a suicide usually yield knowledge that can be applied on behalf of others (Hoff & Resing, 1982).

Team meetings also provide a forum for determining who is best able to make postvention contact with the family. If the counselor who has worked most closely with the victim is too upset to deal with the family, a supervisory person should handle the matter, at least initially. In hospitals or mental health agencies in which no one has had training in basic suicide prevention and crisis counseling, outside consultation with suicidologists or crisis counselors should be obtained whenever possible.

Support and Crisis Intervention for Survivors

Most suicides do not occur among people receiving help from a health or counseling agency. This is one reason many survivors of suicide get so little help. In some communities, there are special bereavement counseling programs or self-help groups, such as widow-to-widow clubs, to help survivors of suicides. Ideally, every community should have an active outreach program for suicide survivors as a basic part of comprehensive crisis services (Hoff & Miller, 1987). Survivors are free to refuse an offer of support, but such support should be available.[1]

A parent survivor, Adina Wrobleski, is one of the pioneers in developing Survivors' Grief Groups, having formed such a group in 1982 following the suicide of her teenage daughter in the metropolitan Minneapolis area. Since then, many similar groups have been established. Wrobleski's work is significant in two respects: (1) following the suicide of her daughter, there were no peer support groups available to her and her husband; (2) survivors of suicide do not necessarily need professional therapy as much as they need support from people who have experienced the same kind of loss. This point has been illustrated by groups such as the Sudden Infant Death Syndrome Foundation and self-help groups for health and social problems, such as Alcoholics Anonymous and groups for mastectomy patients (see Chapters Five, Twelve, Thirteen, and Fourteen).

In the absence of these avenues of help, survivors of suicides can still be reached by police, clergy, and funeral directors, if such caretakers are sensitive to survivors' needs (Grollman, 1977). These key people should take care not to increase guilt and denial, recognizing how strong the suicide taboo and scapegoating tendency can be. The least one can do is offer an understanding word and suggest where people might find an agency or person to help them through the crisis.

Techniques for helping survivors of suicide are essentially the same as those used in dealing with other crises. A survivor should be helped to:

---

[1]A directory listing survivor support groups in the United States and Canada is available from the American Association of Suicidology, 4201 Connecticut Ave. NW Suite 310, Washington, D.C. 20008. The AAS office also has information about a quarterly newsletter, *Surviving Suicide.*

1. Express feelings appropriate to the event
2. Grasp the reality of the suicide
3. Obtain and use the help necessary to work through the crisis (including some-times his or her own suicide crisis)

If a survivor depended on the suicide victim for financial support, he or she may also need help in managing money and housing, for example.

Helping Child Survivors of Parent Suicide

A surviving spouse with young children, including preschoolers as young as three or four, usually needs special help explaining to them that their parent has committed suicide. People tend to hide the facts from children in a mistaken belief that they will thus be spared unnecessary pain. But adults often fail to realize that children usually know a great deal more than adults think they know. Even without knowing all the facts surrounding a death, children are likely to suspect that something much more terrible than an accident has occurred. If the suicide is not discussed, the child is left to fill in the facts alone—and to do it with fantasies even more frightening than the real story would be. For example, a child may fear that the surviving parent killed the dead parent or that the child's own misbehavior caused the parent's death. The child may have unrealistic expectations that the dead parent will return: "Maybe if I'm extra good, Daddy will come back." What children do not create in their fantasy lives will often be filled in by information from neighborhood and school companions. Some child survivors also suffer from jeers and teasing by other children about the parent's suicide.

Survivors should explain the death by suicide clearly, simply, and in a manner consistent with the child's level of development and understanding. The child should have an opportunity to ask questions and express feelings. He or she needs to know that the surviving parent is also willing to answer questions in the future, as the child's understanding of death and suicide grows. A child should never be left with the impression that the issue is closed and is never to be discussed again.

Examples of Discussions with Children. Parents might explain suicide to child survivors as follows:

"Yes, Daddy shot himself. . . . No, it wasn't an accident; he did it because he wanted to."

"Mommy will not be coming back anymore. . . . No, Mommy didn't do it because you misbehaved last night."

"No one knows exactly why your daddy did it. . . . Yes, he had a lot of things that bothered him."

Surviving parents who cannot deal directly with their children about the other parent's suicide have usually not worked through their own feelings of guilt and responsibility. In these cases, parents need the support and help of a counselor for themselves as well as for their children. Parents often do not understand that serious consequences can arise from hiding the facts from children. Counseling should include an explanation of the advantages of talking openly with children about the suicide.

In some cases, a child is completely aware that the parent committed suicide, especially if there were many open threats or attempts of suicide. Sometimes a child finds the dead parent or has been given directions by the other parent to "call if anything happens to Mommy" (Cain, 1972). If the suicidal person was very disturbed or abusive prior to committing suicide, the child may feel relief. In all of these cases, surviving children may feel guilt and misplaced responsibility for the death of their parent. They may become restless and fearful and refuse to sleep in their own beds. Parents will usually need the assistance of a crisis worker or a child guidance counselor to help a child through this crisis. Crisis intervention programs for such children are far too uncommon.

Additional Outreach to Survivors

Help for survivors of suicides has always been one of the goals of the suicide prevention movement. Such work is important but difficult to carry out. Many people, including those in some coroners' offices, tend to cover up the reality of a suicide. The suicide taboo in modern times continues, despite a growing acceptance of the morality of suicide in certain instances (Battin & Mayo, 1980; Hall & Cameron, 1976; see also "Ethical Issues Regarding Suicide" in Chapter Six).

One means of reaching a large number of survivors is through coroners' offices. Every death is eventually recorded there. In Los Angeles County, all suicide deaths as well as equivocal deaths (those in which suicide is suspected but not certain) are followed up by staff from the Los Angeles Suicide Prevention Center. Suicidologists do a "psychological autopsy" (Litman, 1987), that is, an intensive examination to determine whether the death was by suicide, and if it was, to uncover the probable causes. Information for the psychological autopsy is obtained from survivors and from medical and psychiatric records.

Research is the primary purpose of the psychological autopsy; however, it is an excellent means of getting in touch with survivors who are not in contact with a crisis center, physician, or mental health agency. Survivors are, of course, free to refuse participation in such postmortem examinations. Experience reveals, however, that the majority of survivors do not refuse to be interviewed and welcome the opportunity to talk about the suicide. This is especially true if they are contacted within a few days of the suicide, when they are most troubled with their feelings. Many survivors use this occasion to obtain some help in answering their own questions and dealing with suicidal inclinations following a suicide. Some people find the "official" interview an acceptable context in which to talk about an otherwise taboo subject. Thus it provides an ideal opportunity for the interviewer to suggest follow-up counseling resources to the survivor. If weeks or months pass, survivors may resent the postmortem interview. By that time, they have had to settle their feelings and questions on their own and in their own way, which may include denial and resentment. A delayed interview may seem like the unnecessary opening of an old wound.

Various suicide prevention and crisis centers certified by the American Association of Suicidology also conduct survivor counseling programs (Hoff & Wells, 1989). Many communities, however, still do not have formal programs available to survivors of suicides. Obviously, a great deal of work remains to be done in this important area.

Summary

People who get help after a suicide attempt or other self-destructive behavior may never commit suicide. Much depends on what happens in the form of emergency, crisis, and follow-up intervention. However, when suicide does occur, survivors of suicides usually are in crisis and are often neglected because of cultural taboos and the lack of aggressive outreach programs for them. Children, spouses, and parents who lose a loved one by suicide are especially vulnerable if they do not receive support during this crisis. This is an area of great challenge for crisis program staff.

References

Barnes, R. A. (1986). The recurrent self-harm patient. *Suicide & Life-Threatening Behavior, 16*(2), 399–408.

Battin, M. O., & Mayo, D. J. (Eds.). (1980). *Suicide: The philosophical issues.* New York: St. Martin's Press.

Berman, A. L., Coggins, C. C., Zibelin, J. C., Nelson, L. F., & Hannon, T. (1993). Inpatient treatment planning. *Suicide & Life-Threatening Behavior, 23*(2), 162–168.

Berman, A. L., & Cohen-Sandler, R. (1982). Suicide and the standards of care: Optimal vs. acceptable. *Suicide & Life-Threatening Behavior, 12*(2), 114–122.

Blumenfeld, W., & Lindop, L. (1994). *Family, schools, and students' resource guide.* Boston: Massachusetts Department of Education, Safe Schools Program for Gay and Lesbian Students.

Bongar, B., Maris, R. W., Berman, A. L., & Litman, R. E. (1992). Outpatient standards of care and the suicidal patient. *Suicide & Life-Threatening Behavior, 22*(4), 453–478.

Bongar, B., Maris, R. W., Berman, A. L., Litman, R. E., & Silverman, M. M. (1993). Inpatient standards of care and the suicidal patient: Part I: General clinical formulations and legal considerations. *Suicide & Life-Threatening Behavior, 23*(3), 245–256.

Breggin, P. (1994). *Talking back to Prozac: what doctors won't tell you about today's most controversial drug.* New York: St. Martin's Press.

Brown, G. W., & Harris, T. (1978). *The social origins of depression.* London: Tavistock.

Cain, A. C. (Ed.). (1972). *Survivors of suicide.* Springfield, IL: Charles C. Thomas.

Cain, A. C., & Fast, R. (1972). Children's disturbed reactions to parent suicide: Distortions of guilt, communication, and identification. In A. C. Cain (Ed.), *Survivors of suicide* (pp. 93–111). Springfield, IL: Charles C. Thomas.

Clark, D. C., & Kerkhof, A.J.F.M. (1993). No-suicide decisions and suicide contracts in therapy. *Crisis, 14*(3), 98–99.

Cloward, R. A., & Piven, F. F. (1979). Hidden protest: The channeling of female innovations and resistance. *Signs: Journal of Women in Culture and Society, 4*, 651–669.

Danto, B. (1981). *Crisis Behind Bars: The Suicidal Inmate.* Warren, MI: Dale.

Doweiko, H. E. (1993). *Concepts of chemical dependency* (2nd ed.). Belmont, CA: Brooks/Cole.

Dunne, E., Dunne-Maxim, K., & McIntosh, J. (Eds.). (1987). *Suicide and its aftermath.* New York: W.W. Norton.

Extein, I., Gold, M. S., & Pottash, A.L.C. (1984). Psychopharmacologic treatment of depression. *Psychiatric Clinics of North America, 7*(3), 503–517.

Farberow, N. L. (1981). Suicide prevention in the hospital. *Hospital and Community Psychiatry, 32*(2), 99–104.

Farberow, N., Gallager-Thompson, D., Gilewski, M., & Thompson, L. (1992). Changes in grief and mental health of bereaved spouses of older suicides. *Journal of Gerontology, 47*(6), 357–366.

Frederick, C. J., and Farberow, N. L. (1970). Group psychotherapy with suicidal persons: A comparison with standard group methods. *International Journal of Social Psychiatry, 16*, 103–111.

Garrison, C. Z., McKeown, R. E., Valois, R. F., & Vincent, M. L. (1993). Aggression, substance use, and suicidal behaviors in high school students. *American Journal of Public Health, 83*(2), 179–184.

Gordon, V. C., & Ledray, L. E. (1985). Depression in women: The challenge of treatment and prevention. *Journal of Psychosocial Nursing and Mental Health Services, 23*(1), 26–34.

Grollman, E. (1977). *Living—when a loved one has died.* Boston: Beacon Press.

Hall, E., & Cameron, P. (1976). Our failing reverence for life. *Psychology Today, 9*, 104–113.

Halleck, S. (1971). *The politics of therapy.* New York: Science House.

Haycock, J. (1993). Suicide rates in forensic hospitals. *Suicide & Life-Threatening Behavior, 23*(2), 130–138.

Hoff, L. A., & Miller, N. (1987). *Programs for people in crisis: A guide for educators, administrators, and clinical trainers.* Boston: Northeastern University Custom Book Program.

Hoff, L. A., & Resing, M. (1982). Was this suicide preventable? *American Journal of Nursing, 82*(7), 1106–1111.

Hoff, L. A., & Wells, J. O. (1989). *Certification standards manual* (3rd ed.). Denver: American Association of Suicidology.

Joan, P. (1986). *Preventing teenage suicide: The living alternative handbook.* New York: Human Sciences Press.

Johnson, A. B. (1990). *Out of bedlam: The truth about deinstitutionalization.* New York: Basic Books.

Kerkhof, A.J.F.M., & Clark, D. C. (1993). Suicide attempts and self-injury in prisons. *Crisis, 14*(4) 146–147.

Leenaars, A., & Wenckstern, S. (Eds.). (1991). *Suicide prevention in schools.* Washington: Hemisphere.

Litman, R. E. (1987). Mental disorders and suicidal intervention. *Suicide & Life-Threatening Behavior, 17*(2), 85–92.

McGinnis, C. (1993). *Lifeline: A training manual.* Boston: Suffolk County Jail.

McLeavey, B. C., Daly, R. J., Murray, C. M., O'Riordan, J. O., and Taylor, M. (1987). Interpersonal problem solving deficits in self-poisoning patients. *Suicide & Life-Threatening Behavior, 17*(1), 33–49.

Motto, J. A. (1991). An integrated approach to estimating suicide risk. *Suicide & Life-Threatening Behavior, 21*(1), 74–89.

Osgood, M. (1992). Environmental factors in suicide in long-term care facilities. *Suicide & Life-Threatening Behavior, 22*(1), 98–106.

Polak, P. (1967). The crisis of admission. *Social Psychiatry, 2,* 150–157.

Ray, O., & Ksir, C. (1993). *Drugs, society, and human behavior* (6th ed.). St. Louis: Mosby.

Reed, M. D., & Greenwald, J. Y. (1991). Survivor-victim status, attachment, and sudden death bereavement. *Suicide & Life-Threatening Behavior, 21*(4), 385–401.

Richman, J. (1986). *Family therapy of suicidal individuals.* New York: Springer.

Rogers, M. J. (1971). Drug abuse: Just what the doctor ordered. *Psychology Today, 5,* 16–24.

Shaffer, D. (1993). Suicide: Risk factors and the public health. *American Journal of Public Health, 83*(2), 171–173.

Shneidman, E. S. (1993). Some controversies in suicidology: Toward a mentalistic discipline. *Suicide & Life-Threatening Behavior, 23*(4), 292–298.

Shneidman, E. S. (1972). Forward. In A. C. Cain (Ed.), *Survivors of suicide.* Springfield, IL: Charles C. Thomas.

Skorupka, P., & Bohnet, N. (1982). Primary caregivers' perceptions that met their needs in a home care hospice setting. *Cancer Nursing, 5,* 371–374.

Snyder, S., Pitts, W. M., & Pokorny, A. D. (1986). Selected behavioral features with borderline personality traits. *Suicide & Life-Threatening Behavior, 16*(1), 28–39.

Webb, N. D. (1986). Before and after suicide: A preventive outreach program for colleges. *Suicide & Life-Threatening Behavior, 16*(4), 469–480.

Wenckstern, S. (1991). Suicide postvention: A case illustration in a secondary school. In A. Leenaars & S. Wenckstern (Eds.), *Suicide prevention in schools* (pp. 181–196). Washington: Hemisphere.

Williams, J.M.G. (1984). *The psychological treatment of depression: A guide to the theory and practice of cognitive behavior therapy.* New York: Free Press.

Worden, J. W. (1991). *Grief counseling and grief therapy* (2nd ed.). New York: Springer.

CHAPTER EIGHT

THE CRISIS OF VICTIMIZATION BY VIOLENCE

Victimization by violence knows few, if any, national, ethnic, religious, or other boundaries (Levinson, 1989). In the United States—the most violent society in the Western world—the homicide rate is 10 per 100,000, accounting for 25,000 deaths per year. The rate in England is one-tenth of the U.S. rate, although violence there is also increasing. Among African-American males ages fifteen to twenty-four, homicide is the most likely cause of death (Wolfgang, 1986, p. 11). While figures vary, about 20 percent of spouses in Canada and the United States are enmeshed in abuse; one-half of all Canadian women have experienced at least one violent incident since the age of sixteen (Statistics Canada, 1993). Of intrafamilial homicides (about 50 percent of the U.S. total), two-thirds are women killed by their male partners, and one-third are men killed by their female partners (Browne, 1987). Battering accounts for more injuries to women than accidents, muggings, and stranger rape combined; violence is the leading cause of injury to women between fifteen and forty-four (Novello, 1992, p. 3132). While rape in marriage is now legally recognized throughout the United States and Canada, many loopholes weaken the laws. In a random sample of 920 women, 14 percent had been raped by their husband or ex-husband (Russell, 1982, p. 2).

Studies of acquaintance rape and date rape reveal a wide disparity between women and men on what constitutes rape; the majority of men define as "normal" what women call sexual violence (Warshaw, 1988). Even though rape victims know their attackers in the majority of cases, acquaintance rapes are reported least, probably because victims fear being blamed for the attack. Another result of victim-blaming is that almost half of rape cases are dismissed before trial, and half of those convicted of rape serve less than a year behind bars (Lardner, 1993, p. 4).

Among children and adolescents in the United States, up to 3 million are physically or sexually abused or neglected each year, with as many as 1.3 million left homeless in a given year (Gelles & Cornell, 1985; Samaan, 1993, pp. 16–17; Powers & Jaklitsch, 1989). Surveys of women reveal that up to 50 percent report some kind of sexual encounter with an adult male before the age of sixteen (Herman, 1981, p. 12; Wolfgang, 1986, p. 12) and that abuse by stepfathers is seven times more common than by biological fathers (Russell, 1986).

National survey data in Canada and the United States reveal that about 4 percent of elderly people are abused by relatives each year, while only one in six cases is reported (Hudson, 1986, p 152; McDonald, et al., 1991; Podnieks and Pillemer, 1990). Financial exploitation of elderly people is also rising. A random survey in metropolitan Boston, with a population of more than four million, revealed between 8,646 and 13,487 abused and neglected elders (Pillemer & Finkelhor, 1987). In spite of civil rights legislation, violence originating from bias based on race, religion, and sexual identity continues. Abused immigrants usually face triple jeopardy because of social isolation, language barriers, and fear of deportation if they seek help.

Internationally, victimization is also receiving greater attention, although most research on the topic has been conducted in North America and Europe (Hoff, 1992b; Shallat, 1993). For example, the United Nations has convened international meetings on the topic, and the U.N. Decade for Women conferences feature numerous workshops on the worldwide problem of violence against women.[1] In South Africa, for example, for every act of political violence, at least seven women are victimized at home (Dangor, Hoff, & Scott, forthcoming; Counts, 1987; Edgerton, 1976).

Canada has demonstrated extraordinary leadership on this topic, supporting numerous projects as well as five federally funded research centers (Ross & Hoff, 1994). Canada is the first country to pass a federal, mandatory arrest law for wife beaters and the first in which men in the private sector have taken national leadership in a White Ribbon Campaign to end violence against women. In the United States, the Surgeon General's Workshop on Violence and Public Health (1986) was convened in 1985 to emphasize the fact that victims' needs, treatment of assailants, and the prevention of violence should command much greater attention from health and social service professionals than it has until recently. While progress is noted, much is left to be done (Tilden, et al., 1994). The historical neglect of victimization, especially in the domestic arena, underscores the value placed on family privacy and the myth of the family as a haven of love and security. Neglect of victimization also points to several related issues:

[1]The last such conference was in 1985 in Nairobi, Kenya, with about 17,000 women attending; the next one is scheduled for summer of 1995 in Beijing.

- Social values regarding children, how they should be disciplined, and who should care for them
- Social and cultural devaluation of women and their problems
- A social and economic system in which elderly citizens often have no worthwhile place
- A social climate with little tolerance for minority sexual orientation
- A legal system in which it is difficult to consider the rights of victims without compromising the rights of the accused
- A knowledge system that historically has interpreted these problems in private, individual terms rather than public, social ones (Mills, 1959)

This and the following chapter address these issues in the psychosociocultural perspective that informs this book, with a focus on prevention and crisis intervention. This chapter addresses the various categories of abuse and violence primarily from the perspective of the victim. Chapter Nine addresses violence from the perspective of the assailant, as well as that directed against police and health and human service workers. The two chapters are companion pieces, since the topics overlap; for example, many assailants have been victimized themselves.

Reflecting a major theme of crisis theory (Hoff, 1990), the term "victim/survivor" is used to acknowledge victimization but to simultaneously convey an abused person's potential for growth, development, and empowerment—a status beyond the dependency implied by "victim" (Burstow, 1992; Hoff & Ross, 1993/1994; Mawby & Walklate, 1994). The terms "violence" and "abuse" are used interchangeably.

Theories on Violence and Victimization

Earlier theories to explain violence and its prevalence fall into three categories: (1) psychobiological, (2) social-psychological, and (3) sociocultural (Gelles & Straus, 1979). Today, most violence scholars reject analytic frameworks such as sociobiology that serve to maintain violence as a private matter (Davidson, 1977). Instead, violence is now widely interpreted in psychological, sociological, and feminist terms (Gelles & Loseke, 1993). The position taken in this book is that violence is predominantly a *social* phenomenon, a means of exerting *power* and *control* that has far-reaching effects on personal, family, and public health worldwide (Dobash & Dobash, 1979; Hoff, 1990; McLeod, 1989; Surgeon General's Workshop, 1986; Yllo & Bograd, 1987). Further, the book's psychosociocultural framework implies a continuum between so-called family violence and other forms of aggression. Finally, while controversy rages between feminist and mainstream theorists and activists (Gelles & Loseke, 1993; Hoff, 1990), the focus here is on bridge-building and the common concerns of those who teach and practice violence prevention and who work with victim/survivors and their assailants in diverse settings.

An either-or position is rejected in favor of a feminist and sociocultural perspective that emphasizes the intersection between gender, class, race, and other social categories that may figure in the experience of particular victims or assailants.[2]

Accordingly, the term "family violence" is avoided on the grounds that it obscures the fact that most perpetrators within families are men, and most victims are children and women of all ages. One of the continuing controversies about violence concerns the rates of men's and women's violence (Kurz, 1993; Straus, 1993). The argument centers on the alleged methodological flaws of the Conflict Tactics Scale used in the national surveys conducted by Straus and colleagues in 1980 and 1985. "Family violence" also deflects attention from the sociocultural roots of abuse, which extend beyond the family to deeply embedded cultural values and traditional social structures that disempower women and children particularly.

Many professionals and laypersons have accepted psychological or medical explanations of violence (see "The Medicalization of Crime," Chapter Nine). Common sentiments include: (1) "only a sick man could beat his wife"; (2) child abuse is a syndrome calling for "treatment" of disturbed parents; (3) John W. Hinckley should have been "treated," not punished, for violently attacking President Reagan; (4) a "crazed madman" was responsible (and by implication, not accountable) for a series of fatal Tylenol poisonings in the United States; (5) "temporary insanity" sometimes excuses murder (even though juries are becoming more skeptical about this plea); and (6) women who kill their abusers are victims of the "battered woman syndrome."

Public debate about medical approaches to social problems is increasing (Warshaw, 1989). There is growing acceptance of the view that attention to violent persons and their victims in predominantly individual terms is incomplete at best and at worst does little to address the roots of violence. This view is in accord with the crisis paradigm of this book: crises stemming from violence should be treated with a *tandem* approach, taking both individual and sociocultural factors into account. A person in crisis because of violence will experience many of the same responses as persons in crisis from other sources (Burgess & Holmstrom, 1979; Sales, Baum, & Shore, 1984, p. 131). And similar intervention strategies, such as listening and decision counseling, are called for during the acute crisis phase. However, attention to the social and cultural *origins* of crises stemming from violence is important in designing prevention and follow-up strategies that avoid implicitly blaming the victim (Ryan, 1971; Hoff, 1990). Indeed, the implications of a social/cultural framework are even more critical when considering crises originating from vio-

[2]In feminist theory, this approach is called "socialist feminism." As readers examine their own positions vis-a-vis feminist and mainstream theories of violence, it is important to note that there is no such thing as a monolithic feminism. See Breines & Gordon, 1983; Hoff, 1990; Segal, 1987.

lence than when dealing with crises from other sources (see Figure 2.2, Chapter Two). For victims of violence, a strictly individual approach can compound the problem rather than contribute to the solution (Stark, Flitcraft, & Frazier, 1979).

There is no single "cause" of violence. Rather, there are complex, interrelated *reasons* that some individuals are violent and others are not. In cases of violence against children, wives, and elders, for example, psychological, cultural, and socioeconomic factors are often present together, forming the *context* in which violence as a means of control seems to thrive. Children, elders, and often wives are economically dependent on their caretakers and in most cases are physically weaker than their abusers. Caretakers of children and older people are often stressed psychologically by difficult behaviors and socioeconomically by a lack of social and financial resources to ease the burdens of caretaking (Besharov, 1990; Pillemer & Wolf, 1986; Pruschno & Resch, 1989). In cases of wife battering and sex-role stereotyping, psychological and economic factors intersect at both ends of the social class continuum: poor women are less able to survive on their own, while women who earn more than their husbands are more vulnerable to attack than those who earn less (Rubenstein, 1982).

Violence toward others, then, is one way a person can respond to stress and resolve a personal crisis at the same time. For example, a person with low self-esteem who is threatened by the suspected infidelity of a spouse may react with violence (Gondolf, 1987). A violent response is not inevitable, though; it is *chosen,* and may be influenced by such factors as an earlier choice to use alcohol and other drugs. The choice of violent behavior to control another person is influenced by the social, political, legal, and belief and knowledge systems of the violent person's cultural community. The element of choice implies an interpretation of violence as a moral act. That is, violence is social action engaged in by human beings who by nature are rational and conscious. Through socialization, humans become responsible for the actions they choose in various situations.

However, consciousness may be clouded and responsibility mitigated by social and cultural factors rooted in the history of human society. Under certain circumstances, a person may be excused from facing the social consequences of his or her behavior, as in cases of self-defense or when a violent act is considered to be irrational. This does *not* mean that every violent act is a result of illness and that the perpetrator should therefore be "treated," as suggested by a popular conception of violence. Nor does it mean that violence can be excused on grounds of racial or economic discrimination; this would suggest that the moral stature of disadvantaged groups is below the standard of responsible behavior. Given the poverty, unemployment, and other tragic results of social inequalities endured by many people—mostly racial minority groups—perhaps in no other instance is the *tandem* approach to crisis intervention more relevant: violent *individuals* are held accountable for their behavior, while the political and socioeconomic *context* within which much violence occurs is also addressed. In other words, an individual can be held accountable, can be restrained and/or rehabilitated while also addressing the factors contributing to the person's vulnerability to choosing aggressive behaviors in the first place. This principle applies regardless of gender or race.

Another troubling aspect of a simplistic interpretation of the nature of violence is the tendency toward "solutions" in the form of revenge, as suggested, for example, by U.S. voters' choice of capital punishment. To describe violence as a moral act rather than a disease does not imply support of revenge as an appropriate response. As responses to the complex problem of violence, treatment and revenge represent opposite extremes of response. As in the case of race or gender, excusing violent acts on the basis of psychiatric illness suggests that violent human beings are somewhat less than human, generally incapable of judging and acting according to the consequences of their behavior and driven by uncontrollable, aggressive impulses. Revenge, on the other hand—in the form of capital punishment, inhumane prison conditions, or a failure to provide economic and other opportunities for learning to change a violent lifestyle—implies a departure from the moral foundations of society.

Violence and our response to its victims/survivors and perpetrators can be interpreted in a multifaceted perspective: moral, social-psychological, legal, and medical. Violence can be defined as an infraction of society's rules regarding people, their relationships, and their property. It is a complex phenomenon in which sociocultural, political, medical, and psychological factors touch both its immediate and chronic aspects. Functioning members of a society normally know a group's cultural rules and the consequences for violating them. Those lacking such knowledge generally are excused and receive treatment instead of punishment. Others are excused on the basis of self-defense or the circumstances that alter one's normal liability for rule infractions. A moral society would require restitution to individual victims from those not excused and would design a criminal justice system to *prevent* rather than promote future crime. A truly moral approach to violence would also avoid or reform practices that discriminate on the basis of race, gender, class, or sexual orientation—practices that create a climate in which crime flourishes with the implicit support of society (Brown & Bohn, 1989; Dobash & Dobash, 1979; Report, 1986).

Decisions about crisis and follow-up approaches to victims and perpetrators of violence demand a critical examination of the theories and research supporting such practice, an examination not undertaken until recently. This theoretical overview applies to the topics in this and the following chapter. It assumes a continuum between what happens between family members and intimates and the larger sociocultural factors affecting them. In the following discussion, social-psychological and sociocultural theories will be examined as they apply to crises stemming from violence in respect to:

- Prevention
- Intervention during crisis
- Follow-up service

FIGURE 8.1. CRISIS PARADIGM.

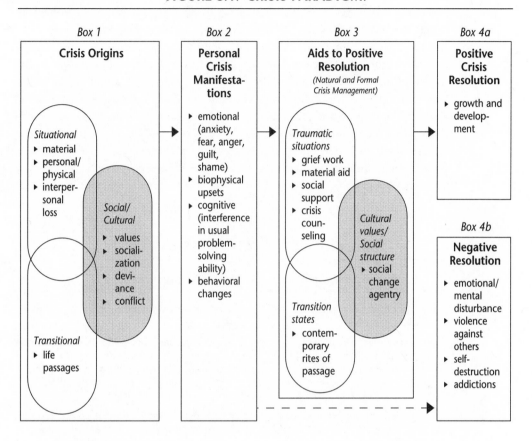

	Box 1	Box 2	Box 3	Box 4a

Box 1

Crisis Origins

Situational
- material
- personal/ physical
- interpersonal loss

Social/ Cultural
- values
- socialization
- deviance
- conflict

Transitional
- life passages

Box 2

Personal Crisis Manifestations

- emotional (anxiety, fear, anger, guilt, shame)
- biophysical upsets
- cognitive (interference in usual problem-solving ability)
- behavioral changes

Box 3

Aids to Positive Resolution
(Natural and Formal Crisis Management)

Traumatic situations
- grief work
- material aid
- social support
- crisis counseling

Cultural values/ Social structure
- social change agentry

Transition states
- contemporary rites of passage

Box 4a

Positive Crisis Resolution

- growth and development

Box 4b

Negative Resolution

- emotional/ mental disturbance
- violence against others
- self-destruction
- addictions

Each of these topics is important, but the discussion in these two chapters will focus on assessment and intervention, with general reference to the preventive and follow-up strategies necessary for a long-range political and social approach that will reduce crises stemming from violence (see Figure 8.1, right circle of Box 3).

Victimization Assessment Strategies

Crisis workers in various entry points to the health and social service system should incorporate questions about possible victimization into their routine assessments. Bell et al. (1994) state that protocols for such assessments should be mandated by law. Table 8.1 presents a Victimization Assessment Scale for use by entry-point workers that is adapted from the Comprehensive Mental Health Assessment Guide discussed in Chapter Three. Exhibit 8.1, Screening for Victimization and Life-Threatening Behaviors: Triage Questions, includes suggested questions for use with this tool as well as with the Homicide/Assault Assessment Scale described in

Chapter Nine (see Hoff & Rosenbaum, 1994). As in the case of suicide risk assessment, *no crisis assessment is complete without ascertaining risk and trauma from victimization and assault.* Work with battered women, for example, has uncovered the repeated revelation by survivors seeking help: "No one asked." As the study by Sugg and Inui (1992) suggests, physicians, nurses, and others must move beyond their traditional fear of opening Pandora's box by inquiring about abuse. Just as health assessments now include routine questions about smoking and drinking, so should victimization and violence assessment be routine for anyone in emotional distress or whose symptoms do not readily suggest a medical diagnosis. Questions about suicide and assault potential and resource depletion should be included in the screening protocol because these problems are often secondary to the primary problem of abuse and may signal the severity of trauma from victimization. As

TABLE 8.1. VICTIMIZATION ASSESSMENT SCALE.

Level of Victimization	Typical Indicators
1 = No experience of physical violence or abuse	No memory of violence recently or in the past
2 = Experience of abuse/violence with minor physical and/or emotional trauma	Currently, verbal arguments that occasionally escalate to pushing and shoving or mild slapping. History *may* include past victimization that is no longer problematic or for which a solution is in process.
3 = Experience of abuse/violence with moderate physical and/or emotional trauma	Abused several times a month in recent years resulting in moderate trauma/emotional distress (e.g., bruises; no threat to life; no weapons). History *may* include past victimization that is still somewhat problematic (e.g., a sexual abuse incident/overture by a parent or stepparent over 2 years ago)
4 = Experience of abuse/violence with severe physical and/or emotional trauma	Violently attacked (e.g., rape) or physically abused in recent years, resulting in physical injury requiring medical treatment. Threats to kill; no guns. History *may* include serious victimization (e.g., periodic battering, incest, or other abuse requiring medical and/or psychological treatment).
5 = Life-threatening or prolonged violence/abuse with very severe physical and/or emotional trauma	Recent or current life-threatening physical abuse; potentially lethal assault or threats with available deadly weapons. History *may* include severe abuse requiring medical treatment; frequent or on-going sexual abuse; recent rape at gun- or knife-point; other physical attack requiring extensive medical treatment.

EXHIBIT 8.1. SCREENING FOR VICTIMIZATION AND LIFE-THREATENING BEHAVIORS: TRIAGE QUESTIONS.

1. Have you been troubled or injured by any kind of abuse or violence? (e.g., hit by partner, forced sex)

   Yes _____ No _____ Not sure _____ Refused _____

   If yes, check one: By someone in your family _____

   By an acquaintance or stranger _____

   Describe:

2. If yes: Has something like this ever happened before?

   Yes _____ No_____ If yes, when? _____

   Describe:

3. Do you have anyone you can turn to or rely on now to protect you from possible further injury?

   Yes _____ No _____ If yes, who? _____

4. Do you feel so badly now that you have thought of hurting yourself/suicide?

   Yes _____ No _____ If yes: What have you thought about doing?

5. Are you so angry about what's happened that you have considered hurting someone else?

   Yes _____ No _____ If yes: Describe briefly: _____

the triage questions in Exhibit 8.1 suggest, such routine inquiry could prevent suicide and/or murder as desperate responses to victimization trauma.

Once victimization status is identified, it should be followed by in-depth assessment (preferably by mental health professionals with backgrounds in victimology who are also sensitive to gender issues) to ascertain the extent of trauma and the victim/survivor's response. (See also Burstow, 1992; Campbell & Humphreys, 1993; Herman, 1992; van der Kolk, 1987.)

Child Abuse

The tragedy of child abuse continues, while public debate about related values and social issues escalates.

The Problem

Child abuse can be physical, emotional, verbal, or sexual—any acts of commission or omission that harm or threaten to harm a child (Cook & Bowles, 1980). The biblical expression "spare the rod and spoil the child" suggests a long history of child abuse. DeMause (1975) has written that the "helping mode" in caring for children is of very recent origin and was preceded historically by infanticide and

CASE EXAMPLE: RICHARD

A young mother with four children felt over-whelmed trying to care for her five-year-old hyperactive child, Richard. The woman's husband was employed as a hospital mainte-nance worker but found it difficult to sup-port the family. The family could not obtain public assistance although their income was just above the level to qualify for food stamps. The mother routinely spanked Richard with a strap several times during the day. By evening, the child was even more hyperactive, so the mother sometimes put him to bed without feeding him. The father and mother mutually approved of this form of disciplining Richard. A neighbor reported the parents of suspected abuse after observ-ing the mother chase and verbally abuse Richard on the street with a strap poised to spank him.

rampant cruelty toward children. The institution of "Good Samaritan" laws is a legal response to those practices. Although the natural helplessness of children in-spires most adults to aid and protect them, societies have found it necessary to have specific laws to protect children. These laws also protect physicians, nurses, and social workers from prosecution for slander when they report suspected child abuse to authorities.

Child abuse happens in well-to-do families and poor families, in cities, sub-urbs, and rural areas. No one knows exactly how many children are abused each year, since many cases are not reported. Besides the estimated two to four mil-lion abused and neglected children, 2,000 to 5,000 deaths occur annually in the United States at the hands of parents and caretakers. One or both parents or sib-lings may be involved. In her study of women who killed their children, Korbin (1987) uncovered a dynamic similar to the "cry for help" noted in suicidal people. If the women's networks of kin and professionals had responded to their behav-ioral pleas for help, they would have been "secretly relieved" and perhaps fatal abuse would have been avoided.

There is disagreement on just what child abuse is. Most people agree that some kind of discipline is necessary and that a swat or controlled spanking for playing with fire or running in front of cars is not the same as child abuse. But it is difficult to persuade the average North American that a child can be brought up without physical punishment, in spite of research supporting the negative ef-fects of such punishment (Greven, 1990; Straus, Gelles, & Steinmetz, 1980).

The tragic reality of child abuse gained national attention in North Amer-ica with the works of Kempe and Helfer (1980) in pediatrics and Gil (1970) in so-cial science. More recent work (e.g., Bagley & King, 1990; Finkelhor, 1984) exposed the extent of sexual abuse, while Newberger and Newberger (1981) challenge single-factor approaches to the issue. They suggest instead an "ecologic" inter-active theory and preventive practice in response to the problem.

A tragedy related to child abuse is that of runaway children: 35 percent of these American runaways leave home because of incest and 53 percent because

CASE EXAMPLE: LINDA

Linda, age fifteen, had never told anyone about her father's repeated visits to her room where he sexually abused her over a four-year period. Linda did not tell her mother because she thought her mother already knew and approved of what was happening. Linda looked forward to leaving home and marrying her boyfriend, age nineteen. One night her boyfriend raped her; afterward, she went into the bathroom and took twenty of her mother's sleeping pills. If her mother had not heard her crying and taken her to the hospital for emergency treatment, Linda would have died.

of physical neglect. The majority are never reported missing by their parents; 80 percent are from white, middle-class families; 150,000 disappear each year, many dying of disease, exploitation, and malnutrition (Powers & Jaklitsch, 1989; Russell, 1986).

When dealing with individual cases of child abuse or neglect, especially if the parents were abused themselves or problems with alcohol are involved, it is easy to lose sight of the evidence that child abuse is rooted in the fabric of many societies:

1. Violence as an appropriate solution to problem solving is a culturally embedded value of U.S. society. There is widespread evidence that the use of violence (such as in harsh discipline) trains a person for violence (Gil, 1970; Straus, Gelles, & Steinmetz, 1980). Thus, when a parent uses violent forms of discipline while interpreting it as an act of love and concern for the child, the child is likely to absorb the value that violence is a socially approved form of problem solving. The embeddedness of the spare-the-rod philosophy was dramatized in the 1994 incident in Singapore of "caning" a U.S. teenager as punishment for vandalism. More disturbing than the incident itself is the expressed view of large numbers of Americans that similar public punishment should be adopted in the United States (Goodman, 1994).

2. Economic hardship and stress can often be traced to unequal social opportunities in the United States. The national survey on domestic violence (Straus, Gelles, & Steinmetz, 1980) suggests a clear association between economic disadvantage and child abuse; the difficulty of providing basic necessities as well as special medical and social services for handicapped or sick children is a source of extraordinary parental stress. Such stress is exacerbated by the homelessness now suffered by millions of women and children (see Chapter Twelve).

3. Child care, though necessary for the continuation of society, is socially devalued, as revealed in several practices: (a) the failure to provide adequate child care for wage-earning parents; (b) the low pay scales for those who do provide child care; (c) the continuing acceptance of child rearing as a predominant responsibility of mothers.

Miller (1986) suggests that if men and women wish to have children, they should also figure out how to take care of them so that the children have the benefit of paternal as well as maternal upbringing (see "Birth and Parenthood" in Chapter Thirteen).

Preventive Intervention

Preventive strategies are always important in crisis intervention, but they are particularly urgent concerning the tragedy of child abuse. A focus on the social origins of this problem is critical. Preventive intervention includes:

1. Critically examining child-rearing practices and incorporating nonviolent approaches to discipline into high school curriculum courses for boys and girls (Brendtro, Brokenleg, & Van Bockern, 1990; Eggert, 1994; Judson, 1984)
2. Instituting social and political action to relieve the economic hardship and poverty of many families
3. Instituting social and political action to address substandard child-care programs and develop family policies appropriate to the resources and ideals of a nation
4. Using consciousness-raising and education to stress the advantages to individuals and to society of having children reared in an egalitarian fashion by mothers and fathers—as well as by extended family, foster grandparents, and others
5. Examining government child-welfare agencies systematically to ensure that children's problems are adequately attended to before abuse occurs
6. Instituting public education programs on child abuse and providing in-service training programs for school nurses, teachers, and others working with children
7. Developing hotlines and drop-in centers for children and adolescents as additional supports and outlets for troubled youth
8. Instructing children that they own the private parts of their bodies and reassuring them that they have no obligation to satisfy the sexual desires of parents, relatives, or others (Conte, Wolf, & Smith, 1987).
9. Renewing commitment to improving the mental health of children as an aid to resisting seduction (Conte, Wolf, & Smith, 1987), for example, by working with police officers to teach children how to detect and resist would-be abductors
10. Examining the societal values and economic arrangements that support the idea so many teenage mothers have absorbed: their most important contribution to society and means of feeling valuable is to produce a baby, irrespective of their emotional, social, and economic ability to care for a child. A related value is the near-disregard of responsibility by teenage, unmarried fathers (Eyre & Eyre, 1993).

All these preventive strategies demand that we take the time to discover why so many of our children are being abused and neglected. A shift "from care to prevention" was highlighted in the Surgeon General's Workshop on Violence (1986). Newberger's (1980) testimony before the U.S. House of Representatives affirmed the importance of addressing exploitive sex, isolation, poverty, and a cultural climate that supports violence if we are serious about preventing child abuse and neglect.

Legal and Crisis Intervention

Everyone should be aware of the signs of possible child abuse:

- Repeated injury to a child with unconcern on the part of the parent(s) or with unlikely explanations
- Aggressive behavior that implies a child's cry for help
- Neglected appearance
- Overly critical parental attitude
- Withdrawal, depression, and self-injury (especially with incest)

Serious effects of child abuse include physical handicaps, emotional crippling—an abused child may never be able to love others—homelessness, psychiatric illness, antisocial or violent behavior later in life, and death (Carmen, Rieker, & Mills, 1984; Helfer & Kempe, 1987).

Suspicions of child abuse must be reported to child protection authorities, although we should be cautious about making unsubstantiated accusations. A related concern, primarily in longer-term therapy situations, is the controversial "false memory syndrome" and "therapist-induced memories." Despite this controversy, it is important to *believe* children's stories about abuse. All parents make mistakes; it is the crisis of child abuse and the *pattern* of abuse that must be reported. In cases of incest, the crisis for the child as well as for the entire family occurs when "the secret" is revealed (Herman, 1981).

We can assume that most parents have the welfare of their children at heart. When parents do not appear to be concerned for the welfare of their children, they must be confronted with the reality that children as well as parents have rights. When abuse is suspected, everyone who knows the child must realize that a parent's rights are not absolute. "Minding one's own business" is inappropriate when child abuse is involved, although many people use that as an excuse for not reporting what they suspect.

Teachers are in a strategic position to help an abused child; the school is often the only recourse open to the child (Hillman & Solek-Tefft, 1988). Although teachers are not trained to deal with disturbed parents, they are responsible for reporting suspected child abuse to child welfare authorities. Parents who think they are abusive or who are afraid of losing control should be encouraged to seek help on their own by contacting Parents Anonymous, a self-help organization in the United

States and England. Hotlines for parents, children, and others concerned about child abuse can be contacted through any crisis or mental health agency or by simply dialing the operator. In mental health and social service settings, early signs of child abuse can often be uncovered through family-focused assessment as discussed in Chapters Three and Five. The Child Screening Checklist (Exhibit 3.3) can guide such assessment.

Child abuse is a crisis for the parent as well as the child; the abused child is often one whose behavior causes extreme stress, even for the most forebearing parent. Parents in crisis are, unfortunately, sometimes overlooked by health personnel attending a battered child. The tragic situation of treating a helpless, beaten child makes it very difficult for nurses and physicians to recognize the equally great need of the battered child's parents. Whether parents bring the abused child to the hospital themselves or whether they are reported by nurses, teachers, or neighbors, parents are usually guilt-ridden and shaken by the experience. In most cases, they are fearful for the child's life, remorseful about their uncontrolled rage, fearful of treatment at the hands of the law, and fearful of future outbursts of uncontrollable anger.

If nurses, physicians, and social workers can overcome their own aversion and feelings of rejection, the crisis can become a turning point in parents' lives. Understanding the emotional needs of abusive or neglectful parents is important for doing crisis intervention with them; abusers often have the following characteristics:

- Inability to understand and communicate with children
- Emotional immaturity
- Generally disturbed lives
- Unhappy marriage
- Stress related to economic, unemployment, and housing problems
- Feelings of inadequacy in their role as parents
- Frequent life crises as well as drug and alcohol problems
- Deprived or abused childhood
- Unrealistic and rigid expectations of their children
- Minimal or inadequate parenting skills

Crisis intervention in instances of child abuse includes:
1. Encouraging the parent to express feelings appropriate to the event.
2. Actively engaging the parent in planning medical care for the child—a corrective emotional experience that moves the parent in the direction of doing something constructive for the child, as would be appropriate in Richard's case.
3. Enlisting the parents' cooperation with child welfare authorities who have been appropriately informed by a health professional. This includes correcting the parents' probable perception of child welfare authorities as punitive. In reality, the people representing such authorities generally are concerned and will help parents carry out their parental responsibilities. This point is important

for preventing further tragedies such as murder of the children by a father accused of incest, as is possible in the case of Linda.

4. Avoiding the removal of an incest victim instead of her assailant from the home. Removing the victim perpetuates the notion that she is responsible for the abuse and for the breakup of the family and also alienates her from her mother (Herman, 1981).

5. Referring the parent to self-help groups such as Parents Anonymous or Parents in Crisis where they can share their feelings and get help from other parents in similar situations—as would be helpful for the parents of both Richard and Linda (see Chapter Five).

6. Instituting job training and day-care services in cases of economic strain and when a mother is overwhelmed with the care of several children at home by herself, as is Richard's mother.

7. Providing concrete suggestions of nonviolent alternatives to discipline such as isolation or thinking time for the child and nonviolent stress management techniques for parents. There are excellent books on this topic written specifically for parents (e.g., Canter & Canter, 1988; Hillman & Solek-Tefft, 1988; Judson, 1984).

Follow-Up Service

Follow-up for child-abusing parents should include referral to a counseling agency where they can receive more extensive help concerning the underlying emotional problems that led to the crisis. Child welfare departments can facilitate parent counseling if they do not offer it themselves. Role modeling, home supervision, and parent-effectiveness training are other services that should be available to these parents.

These suggestions for prevention should be considered even if abuse has already occurred. It is never too late to consider ways to eliminate pain and the unnecessary death of our children and to reduce this tragic waste of a nation's most precious resource.

Rape and Sexual Assault

Rape is a violent crime, not a sexual act. Because of people's attitudes toward the crime of rape, the crisis of rape victims has not received appropriate attention until recently. Feminists and others who have become sensitized to the horrors of this crime against women are slowly bringing about necessary changes in a legal system that often causes double victimization of the person who has been attacked. Although most rape victims are female, male rape also occurs, leaving its victims with crisis manifestations similar to those of women victims and sometimes with even more reluctance to report the rape and seek help.

In a widely publicized rape conviction, the rapist's defense attorney outraged

public opinion by declaring on national television that the convictions would never
have occurred if he had been allowed to enter into testimony the history of the
victim's sex life. Similarly, there was public outcry against a judge who let an admitted rapist off with a light sentence for raping a five-year-old girl because of the
girl's "precocious sexual behavior." If a woman is sexually abused or raped by her
physician, the chances of successful prosecution are further reduced because (1)
the social and political influence of the medical profession is enormous; (2) the average woman thus abused has been seduced into believing the action is part of
medical practice; (3) the woman is often afraid to report the incident and cannot
imagine that this could happen to anyone but herself; (4) she may have absorbed
the message that she invited the rape or did something wrong. This point applies
to any professional who violates a position of trust and power (Burgess & Hartman, 1989).

Only recently in North America has rape in marriage been recognized legally
as an offense. The cultural notion of woman as the property and appropriate object of man's violence and pleasure still lingers (Russell, 1982). Rape as a common
crime of war also still goes unpunished, while in Bosnia the crime extends to children and men as well.

The criminal justice system is not the only arena in which rape victims are
blamed. Holmstrom and Burgess (1978) found that attitudes of hospital personnel
(physicians and nurses) were the same as those of the police: there was considerable sympathy for the victim with obvious physical injuries but general blaming
and skepticism regarding victimization in less brutal rapes. This is significant when
considering the threat to life accompanying many rapes and the great number
of acquaintance rapes (47 percent of all rapes). In date rape, it is often assumed
that if a woman says no she does not mean it and that in some way she invited the
attack (Levy, 1991). This issue is complicated when women have drunk too much
and are victimized by a gang of rapists. The woman's intoxication is used as an
excuse to exploit her; college women are particularly vulnerable to such attacks.
These are reported least often because of the continued tendency to excuse rapists
on grounds of their *victims'* behavior. A survey of thousands of college students revealed that one-quarter of college women have been victims of rape or attempted
rape and almost 90 percent of the women knew their assailants (Warshaw, 1988).
In two recent campus gang rapes, women made public, victim-blaming statements,
for example, "If she hadn't stayed out so late, it probably wouldn't have happened." One interpretation of such behavior is that it is a potential victim's means
of gaining some control and reducing her own vulnerability: "If *I* don't stay out
too late or drink too much, I won't get raped." In Warshaw's study, 50 percent of
the men had forced sex on women but did not define it as rape, while only 33 percent said that under no circumstances could they rape a woman.

We should not, however, be surprised at these responses in a culture in which
women are often considered fair game. Recently, psychiatric and general health
personnel have responded to the research regarding attitudes of health profes-

sionals toward rape victims. These workers are developing rape crisis intervention programs in hospital settings based on principles of equality and a rejection of popular myths about rape.

The fallacy of blaming a woman for her attack because she was "dressed too provocatively" or "out on the street alone" becomes clear in the analogy of a well-dressed man who is robbed of his wallet: no one would say he was robbed because of what he wore. Regarding women who are raped while out at night, we might attend to Golda Meir's response to the curfew proposal for Israeli women at risk of attack: let the men who are raping be curfewed instead.

Another popular myth about rape is that the victim "enjoys rape" and that the average woman entertains fantasies of being raped. This notion is reinforced by popular movies such as "Last Tango in Paris," by hard- and soft-core pornography, and by advertising images in which women are depicted as appropriate objects of male violence. These myths about rape stem from the persistent interpretation of rape as a sexual event rather than an act of violence.

Societal attitudes, then, play a major part in the outcome of a rape crisis experience. When rape victims are blamed rather than assisted through this crisis, it is not surprising that they blame themselves and fail to express feelings appropriate to the event such as anger. Such attitudes also impede the process of long-term recovery (Braswell, 1989; Sales, Baum, & Shore, 1984).

There is still much to be done to change public attitudes, reform institutional responses to rape victims, and dismantle the widespread belief that women and girls who are raped are "asking for it." It is instructive to note that many victims fail to report rape because of fear, their perception that police are ineffective, and the threat of further victimization by authorities (Kidd & Chayet, 1984). Another study revealed that those victims who sought compensation were even more dissatisfied than those who did not, because payment was either inadequate or denied altogether (Elias, 1984, p. 113).

Preventing Rape and Sexual Assault

Long-range strategies to prevent rape include dismantling the myths that promote the double victimization of women. Such a campaign should cover education, health, social service, and criminal justice systems as well as the public at large.

At the individual level, a woman whose life is threatened can do little or nothing to prevent sexual assault. In some cases, however, women can lessen their chances of attack by training themselves to be street-smart—alert at all times to their surroundings when outside. Potential victims should remember that even though crime may *appear* to be random, the would-be criminal has a plan. That plan includes attacking a person who *appears* to present the greatest chance of success at the crime with the least amount of trouble. Therefore, women on the street who are alert and make this evident have, to some extent, equalized the criminal-victim relationship. Signals of an escape plan may be as simple as looking around frequently or carrying a pencil flashlight—cues that alert a would-be attacker that you are not an easy target. Also, the attacker does not know what else you may possess—perhaps mace or karate expertise—and generally will not take unnecessary chances with people who appear prepared to resist. Alertness at home is also important. For example, a fifty-six-year-old woman was raped in her home by a man posing as a delivery man in spite of a highly organized neighborhood patrol on her street.

Self-defense training is also useful as an immediate protection strategy (Kidder, Boell, & Moyer, 1983). It provides physical resistance ability as well as the psychological protection of greater self-confidence and less vulnerability. However, women should not rely on self-defense excessively because (1) it may lead to a false sense of security and neglect of planning and alertness, and (2) some attackers are so fast and overpower the victim so completely that there may be no opportunity to put self-defense strategies to work.

Preventing the sexual assault of children includes not leaving children unattended, instructing them about not accepting favors from strangers, and keeping communication open so that a child will feel free to confide in parents about a threat or attack.

Crisis Intervention

There is no question that people who have been raped are in crisis (Burgess & Holstrom, 1979). They are in shock; they fear for their lives and feel dirty and physically violated. Sometimes they feel shame and blame themselves for being attacked. They may or may not feel angry, depending on how much they feel responsible for their victimization. These feelings lead to a temporary halting of their usual problem-solving ability and often to delay in reporting the crime. Rape is sometimes accompanied by robbery and abandonment at the location where the victim was taken by the rapist. Such a series of events further reduces the victim's normal problem-solving ability. Holmstrom and Burgess (1978) have described the crisis and treatment of rape victims; Brownmiller (1975) deals with the historical and anthropological aspects of rape. Emergency and police personnel are referred to these works for more information about rape—that it is a serious crime, that the *victims* of this crime should not also be the defendants, and that medical center protocols should reflect these concepts.

If a sexual assault has occurred, friends, family, strangers, the police, and agency staff may be in a position to offer immediate crisis assistance to the victim. The rape victim is sometimes hesitant to ask family and friends for help, especially in cases of date or acquaintance rape. Helpers should actively reach out in the form of crisis intervention in every instance of sexual assault, regardless of type. The chance of being asked for such help and our success in offering it during crisis depend on our basic attitudes toward rape and our knowledge of what to do. The following is quoted from the public information card of the Manchester, New

Hampshire, Women's Crisis Line. It contains essential information that anyone (including victims themselves) can use if someone has been raped. Similar information cards are available at hospital rape crisis intervention programs and in police departments:

What to Do If You Have Been Raped

Emotional considerations: A rape is usually traumatic. Call a friend and/or Manchester Women Against Rape (MWAR) for support. A trained MWAR volunteer can provide information, support, and referral, and is willing to accompany you to the hospital, police, and court.

Medical considerations: Get immediate medical attention. Take a change of clothing along to the emergency service of a hospital or to a private physician (the police will provide transportation if you need it). The exam should focus on two concerns: medical care and the gathering of evidence for possible prosecution. You will have a pelvic examination and be checked for injuries, pregnancy, and venereal disease. Be prepared to give enough details of the attack for the exam to be thorough. Follow-up tests for venereal disease about six weeks later and pregnancy are also important.

Legal considerations: Do not bathe, douche, or change clothes until after the exam; that would destroy evidence you will need if you should later choose to prosecute. Try to recall as many details as possible. Call the police to report the crime. Be prepared to answer questions intended to help your case, such as: Where were you raped? What happened? Can you identify the man?

If the victim does come to an emergency medical facility, emergency personnel should listen to the victim and support her emotionally while carrying out necessary medical and legal procedures. Victims should be advised that there are standard protocols for these procedures that are legally required if charges are to be filed. The victim should be linked with crisis counseling services. Some hospital emergency departments are staffed with such counselors, and many cities have rape crisis services with crisis hotlines or women's centers. Where specialized services do not exist, rape victims should be offered the emergency services of local mental health agencies, which exist in nearly every community.

Crisis counseling by telephone for the rape victim is illustrated in Table 8.2, an interview example.

Follow-Up Service

Women who have been raped usually describe it as the most traumatic experience of their life. It should not be assumed, however, that the experience will damage

TABLE 8.2. TELEPHONE CRISIS COUNSELING FOR
THE RAPE VICTIM.

Characteristics of Crisis and Intervention Techniques	Telephone Interview Between Victim and Crisis Counselor Case Example: Elaine	
	Counselor:	Crisis Center, May I help you?
	Elaine:	I just have to talk to somebody.
Establishing personal human contact	*Counselor:*	Yes—my name is Sandra. I'd like to hear what's troubling you. Will you tell me your name?
Upset, vulnerable, trouble with problem solving	*Elaine:*	I'm Elaine. . . . I'm just so upset I don't know what to do.
Identifying hazardous event	*Counselor:*	Can you tell me what happened?
	Elaine:	Well, I was coming home alone last night from a party. . . . It was late (chokes up; starts to cry).
	Counselor:	Whatever it is that happened has really upset you.
	Elaine:	(continues to cry.)
Empathy, encouraging expression of feeling	*Counselor:*	(waits, listens—Elaine's crying subsides.) It must be really hard for you to talk about.
Self-blaming	*Elaine:*	I guess it was really crazy for me to go to that party alone. . . . I should never have done it . . . on my way into my apartment, this man grabbed me (starts to cry again).
Identifying hazardous event	*Counselor:*	I gather he must have attacked you.
Self-blame and distorted perception of reality	*Elaine:*	Yes! He raped me! I could kill him! But at the same time, I keep thinking it must be my own fault.
Encouraging appropriate expression of anger instead of self-blame	*Counselor:*	Elaine, I can see that you're really angry at the guy, and you should be. Any woman would feel the same, but Elaine, you're blaming yourself for this terrible thing instead of him.
Self-doubt, unable to use usual social support	*Elaine:*	Well, deep down I really know it's not my fault, but I think my parents and boyfriend might think so.
Obtaining factual information, exploring resources	*Counselor:*	In other words, you haven't told them about this yet, is that right? Is there anyone you've been able to talk to?
	Elaine:	No, not anyone. I'm too ashamed (starts crying again).
Empathy	*Counselor:*	(listens, waits a few seconds.) I can tell that you're really upset.
Failure in problem solving	*Elaine:*	(continues crying.) I just don't know what to do—I feel like maybe I'll never feel like myself again.
Empathy Suicide risk assessment Feels isolated from social supports	*Counselor:*	This is a serious thing that's happened to you, Elaine. I really want to help you. Considering how upset you are, and not being able to talk with your family and your boyfriend, is there a possibility that you've thought of hurting yourself?

Suicidal ideas only, is reaching out for help	*Elaine:*	Well, the thought has crossed my mind, but no, I really don't think I'd do that—that's why I called here. I just feel so dirty and unwanted—and alone—I know I'm not really a bad person but you just can't believe how awful I feel (starts crying again).
Empathy Involving Elaine in the planning	*Counselor:*	Elaine, I can understand why you must feel that way. Rape is one of the most terrible things that can happen to a woman (waits a few seconds). Elaine, I'd really like to help you through this thing—can we talk about some things that you might do to feel better?
Feels distant from social resources	*Elaine:*	Well, yes—I know I should see a doctor, and I'd really like to talk to my boyfriend and my parents, but I just can't bring myself to do it right now.
Supporting Elaine's decision, direct involvement of counselor, exploring resources	*Counselor:*	I'd recommend, Elaine, that you see a doctor as soon as possible. Do you have a private doctor?
Decision	*Elaine:*	Yes. I'll call and see if I can get in.
	Counselor:	And if you can't get in right away, how about going to a hospital emergency service as soon as possible?
	Elaine:	OK—I'll do that.
Obtaining factual information	*Counselor:*	Elaine, I gather you didn't report this to the police. Is that right?
Helplessness, feeling isolated	*Elaine:*	I didn't think it would do any good, and besides, just like with my boyfriend, I was too ashamed.
Obtaining factual information	*Counselor:*	Were your clothes torn and do you have any bruises from the rape?
	Elaine:	No, not that I'm aware of. I just feel sore all over, so maybe I do have some bruises I can't see. I probably shouldn't have taken a bath before going to the doctor, but, I felt so dirty, I just couldn't stand it.
Reinforcing decision, suggestion to reconsider reporting	*Counselor:*	It's really important, Elaine, that you see your doctor soon. You may also want to reconsider reporting the rape to the police.
	Elaine:	I guess maybe you're right.
Exploring continued crisis counseling possibility	*Counselor:*	Elaine, considering how badly you feel about this and that you don't feel up to talking with your parents and your boyfriend yet, would you like to come in to see a counselor and talk some more about the whole thing?
Needs help in reestablishing contact with significant people in her life	*Elaine:*	Not really . . . anyway, I really feel better now that I've talked with you. But, I still can't really face my parents and boyfriend.
Encouraging further expression of feeling with significant others; paving way for this through crisis counseling	*Counselor:*	This is a lot to handle all at one time. I'm sure you're going to be more upset about it, especially until you're able to talk with your boyfriend and parents about it. That's one of the things a counselor can help you with. . . . A counselor can also help you take a second look at the pros and cons of reporting or not reporting the rape to the police.

TABLE 8.2, CONT.

Mutually agreed-on plan	*Elaine:*	I guess maybe it's a good idea. I do feel better now, but I've been crying off and on since last night—and maybe I'll start crying all over again after I hang up. Besides, I called in sick today because I couldn't face going to work. So I guess I'll stay home tomorrow too and come in and talk to some-body. What time?
Concrete plan mutu-ally arrived at by Elaine and counselor	*Counselor:* *Elaine:* *Counselor:* *Elaine:*	How about 10 o'clock? That's OK, I guess. How are you feeling right now, Elaine? Like I said before, quite a bit better.
Reinforcement of plan	*Counselor:*	Elaine, I'm really glad you called and that you're going to see a doctor and come here to see someone too. Mean-while, if you get upset and feel you want to talk to someone again, please call, as there's always someone here, OK?
	Elaine:	OK, I will—thanks so much for listening.

the woman for life. Whether or not permanent damage occurs depends on two factors: (1) the resources available to the woman for working through the crisis and not blaming herself for the crime; and (2) the woman's precrisis coping ability. If the woman has a supportive social network and a healthy self-concept, she will probably work through the crisis successfully. For women in such circumstances, crisis counseling will usually suffice, and long-term therapy is not indicated. With-out support and healthy precrisis coping, though, psychological scarring can occur, for example, becoming paranoid about all men or unable to relate sexually to one's husband or lover. This danger is increased by a rape trial in which the defense lawyer succeeds in making the victim rather than the rapist appear to be the crim-inal or by her husband and others joining the defense in blaming her for the attack (Estrich, 1987). In these cases, rape victims will probably need longer-term therapy.

In an era of cutbacks in funding for social services, vigilance and advocacy are indicated to assure the continuation of special services to rape victims. In fact, with the current AIDS crisis, additional services are needed to assist the victim through not only the trauma of rape but also the additional crisis of the threat of infection by HIV (see Chapter Fourteen). Peer support groups of other abused women are also helpful. The difficulty of undoing the damage of sexual assault highlights the importance of preventing rape in the first place.

Finally, in regard to child victims, it is important not to project our own shock and horror about the crime onto the child. The child should be treated and sup-ported in proportion to her or his own trauma and perception of the event—phys-ical and psychological—not in proportion to our adult view of the attack. Protection, sympathy, and anger are in order but should not be expressed in a way that might cripple a child's future development and normal interaction with others.

Woman Battering

Abused women say they do not expect us to rescue them. Rather, they want health and crisis workers to be there for them and offer support as they seek safety, healing, and a life without violence. They want us to listen to their terror and dilemmas, as the following vignettes depict:

Vignettes from the Lives of Battered Women

One time when he beat me I started to fight back. . . . He threw kerosene around me and threatened to put a match to it. . . . I never fought back again . . . just kept trying to figure out what I was doing wrong that he would beat me that way. There were some good times together, like when we talked about going to college, and somehow I just kept hoping and believing he would change.

Before I came to this shelter, I had no idea so many other women were going through the same thing I was. . . . I used to think the only way out of my situation would be a tragic one—to kill either myself or him. I'd go to my friend's or mother's house, but I just couldn't make ends meet. I didn't have a baby-sitter, money, or the physical and mental strength. . . . I was depressed about everything. My mother stuck it out for forty years. I didn't believe in divorce; I believed in marriage. Basically, it was my religion and need for financial support [that kept me from leaving earlier] (Hoff, 1990).

Traditionally, it was often assumed that a woman was beaten because the man was drinking, unemployed, or otherwise under stress, or the woman provoked his behavior by saying the wrong thing or failing to meet his whimsical demands. If, for example, a man beat his wife while she was pregnant, it was because "women are so emotional during pregnancy." It was also claimed that women did not leave violent relationships because they were not sufficiently motivated, and they ignored the resources they had. Such conclusions were drawn in spite of the fact that when the same women sought help from the police, family, friends, or health or social service professionals, they received little assistance or were blamed by their confidantes. A "resource" is hardly a resource if it provides a negative response to a woman in crisis.

More recent research (Dobash & Dobash, 1979; Hoff, 1990; Schechter, 1982; Stark, 1984) provides overwhelming evidence that legal, healthcare, and religious institutions support and give tacit approval to woman battering by such actions as:

1. *Defining assault on one's wife as a misdemeanor while the same assault on a stranger is a felony* and then failing to hold violent men accountable even at this level. This

situation is changing with better police training (MacLeod, 1989). Several class action suits brought against large police jurisdictions for failure to arrest and act on abuse prevention laws have also helped to effect change (Gee, 1983).

2. *Diagnosing a battered woman as mentally ill and psychiatrically excusing a violent man.* This practice was uncovered in 1979 by Stark, Flitcraft, and Frazier in a study of 481 battered women using the emergency service of a metropolitan hospital. In this study, "medicine's collective response" to abuse was found to contribute to a "pathological battering syndrome," actually a socially constructed product in the guise of treatment (pp. 462–463). Problems such as alcoholism and depression were treated medically, masking the political aspects of violence. Thus, the abused woman was psychiatrically labeled, suggesting that she was personally responsible for her problems, and violent families were treated to maintain family stability. The researchers state that medical and psychiatric agencies play a major role in the violence related to the political and economic constraints of a patriarchal authority structure (see also, Firsten, 1990; Gondolf, 1987; Hilberman, 1980; Warshaw, 1989). Battered women can relate numerous instances of efforts by professional counselors to uncover "what the woman is doing to provoke her husband to beat her" (Hoff, 1990).

3. *Counseling a woman to stay in a violent relationship "for the sake of the children"* instead of examining the damaging effects of the violence on the children as well (see Bograd, 1984; Warshaw, 1989).

4. *Failing to enforce laws requiring equal pay and job opportunities,* thus making it very difficult for women to support themselves and their children alone.

5. *Failing to provide enough refuge facilities and emotional support for battered women in crisis,* claiming that battering is a private matter between the woman and her husband.

6. *Failing to consider the powerful and complex obstacles a woman faces* when she tries to free herself from violence and blaming the victim instead (Hoff, 1992a, 1993).

While traditional responses to wife battering are damaging enough to women, they are not complimentary to men either. Maintaining simplistic explanations of this complex problem implies that men are less than moral beings. It suggests that they are essentially infants, driven largely by impulse and not responsible for their actions. A recent study (Hoff, 1990), supports earlier research (Dobash & Dobash, 1979; Stark, Flitcraft, & Frazier 1979) and provides new insights into the *process* of violence between spouses. It suggests that violence occurs not merely as a stress response but as a complex interplay between conditions of biological reproduction and economic, political, legal, belief, and knowledge systems of particular historical communities. These interacting systems produce a *context* in which cultural values, the division of labor, and the allocation of power operate to sustain a climate of oppression and conflict. In such a climate, violence against women flourishes, suggesting a link between the *personal* trouble of individual battered women and the *public* issue of women's status.

Prevention

This sociocultural interpretation of why men are violent with their mates and why battered women stay in abusive relationships aids our understanding of the problem. How, though, can this understanding help us deal constructively with the woman who repeatedly calls police and repeatedly receives emergency medical treatment but does not leave the relationship? This cyclic aspect of violence is one of the most complex issues facing police, nurses, physicians, and others trying to help abused women. There is probably nothing more frustrating for a concerned helper than the situation illustrated in the following case example.

CASE EXAMPLE: STAYING IN AN ABUSIVE RELATIONSHIP

A woman calls a hotline, afraid for her own life and worried that she might kill her husband if he returns. She says she wants to come to the shelter and wants to know how she can get there since she has no money. She agrees to a plan to have police come and bring her to a designated place to meet a shelter staff member. The woman never shows up. On follow-up, the shelter volunteer learns that when the police arrived, the woman had changed her mind.

Even people who are sympathetic to the plight of women and eager to help are ready to give up in the face of such apparent resistance to being helped. Such situations make it tempting to blame the victim and assume that if a woman did not like to be beaten she would take advantage of available help. A helper can avoid falling into this trap by (1) remembering that the issue is much larger than the immediate crisis of a particular woman, and (2) realizing that the woman has reasons for staying, whether or not the helper understands or agrees with those reasons. Some of these reasons might be (1) fear of the unknown and how she can manage without her husband's financial support, (2) continued hope and belief that the man will act on his frequent promises and stop beating her, and (3) fear of retaliation—even murder—after she leaves the shelter unless she leaves the area permanently. The experience of women in shelters reveals that some men employ elaborate detective strategies to find a woman who has left. Some who find a woman in a shelter threaten to harm all the shelter residents unless the woman returns. This is why many shelters maintain a secret location.

The complexity of the problem is illustrated further by an analysis of what happens after the *first* time a woman is beaten. She faces a difficult situation: the first violent incident usually is very shocking to her ("How could he do this to me?") and is followed by the man's elaborate promises never to do it again. The woman believes him and decides not to leave. This apparently rational decision is reinforced by positive, valued aspects of the relationship that the woman wishes to salvage. When the man beats her a second time, he not only has broken his promise but has distorted her trust and belief in his word into justification for beating her again ("If she didn't think it was all right for me to beat her, she'd leave."). The cycle is reinforced by the man's blaming his behavior on the woman—she doesn't cook right, dress right, or respect him—which she increasingly absorbs and believes. This complex interactional process underscores the importance of preventing violence in the first place. Once this cycle begins, it is very difficult to interrupt. Thus, our prevention efforts should focus on the following:

1. *Reinforcing and educating police, health, and social service workers about the Abuse Protection Acts,* which define wife abuse as a crime punishable by law. Through the battered women's movement, these laws have been updated in North American states and provinces. Recent crime legislation in the United States also describes battering as a gender-based civil rights violation. Legal information about battering can be obtained from local shelters, the police, and government offices concerned with this issue.

2. *Examining educational, social, and religious programs for their implicit support of violence* through socialization of boys and men to aggressive behavior and girls and women to passive, dependent behavior (Broverman, et al., 1970; Sadker & Sadker, 1994). This process reinforces the view of wives as appropriate objects of violence.

3. *Instituting campaigns to end the marketing of pornography* and other products of popular culture that portray women as objects and glorify violence against them.

4. *Enforcing the Equal Pay Act,* passed in the United States in 1967, and *improving child care and economic and educational services* for women so that financial and educational disadvantages do not prevent them from leaving violent relationships.

5. *Instituting community-wide consciousness-raising groups* for men and women and focusing on ways to promote egalitarian marriage and break out of dominant or excessively dependent behavior patterns.

These and other "upstream" preventive strategies should be carried out in tandem with immediate intervention for women in acute crisis (see Figure 8.1, Box 3). (For a detailed discussion of the obstacles faced by abused women and ways these can be removed, see Hoff, 1992a; 1993.)

Crisis Intervention

Assistance during crisis should be available to women from family and friends. However, relatives and friends often view marital violence as a private issue and are reluctant to get involved. They may also be afraid of getting hurt themselves or making things worse.

Vignette from the Life of a Battered Woman

Until I found out about and came to the shelter, I kept thinking I was the only one. I didn't have any idea so many other women were in the same boat. I was so ashamed and kept thinking that it somehow must have been my fault. He told me it was my fault and I believed him—though I still don't know what I did wrong because I was always trying to second-guess and please him so I wouldn't get beaten (Hoff, 1990).

The least a relative or friend can do is to put a woman in touch with local crisis hotlines, which have staff prepared to deal with the problem. Since many battered women call the police and contact emergency medical resources, putting these women in touch with crisis workers is the first and most important thing emergency workers can do after providing medical treatment and safety planning.

Two factors, however, may impede the accomplishment of this task: some women do not acknowledge the cause of their physical injuries, or they provide a cover-up story. There are several reasons for this: (1) the woman may have been threatened by her mate with a more severe beating if she reveals the beating; (2) she may simply not be ready to leave for her own reasons; (3) she may sense the judgmental or unsympathetic attitude of a physician or nurse and therefore not confide the truth. Because of social isolation, prejudice, and fear of deportation, immigrant minority and refugee women who are abused usually face additional impediments to receiving help (Jang, Lee, & Morello-Frosch, 1991).

Sensitivity to these factors will help us interpret a woman's evasiveness about her injuries and recognize the implausibility of a cover-up story. Besides physical injuries, a battered woman will show other signals of distress or emotional crisis (Hollenkamp & Attala, 1986; Sugg & Inui, 1992). Medical and nursing staff who use a crisis assessment tool such as discussed earlier in this book can more accurately identify and appropriately respond to a battered woman in crisis (Hoff & Rosenbaum, 1994). As is true in dealing with a person at risk of being suicidal, it is appropriate to question a woman directly, which will probably result in her being relieved to know that someone is caring and sensitive enough to discern her distress. And, like suicidal people, if a woman refuses to acknowledge the battering, her refusal may have more to do with our attitude than with her willingness to disclose (Hoff, 1992a).

The important techniques to remember in these situations are: (1) withhold judgment, (2) assist the woman with safety planning, and (3) provide the woman at least with written information—a card or brochure with the numbers of hotlines and women's support groups. This seemingly small response is central to the process of the woman's eventual decision to leave the violent relationship (Hoff, 1993). The reason to have confidence in the value of such a response is that a woman feels empowered if she believes others respect her decision, even if it is to stay in the violent relationship for the time being. She also needs explicit recognition from us that ultimately it is *her* decision that makes the difference and that she can take credit for the decision. Since battered women often feel powerless and unrespected, we should convey to them that they are in charge of their lives. When a woman *believes* this, it becomes a premise for her eventual action. Thus, while a woman may not be ready for more than emergency medical treatment, she at least has the necessary information if she decides to use it in the future. These principles apply to police officers as well as health workers.

It is also important to assure abused women that they are not responsible for their victimization, no matter what the person who battered them says to the contrary (see Figure 2.2 in Chapter Two). In order to do this, we must be convinced that, except in self-defense, violence is not justified no matter what happens in the interaction or the relationship. Even when used in self-defense, a return of violence often escalates rather than decreases the violence (see "Assessing the Risk of Assault and Homicide," Chapter Nine). In addition, we should not assume that battered women are routinely in need of therapy; this could add a psychiatric label to an already heavy burden (Stark, Flitcraft, & Frazier, 1979). If a woman is suicidal, the principles and techniques discussed in Chapters Six and Seven apply.

Once a woman is treated for physical trauma and resolves the dilemma of what to do next, she may be faced with the crises of finding emergency housing, caring for her children, and obtaining money. If a community does not have a safe home network or emergency shelter, if a woman cannot stay with relatives, and if she has no money, she may have little choice but to return to the violent situation. When a woman decides to leave, up-to-date abuse prevention laws require police to accompany her to her home to get her children, legal documents, and whatever possessions she can bring to an emergency housing situation. Once the woman is in a shelter or linked to a support group network, further assistance is available to deal with legal, housing, and other aspects of the crisis (NiCarthy, 1989).

When a woman is battered, her children are affected as well. Often, the children have either observed the abuse or have been abused themselves (Ericksen & Henderson, 1992; Jaffe, et al., 1990). An important element of helping a mother in crisis, as well as her children, is making child care services available. The mother needs time away from children to deal with housing and other problems. The children, on the other hand, are often highly anxious and in need of a stable, calming influence as well as appropriate physical outlets and nonviolent discipline.

Follow-Up Service

When a battered woman has successfully dealt with the crisis aspect of her situation, the biggest decision she faces is whether or not to leave her partner permanently. Some women take months to make this decision, even after living in a safe environment for some time. Peer support groups of other women who have been battered and have broken out of violent relationships are probably the most valuable resource for a woman at this time. Such groups are important for several reasons:

1. If a woman decides to return to her partner, hoping for a change, and the battering continues, it is important that she know there are people who will not judge her for her decisions.
2. Many women come to shelters convinced that they are psychologically disturbed and in need of a therapist. They have absorbed the message that the battering occurred because of something wrong with them. When they begin

to feel strong and in charge of their lives, they may discover that a therapist is not needed after all and that other women can help them in ways they had not imagined. This discovery is a significant contrast to the traditional view of other women as "competition" in what many perceive as the all-important life task of catching and holding a man. Finding alternatives to therapy occurs most often in shelters that actively encourage women to assume charge of their lives. It also happens through the process of decision making and taking action to obtain housing, money, and legal services. Observing women in responsible, independent, collaborative, and caring roles in shelter staffing also seems to help. After feeling powerless for so long, a woman does not need a program that dictates every hour and detail of her life.[3]

3. These support experiences may provide the basis for battered women to join, if they wish, a wider network of women working on the larger social, political, and economic aspects of stopping violence against women. A woman's positive experience of support while in crisis is the best preparation for such possible involvement.

If women request therapy, referrals should be made to therapists working from a woman's perspective (e.g., Burstow, 1992; Greenspan, 1983; Mirkin, 1994). Therapy may be indicated if, after crisis intervention and social network support, a woman continues to be depressed and suicidal or finds herself unable to make decisions and break out of patterns of dependency and self-blame. When the violent marriage and abuse of the children have left damaging scars, family therapy is indicated.

Other aspects of follow-up include:

- An opportunity for the woman to grieve and mourn the loss of a relationship if she finally decides to leave (see "Loss, Change, and Grief Work" in Chapter Four)
- For women who wish to marry again, a group in which to examine and share with others the complex aspects of avoiding relationships that may lead to a repeat of excessive dependency and violence (Campbell, 1986)
- Parent effectiveness groups to explore nonviolent ways of dealing with children

The preventive, crisis, and follow-up aspects of helping battered women should be practiced with a view to their vital connectedness. This triple approach to the problem may not only help to end the pain and terror of women who are attacked but may also remove the negative consequences of violence for children, men, and the entire society (Hoff, 1990). Exhibit 8.2 presents an example of

---

[3]Information about local shelter services can be obtained from a crisis or community mental health center, a hospital emergency department, or the police. Information about programs for men who batter can be obtained from Emerge, 2380 Massachusetts Avenue, Suite 101, Cambridge, MA 02140; telephone (617) 422–1550; fax (617) 547–0904.

EXHIBIT 8.2. CASE ILLUSTRATION: CRISIS COUNSELING WITH A BATTERED WOMAN.

CASE ILLUSTRATION: SANDRA LECLAIRE

Mrs. Sandra LeClaire is a twenty-two-year-old woman who is currently separated from her abusive husband of five years. She is the mother of two small children, ages two and five. She does not work for pay and is in the process of applying for welfare. Her husband has been her sole source of financial support, and since their separation nine months ago, his support has been sporadic at best. Mrs. LeClaire's visit today is one of several she has made to an emergency department. She presented today with cuts and bruises about her face and across her chest, and two black eyes that are swollen shut—all as a result of a beating by her husband. Mrs. LeClaire says this beating was the culmination of an argument over her husband's lack of financial support to her and her children. She has never been willing to press charges against her husband out of fear, since he has threatened to kill her. She has been drinking more frequently and heavily and is becoming increasingly depressed and despondent about her situation. Mrs. LeClaire has suicidal ideation, but denies having a specific plan, although in the past she has thought of taking Tylenol when upset with her husband.

Mrs. LeClaire became pregnant at age sixteen. She quit high school and married her present husband. She grew up in poverty, the youngest of five children with an alcoholic father and a "born-again" church-going mother. She viewed her marriage as a way out.

Although her father worked steadily, he did not earn enough money to support both his family and his drinking. Her mother did not believe in divorce. She raised the children and largely ignored her husband's drinking, sustaining many beatings herself at his hands. While Mrs. LeClaire feels supported by her mother, who helps her with child care, she does not feel understood. Her mother believes God will provide. She tells Sandra it is just a phase men go through and that things will improve for Sandra as they have for her, since Sandra's father has grown less violent over the years; Sandra is not sure she can wait.

Sandra's first language is Haitian Creole; her second is English. She has problems with getting welfare—she cannot complete the forms. Her abusive husband is also a drinker. Sandra had no drinking problem prior to her abuse.

how crisis counseling with a battered woman might proceed; Exhibit 8.3 depicts a service contract drawn up in a counseling session.

Session One

Using an extended version of the Comprehensive Mental Health Assessment Guide discussed in Chapter Three, the problems and issues Mrs. LeClaire faces could be summarized as follows:

EXHIBIT 8.3 SERVICE CONTRACT: A BATTERING SITUATION.

1. Physical Health	7. Feeling Management	13. Immediate Family/Household	19. Suicide Risk
2. Violence Experienced	8. Decision-Making/Empowerment	14. Caretaking/Leisure Time	20. Assault/Homicide Risk
3. Relationship with Abuser	9. Problem Solving	15. Residential	21. Legal
4. Composite Victimization Rating	10. Agency Use	16. Safety—Self	22. Substance/Use/Abuse
5. Self-Esteem	11. Vocational/Occupational	17. Safety—Children	
6. Life Goal Satisfaction	12. Intimacy/Significant Other	18. Financial Security	

Item/Stress Rating	Problem/Issue Specification	Strategies/Techniques (planned actions of client and crisis worker)
16. Safety–Self (5)	Husband threatened to kill her	*Explore* (a) shelter option; (b) changing locks; (c) restraining order (d) feelings regarding use of these options.
4. Victimization (4)	Does not seem clear about extent of danger	*Provide information about* (a) shelter number and admission process (brochures/cards); (b) emergency phone number.
19. Suicide Risk (3)	Suicidal ideation	*Discuss/listen* to feelings of hopelessness and reluctance to confide in close friend.
	No specific plan or past attempts	*Provide* number of suicide prevention/crisis hotline.
5. Self-Esteem (4)	Increasingly depressed	Sandra agrees to (a) call/reconnect with friend within 3 days; (b) dispose of her supply of Tylenol; (c) call hotline if very despondent and feeling impulse to take pills.
18. Financial Security (4)	Husband/abuser is sole source of support	*Review* the welfare application forms to ascertain Sandra's understanding.
	Has language trouble with welfare forms	*Explore* Sandra's ambivalence regarding financial aid vs. continued attempt to obtain support from husband.
22. Substance Use/Abuse (3)	Never drank before battering	*Discuss* feelings, etc., about referral to substance abuse treatment program.
	Now drinking more frequently	*Provide* names, dates, places of local accessible programs.
		Sandra agrees to (a) choose and phone one source; (b) keep a journal record of drinking context and other possible options when upset.
		Agree to discuss other 2 priority items (goals/decisions about marriage and social support) during second or later session.

Signatures: Client _____   _____ Crisis Worker

Stress Rating Code: 5 = very high stress; 1 = very low stress

- Safety
- Suicidality
- Financial support
- Substance use/abuse
- Goals/decisions regarding marriage
- Social support

Exhibit 8.3 illustrates these issues and the action plan Sandra and the crisis worker developed as a Service Contract in her first crisis counseling session. Such a session would occur following initial assessment and referral by a triage nurse and the physician treating Mrs. LeClaire's injuries. Typically, the full crisis assessment is done by a crisis team member, usually in liaison with triage nurses and physicians. At Boston City Hospital, for example, this function is carried out by psychiatric nurses; at the Ottawa General Hospital, crisis counseling is done by social workers. Crisis counseling as illustrated here is also done by family practice physicians and advanced practice nurses across specialties.

Following are illustrations of how crisis counseling might proceed on behalf of Mrs. LeClaire. In general, the sessions are balanced between structure, an aid to making order out of the chaos of trauma, and openness, which facilitates compassionate regard and empowerment. Typically, there would be six to ten sessions, with attention to the interface between crisis and chronic problems as discussed in Chapter Five.

Session Two

The second session would focus on the following:

- Explore feeling state and urgent issues
- Review safety and progress with action planned from last session
- Examine barriers to progress with planned action
- Identify any new problems
- Negotiate new or revised action plan

Progress notes and an action plan following Session Two might include:

Progress Notes

- Feels less despondent and suicidal
- Does not want to go to a shelter, at least not now
- Discussed women's support group as alternative
- Feels ambivalent about restraining order on husband
- Drinking about the same
- Did not call substance abuse treatment source
- Did not go to welfare office; would like someone to go with her

Action Plan

- Continue suicide crisis plan.
- Continue journal regarding drinking pattern; re-think calling AA or other treatment source.
- Call advocate and arrange visit to welfare office; also, discuss nature of battered women's support group during outing to welfare office with advocate.

Remaining Sessions

Each of the remaining sessions would include:

- Identification of any urgent issues, particularly safety
- General review of mood
- Review of progress with previous action plan
- Identification of any new problems/barriers to progress
- Decision counseling around any issues identified
- Negotiated plan for next steps, strategies, and actions regarding problems, including time and place of next appointment

Possible Problems, Issues, and Barriers to Progress

As crisis counseling proceeds with Mrs. LeClaire, new problems and issues may emerge, for example:

1. *Indecision/ambivalence about divorce.* Sandra may say, "I don't want to be one of those welfare mothers," or "if only he'd get some help for his drinking," or "maybe if I were just more patient when he gets angry."

Action plan: Listen to feelings, fears; discuss pros and cons regarding separation, divorce, and future safety; explore level of financial support (husband, welfare, self); consider possibility of job training; discuss self-blame and issue of accountability for violence.

2. *Need for social support.* Sandra feels lonely, wishes her mother were more understanding; advocate gave her information about a battered women's support group, but she does not feel like going—would rather be able to communicate better with her mother; feels ashamed to have her problem known beyond her family.

Action plan: Explore feelings of shame; reconsider calling AA as an alternative source of support; explore possibility of a joint session with mother to air issues, goals and possible further support.

Husband Beating

This discussion is incomplete without attention to the controversial issue of husband beating. Women as well as men can be violent; not to acknowledge this fact is equivalent to viewing women as less than moral beings, in the same way that excusing male violence implies that men are less than moral beings. Women, like men, should be held accountable for their behavior.

It has been suggested that the "real" domestic problem is husband battering, and that the reason it is still hidden is that it is too much of an assault on the male ego to acknowledge the shame of having been beaten by a woman. A national survey on domestic violence revealed that in *numbers* of violent acts—*not in quality or context*—women and men were approximately equal (Straus, 1993; Straus, Gelles, & Steinmetz, 1980). This statistical finding, however, needs to be qualified: when women are violent, it is primarily in self-defense, and their attacks are not as dangerous or physically injurious as are those of men (Kurz, 1993). Also, when women kill their mates, it is usually after years of abuse, and they do so less frequently than men kill their wives (Browne, 1987; Jones, 1980). Considering also the fact that at least 25 percent of pregnant women have a current or past history of being battered, the contrast is even more dramatic (Stark, 1984).

The pattern of injustice and violence used primarily in self-defense should be kept in mind in trials of women who kill abusive husbands. Rather than medicalizing the woman's case by a contrived "insanity plea," women should have a fair trial on self-defense grounds when the evidence points in that direction. The suggestion that husband beating is more rampant than wife battering covers up the roots of violence against women in traditional social structures and the low socioeconomic status of women that allows violence to flourish. To claim an equal problem of husband battering belies reality, especially as it is revealed in emergency settings and in the differences in physical strength between most men and women. The majority of men are physically more capable of inflicting injury than are women. In addition, men who are beaten have much more freedom to leave because of their socioeconomic advantage in society and relative freedom from child care.

Battering of Lesbian, Gay, and Bisexual Partners

Prevention and intervention strategies for battered women apply to those in lesbian, gay, or bisexual relationships. Additional factors to be considered arise from the bias and social isolation faced by most of these couples; individuals in these relationships usually rely more heavily than others on their partners for emotional support and companionship. As discussed in Chapter Five, excessive dependency in any intimate relationship may be the source of additional stressors that constitute the context in which abuse occurs. In addition, gay men are more vulnerable than lesbian women to violence from strangers or associates motivated explicitly by antigay bias or homophobia.

The extraordinary stress experienced by couples in alternative lifestyles is compounded by stereotypes and the bias that keeps them isolated in the first place. One such stereotype is that "all lesbians are feminists," and since a battering lesbian partner has violated the feminist agenda of nonviolence, she is thus deemed less deserving of help. Another stereotype is that women become lesbians because they have been victims of sexual abuse. In reality, all lesbian women are not feminists, and some feminists are just as homophobic as others might be. Also, many women have been sexually abused as children; most are heterosexual. Finally, since lesbian, gay, and bisexual people are members of a larger cultural community just as others are, why would they be exempt from having absorbed the pervasive message of violence as a control strategy and a solution to conflict resolution? Their disadvantaged social position may result in greater sensitivity to issues of abuse generally, but they face even greater odds in avoiding violence than the general population.

To provide appropriate service for victims in alternative lifestyles, it is imperative that crisis workers examine attitudes that can prevent a battered lesbian woman from disclosing her plight and receiving the help she needs. In general, the legacy of victim-blaming experienced by battered women is exacerbated with regard to lesbian women (Lobel, 1986; Renzetti, 1992).

Abuse of Older Persons

Attention to abuse of older people is gaining increasing international attention (MacLean, 1995; McDonald, et al., 1991; Pillemer & Wolf, 1986). Elder abuse includes the willful infliction of physical injury or debilitating mental anguish, financial exploitation, and unreasonable confinement or deprivation of necessary care and services. Earlier, public attention was focused on abuse and substandard care in nursing homes. In spite of the prevalence of institutional care of the elderly in U.S. society, the majority of elders (95 percent) live alone or with family or other caretakers. The victims are overwhelmingly female, with 58 percent of women victims naming their spouse as the attacker and 24 percent naming a son or daughter as the aggressor (Pillemer & Finkelhor, 1987). Although abuse and neglect may occur in institutions, legal protections limit such abuse. In private settings, legal protections are more difficult to enforce because of civil rights and family privacy issues (*Elder Abuse*, 1991). This discussion is particularly relevant to community health nurses, home health aides, pastors, and other professionals offering consultation and supervision on behalf of older people cared for at home.

Why are elders abused? As already noted, there are parallels between battered children and elders: (1) they are in a dependent position for survival; (2) they are presumed to be protected by love, gentleness, and caring; (3) they are a source of emotional, physical, and financial stress for the caretaker, particularly if the older person is physically or mentally impaired (Sommers & Shields, 1987).

Several other factors can be identified in tracing the roots of elder abuse. Inattention to these factors can form obstacles to prevention, crisis intervention, and follow-up service for older people at risk:

1. *Social:* In the nuclear family structure, there is often no social, physical, and economic room for elders. For example, death rituals in traditional African societies include transfer of social responsibility held by the deceased (Goody, 1962; Chapter Thirteen). In modern societies, an older person's body may linger long after social death occurs. Responsibility for the care of older people is complicated by the trend of women working outside the home while maintaining their traditional home responsibilities as well.

2. *Cultural:* U.S. society is noted for idolizing youth and devaluing the elderly. The cultural emphasis on economic productivity tends to eclipse elders' contributions of wisdom, life experience, and often, continued work. Consequently, elders often lack status, respect, and similar rewards that are taken for granted in other societies. The culture of violence as it affects children and women flows over to the elderly as well; older, abused women are referred to as "forgotten victims" (McLeod, 1994, p 1). In spite of elders' increasing political influence, ageism is still rampant, particularly with respect to older women (Doress & Siegal, 1987).

3. *Economic:* The poverty of many old people is an almost inevitable result of the social and cultural factors noted above. Strong economic motives for protecting children often do not extend to the elderly. In addition, spiraling inflation for caretakers and inadequate home care services increase further the risk of elder abuse (Estes, 1986).

4. *Psychological:* One of the normal features of growing old is a decreased capacity to control impulses and adjust to change. A lifelong pattern of inflexibility can result in a demanding, unpleasant personality in old age. Considering also the interaction between physical dependence and fear of retaliation, elder abuse can remain hidden for some time. Elders abused by adult children—not unlike battered women—will feel deep shame and try to account for the abuse in terms of their own failure as parents. They say, in effect, "What kind of a parent am I that my own child would turn on me in my helplessness and old age?"

5. *Legal:* Civil liberties in democratic societies protect one's right to privacy, self-determination, and the refusal of services. Although most jurisdictions now have Adult Protective Service authorities, all do not require mandatory reporting of suspected elder abuse cases as in cases of suspected child abuse. These factors, combined with an abused elder's shame and fear of retaliation, constitute formidable barriers to dealing effectively with elder abuse.

Prevention, Crisis Intervention, and Follow-Up Service

As with crises discussed earlier, prevention, crisis intervention, and follow-up are interrelated and demand awareness of the origins of the crisis. Preventive measures related to the sociocultural and economic aspects of elder abuse suggest an examination of values regarding old people. Social and political changes affecting the elderly are also needed, such as provision of tax and insurance benefits for families who would care for an older person at home if they could add a room to their house and obtain home health-care assistance without serious financial hardship. Psychologically, we can reduce the risk of elder abuse by preparing for the social, economic, and physical realities of later life (see Chapter Thirteen for a detailed discussion). As we prepare for old age, it is wise to remember that old people with unpleasant personalities are the same as young people with unpleasant personalities, only in exaggerated form.

Crisis intervention for older people at risk of abuse demands careful application of the assessment, planning, and intervention strategies discussed in Chapters Three, Four, and Five, with particular attention to social network approaches. Emergency medical care and crisis intervention for abused elders are complicated for two reasons:

1. *Mental incapacity or confusion on the part of the elder.* State and provincial departments of mental health and elder affairs have standard protocols for these cases. Involuntary commitment or appointment of a legal guardian requires clear and convincing evidence that the adult in question is incapacitated mentally and that an emergency exists. When these legal actions are taken, they should be based on the principle of "least restrictive alternative" and the guarantee of civil liberties.
2. *Misplaced emergency care or crisis intervention.* Carelessness in this area of care for elderly people or the use of inappropriate "savior" tactics can alienate family members who may be needed in the long term. Considering shame, possible retaliation, and the dynamics of family loyalty, follow-up after the emergency as well as future crisis intervention will be very difficult if family members are alienated. Unless foster care is readily available, great care must be taken to prevent complicating further an already difficult situation. Thus, while laws now exist for reporting elder abuse—similar to the Good Samaritan laws protecting children—overzealous action on these laws should not become the occasion for precipitating more trouble.

Application of Intervention and Follow-Up Principles

The following example reveals the intersection of caretaker stress and elder abuse. It also shows the importance of careful teamwork in responding to such abuse.

CASE EXAMPLE: MARTHA

Martha, age eighty-two, suffered crippling arthritis and heart disease. She was visited regularly in her daughter's home by a home health aide who bathed her three times a week. The rest of the time, her daughter Jane, age fifty-five, gave her medicine and helped her out of bed and into a chair when she had time. Jane worked full-time as a legal secretary. Jane's husband Robert, age sixty-three, was at home most of the day. He had been on disability support for ten years after seriously injuring his back doing construction work. For the most part, Robert felt useless, although he did help with shopping and laundry. The disabilities of both her mother and husband left Jane feeling very stressed.

The home health worker discovered black and blue marks on Martha's chest and back and suspected that abuse was occurring. Her attempts to talk to Martha about

this were met by silence. The aide reported her observation to the visiting nurse, who in turn consulted a social worker. (The nurse had known this family for over a year and visited the home approximately once a month in a supervisory, coordinating, and teaching capacity.) The nurse then called Jane and suggested that she be seen by the social worker to discuss the problems of taking care of her mother. Even though the nurse did not directly mention the suspicion of abuse, Jane felt threatened, refused to act on the suggestion, dismissed the nurse and home health aide, and hired a private nurse to care for Martha around the clock to "prove" she was not neglectful of her mother. This move was a great financial burden for the family. Three months later, Jane again requested service for her mother from the home health agency.

Several things seem very clear in this example: (1) everyone concerned appeared to be well-intentioned; (2) Jane was alienated by the approach used by the nurse; (3) the problem was complicated by an inappropriate intervention strategy. The nurse seemed to lack confidence in her ability to take on a key role in intervention; she assumed that a social worker was the more appropriate person to act, in spite of her own year-long relationship with the family.

Success in dealing with sensitive issues like these depends very much on the quality of the relationship between the caregiver and receiver. If the nurse had recognized this, she would not have suggested what Jane interpreted as an accusation that she neglected her mother. Instead, the nurse might have used other intervention and follow-up strategies:

1. After hearing the aide's report, the nurse could have planned an extra visit to the home to spend some time with Martha and Jane individually to further assess the situation. To facilitate communication about the issue, the nurse might have bathed Martha herself once as a way of gaining her confidence. A concerned rather than accusatory approach to Jane might have resulted in Jane's revealing voluntarily the stress and exasperation she experienced in carrying out her multiple responsibilities. Their conversation might have proceeded as follows:

Nurse: How are things going, Jane, with all the things you have to juggle these days? I know that Terri, the aide, has been coming in three times a week. Do you think you're getting all the help you need?

Jane: Well, it's hard, but somehow I'm managing. On the days I have to get Mother out of bed myself I sometimes feel like a nervous wreck—she screams with pain when I touch her. I can't stand the thought of putting Mother in a home, but sometimes I don't know.

Nurse: So, it seems things are pretty rough for you, Jane? I was in to see your mother this week while Terri was bathing and dressing her, and I noticed several black and blue marks. (Nurse tries to keep the aide's relationship with the family intact.) She wouldn't talk about it though, so I'm wondering whether things are getting too difficult for you and if maybe we could be of more help to you.

Jane: If you're thinking I hit my mother, well, I didn't. A couple of times I might have handled her kind of roughly; she's really frail and thin, you know. But I certainly never hit her—after all, she's my mother.

Nurse: This is a really touchy thing to talk about, Jane, and I don't mean to accuse you of anything. I know it must be very difficult at times. What I'm suggesting is that we work on this together to be sure both you and your mother get what you need. I know that you want the best possible care for your mother, and it seems like Robert's disability might wear on you, too. Can you tell me more about the problems you have in taking care of your mother?

Problem exploration continues in this vein; the session ends with agreement to talk again the next week to work on the problem uncovered. It never becomes explicit whether Jane did or did not abuse her mother. It is not a good strategy to try to prove that abuse occurred when the old person is refusing to talk and the caretaker is denying it. It is more important to focus on the underlying issues related to abuse.

2. If, after this, the nurse still does not feel confident about proceeding, she might consult the social worker but not turn the problem over to her.

3. The nurse might also talk with Jane's husband to see whether he might become more helpful with household tasks.

4. After exploring the problem with everyone concerned, a social network conference might be indicated (see Chapter Five). This would include Martha, Jane, Robert, Terri, and possibly a social worker consultant and a representative from Respite Services, which should be discussed as one avenue of relief for Jane.

As the proportion of elders in the population increases, there is hope for favorable political change for elder affairs. With increasing public sensitivity to the problems of elders, we may devise more creative ways to foster the conditions for peace, safety, and health and social services during the later years. Changes are already occurring with New Age families, the Foster Grandparent Program, intergenerational housing experiments, and comprehensive health and other services delivered in home settings. The latter include, for example, around ten people of various ages, with 60 percent over sixty, living in a large, ordinary family home. Each person has a separate room; other areas and general tasks are shared communally. Elders who participate in these programs feel socially useful, with beneficial effects for physical and mental health and less chance of violence directed against them.

Battering of Parents and Teachers by Children

The abuse of infirm and dependent elders by adult children differs from another aspect of violence in families: the physical abuse of parents by their children. A national survey by Straus, Gelles, and Steinmetz (1980) revealed that almost 10 percent of children ages three to eighteen attacked their parents. A pilot psychiatric study by Harbin and Madden (1979, p. 1288) uncovered repeated attacks on, or threats against, parents by more than half the adolescents in fifteen families. Parricide, the most extreme form of parental assault, is usually associated with severe parental sexual and physical abuse of the child (Mones, 1993). Research suggests that in less lethal assaults, the teenagers may "want to punish their parents for having exploited them through permissiveness and lack of leadership" (Harbin & Madden, 1979, p. 1290). The adolescent feels insecure and entrapped when forced, through lack of parental authority, to assume an independent role before feeling developmentally ready.

Parents experiencing abuse by their children are in a "Catch 22" dilemma: like their elder counterparts, confronting the situation implies an admission of failure at parenting; not confronting it reinforces the child's misplaced sense of omnipotence and need to control others (Harbin & Madden, 1979, p. 1290).

Preventive strategies are similar to those discussed for child and elder abuse: at the societal level, fostering nonviolent solutions to child rearing and greater respect for the elderly can reinforce parental authority. Crisis and follow-up strategies include parent effectiveness training or, if necessary, family therapy. In addition, parents should have access to help during crisis without shame or denial of the problem. Crisis intervention planning with such families should feature nonviolent tactics that a child can use when angry at a parent. Parents, too, need alternatives to giving in to children who behave like dictators (Charney, 1993; Judson, 1984).

Parents, however, are not the only ones abused by violent children. For years, teachers have been terrorized, raped, knifed, and attacked in other ways (Walker, 1993). The same issues are at stake here: social and cultural approval of violence, poverty, racism, loss of respect for parental and other authority, and the need to listen to children. The widespread neglect of inner-city public schools and the disadvantages to students who attend them must also be remedied if we wish to stem the large-scale loss of disaffected, traumatized, and burned-out teachers. Poorly supported schools cannot be solely responsible for the intellectual and moral training of children (Long & Wilder, 1993).

In many communities, a violence-prevention curriculum has been instituted (Eggert, 1994; Prothrow-Stith, 1986). Teens are taught nonviolent approaches to conflict resolution, and troubled teens and their families are referred to hotlines and other crisis intervention services.

Other Sources of Victimization

Besides abuse from one's own family or spouse, there are many other sources of violent crime. During 1992, 6.6 million people in the United States were victims of crimes such as assault or rape. Of these, nearly one in four were between twelve and seventeen, with African-American male teens at highest risk. Public opinion polls reveal continued concern about crime, even though the U.S. Justice Department crime statistics show declining rates. People are angry and afraid. They blame their unease on the media, the courts, television, pornography, the economy, drugs, poor housing conditions, indifference to the poor, racial tension and discrimination, poverty, youth gangs, the police, handguns, and the disintegration of the American family. In the United States, there are nearly as many firearms as there are people, along with widespread denial of scientific evidence showing that the presence of guns *decreases* rather than increases safety. The significantly lower rates of homicide and other assaults in Canada and Western European countries are attributed to stringent gun control laws and related cultural factors. As Jackson (1994, p. 13) notes, nothing will come of public outrage over children killing children "unless the grownups have had enough of guns."

No doubt, each of the factors mentioned plays some part in this complex problem. Fear of crime seems to generate chronic stress, worry, paranoia, and a sense of helplessness. If no arrests are made and criminals receive light sentences or acquittals, victims and the general public often feel that no one cares or that there is no justice. These feelings can lead to alienation, revenge, and a sense of callousness and insensitivity to others. This may account for the returning popularity of the death penalty and for the widespread public support of caning in Singapore and of Bernhard Goetz, who felt entitled to take the law into his own hands when he felt threatened and shot people on the New York subway system.

Victim Assistance After a Crime

What is the ordinary citizen's role in assisting victims of crime? In France, such assistance is mandated by law; in the United States it is not. Should we intervene on the victim's behalf or ignore a crime? In a frequently cited case in New York

City, Kitty Genovese was attacked more than twenty years ago late one night while people in at least a dozen households listened to her screams. Nobody went to help or even bothered to call the police from the safety of their own homes. In contrast today, many groups of people are organizing neighborhood patrols and other means of coming to the aid of people victimized by crime. Every would-be helper faces the dilemma of whether and how to intervene in a crime. A basic principle of crisis intervention is to protect oneself from getting hurt while assisting others. While some people voluntarily sacrifice their lives for others, such a sacrifice is neither expected nor demanded. Not intervening out of fear for one's own safety is fair enough. But not to mobilize police on behalf of a victim is a failure to meet the obligations implicit in our common humanity.

There is now a specialty field called "victimology," complete with journals and professional conferences. Yet at the practical level, victims of crime seem cruelly shortchanged in the criminal justice, emergency medical, and crisis service systems (Surgeon General's Workshop, 1986). Through federal task forces (President's Task Force on Victims of Crime, 1982; Attorney General's Task Force on Family Violence, 1984) and the advocacy and lobbying of the National Organization for Victim Assistance (NOVA), many communities now have victim assistance programs, as do some crisis centers. In general, however, there are no constitutional protections for victims, nor is there much special training for police and emergency medical personnel in meeting the special needs of victims. NOVA has been instrumental in improving this situation, particularly through its Crisis Response Team, which offers service in instances of community-wide trauma such as the massacre of fourteen postal employees in Edmond, Oklahoma.[4]

Funding of victim assistance programs is a continuing struggle; funding has often been focused on programs that try to understand and reform the criminal. This is not to say that criminals' needs should be ignored, but, as stated in the Presidential Task Force (1982, p. vi) hearing on victims of crime, "If we take the justice out of the criminal justice system, we leave behind a system which serves only the criminal." Indeed, the visibility of victims and their needs should benefit even the criminal.

Since the Presidential Task Force and the Attorney General's hearings, federal legislation has supported the development of victim witness and assistance programs in the states. These include the development of self-help groups, training of victim advocates, and a plan for financial assistance to victims. Similar programs have been instituted in Canada, England, and other countries.

Meanwhile, greater attention should be focused on the needs of victims in emergency medical, police, and criminal justice systems. Victims are people in cri-

[4]For further information, contact NOVA, 1757 Park Road, NW, Washington, DC 20010; telephone (202) 232–6682; fax (202) 462–2255. Omega Emotional Support Services, Inc., is an example of a local agency offering special assistance to people who have lost loved ones through violence. This group can be contacted at 34 Heath Street, Somerville, MA 02145; telephone (617) 776–6369.

sis who should have the advantage of being listened to and helped by workers who are sensitive, knowledgeable, and skilled in crisis intervention. The report of the Surgeon General's Workshop on Violence and Public Health (1986) recommends that information about the care of victims be included in the curricula for preparing all health and social service professionals, that board examinations of those practicing with a license (e.g., nurses, physicians, social workers, psychologists) include questions on such content, and that practicing professionals who did not have preparation in the care of victims be offered appropriate in-service education programs. The Canadian government has gone a step further in supporting formal curriculum development on violence issues for all health professionals (Hoff, 1995). However, emphasizing crisis service does not mean that we should neglect life-saving physical treatment in a hospital trauma unit. Even the victims' relatives expect appropriate priorities. While medical and legal needs are met, psychosocial needs can be addressed as well. Thus, victims need a bill of rights, for example, the right to:

- Be informed of the release of a prisoner who previously harmed them. Most jurisdictions now oblige psychotherapists, for example, to warn potential murder victims of would-be assailants' plans (VandeCreek & Knapp, 1993).
- Receive information about protection services.
- Be secure in a court waiting room that is separate from defendants.
- Receive restitution of stolen or damaged property.
- Receive social and psychological support in working through the crisis.

Perhaps the international attention currently focused on this problem will help to remedy this neglected area of crisis intervention.

Summary

People in crisis because of the violence of others suffer emotional and physical injury and have their place in society disrupted if the violence is from a family member or intimate. In addition to assistance for individual victims of violence, social change strategies are paramount in addressing the culturally embedded values and social practices from which so much violence originates worldwide. Such a tandem approach may eventually reduce the tragic effects of violence for individuals, their family, and society as a whole.

References

Attorney General's task force on family violence: Final report. (1984). Washington, D.C.: U.S. Department of Justice.

Bagley, C., & King, K. (1990). *Child sexual abuse: The search for healing.* New York: Routledge.

Bell, C. C., Jenkins, E. J., Kpo, W., & Rhodes, H. (1994). Response of emergency rooms to victims of interpersonal violence. *Hospital and Community Psychiatry, 45*(2), 142–146.

Besharov, D. (1990). *Recognizing child abuse: A guide for the concerned.* New York & Don Mills, Ontario: Collier MacMillan.

Bograd, M. (1984). Family systems approaches to wife battering: A feminist critique. *American Journal of Orthopsychiatry, 54*(4), 558–568.

Braswell, L. (1989). *Quest for respect: A healing guide for survivors of rape.* London: Pathfinder Press.

Breines, W., & Gordon, L. (1983). The new scholarship on family violence. *Signs: Journal of Women in Culture and Society, 8*, 490–531.

Brendtro, L. K., Brokenleg, M., & Van Bockern, S. (1990). *Reclaiming youth at risk.* Bloomington, IN: National Educational Service.

Broverman, I. K., Clarkson, F. E., Rosenkrantz, P. S., & Vogel, S. R. (1970). Sex-role stereotypes and clinical judgments of mental health. *Journal of Consulting and Clinical Psychology, 34*, 1–7.

Brown, J. C., & Bohn, C. R. (1989). *Christianity, Patriarchy, and Abuse: A Feminist Critique.* New York: Pilgrim Press.

Browne, A. (1987). *When battered women kill.* New York: Free Press.

Brownmiller, S. (1975). *Against our will.* New York: Simon & Schuster.

Burgess, A. W., & Hartman, C. (Eds.). (1989). *Sexual exploitation of patients by health professionals.* New York: Praeger.

Burgess, A. W., & Holmstrom, L. L. (1979). *Rape: Crisis and recovery.* Englewood Cliffs, N.J.: Brady.

Burstow, B. (1992). *Radical feminist theory: Working in the context of violence.* Newbury Park, Calif.: Sage.

Campbell, J. C. (1986). A support group for battered women. *Advances in Nursing Science, 8*(2), 13–20.

Campbell, J. C., & Humphreys, J. H. (1993). *Nursing care of survivors of family violence.* St. Louis: Mosby.

Canter, L., & Canter, M. (1988). *A proven step-by-step approach to solving everyday behavior problems* (Rev. ed.). Santa Monica, Calif.: Lee Canter & Associates.

Carmen (Hilberman), E., Rieker, P. P., & Mills, T. (1984). Victims of violence and psychiatric illness. *American Journal of Psychiatry, 141*(3), 378–383.

Charney, R. (1993). Teaching children nonviolence. *Journal of Emotional and Behavioral Problems, 2*(1), 46–48.

Conte, J. R., Wolf, S., & Smith, T. (1987). What sexual offenders tell us about prevention: Preliminary findings. Paper presented at the Third National Family Violence Conference, Durham, N.H.

Cook, J. V., & Bowles, R. T. (Eds.) (1980). *Child abuse.* Scarborough, Ontario: Butterworth.

Counts, D. (1987). Female suicide and wife abuse: A cross-cultural perspective. *Suicide & Life-Threatening Behavior, 17*, 194–204.

Dangor, Z., Hoff, L. A., & Scott, R. (forthcoming). *Violence against South African women.* Johannesburg: NISAA, and Boston: Free South Africa.

Davidson, T. (1977). Wifebeating: A recurring phenomenon throughout history. In M. Roy (Ed.), *Battered women: A psychosociological study of domestic violence* (pp. 2–23). New York: Van Nostrand Reinhold.

DeMause, L. (1975). Our forebears made childhood a nightmare. *Psychology Today, 8*, 85–88.

Dobash, R. P., & Dobash, R. E. (1979). *Violence against wives: A case against the patriarchy.* New York: Free Press.

Doress, P. B., & Siegal, D. L. (1987). *Ourselves, growing older.* New York: Simon & Schuster.

Edgerton, R. B. (1976). *Deviance: A cross-cultural perspective*. Menlo Park, Calif.: Benjamin/Cummings.

Eggert, L. L. (1994). *Anger management for youth: Stemming aggression and violence*. Bloomington, Ind.: National Education Service.

Elder abuse: The hidden crime. (1991). Toronto: Advocacy Centre for the Elderly and Community Legal Education Ontario.

Elias, R. (1984). Alienating the victim: Compensation and victim attitudes. *Journal of Social Issues, 40*, 103–116.

Ericksen, J., & Henderson, A. D. (1992). Witnessing family violence: The children's experience. *Journal of Advanced Nursing, 17*, 1200–1207.

Estes, C. L. (1986). Older women and health policy. Paper presented at the Women, Health, and Healing Summer Institute. Berkeley: University of California.

Estrich, S. (1987). *Real rape: How the legal system victimizes women who say no*. Cambridge: Harvard University Press.

Eyre, J., & Eyre, R. (1993). *Teaching your children values*. New York: Simon & Schuster.

Finkelhor, D. (1984). *Child sexual abuse: New theory and research*. New York: Free Press.

Firsten, T. (1990). *An exploration of the role of physical and sexual abuse for psychiatrically institutionalized women*. Toronto: Ontario Women's Directorate. Ministry of Health.

Gee, P. W. (1983). Ensuring police protection for battered women: The Scott v. Hart suit. *Signs: Journal of Women in Culture and Society, 8*, 554–567.

Gelles, R. J., & Cornell, C. P. (1985). *Intimate violence in families*. Beverly Hills: Sage.

Gelles, R. J., & Loseke, D. R. (Eds.). (1993). *Current controversies on family violence*. Newbury Park, Calif.: Sage.

Gelles, R. J., & Straus, M. A. (1979). Determinants of violence in the family: Toward a theoretical integration. In W. R. Burr, et al. (Eds.), *Contemporary theories about the family* (Vol. 1) (pp. 549–581). New York: Free Press.

Gil, D. (1970). *Violence against children*. Cambridge, Mass.: Harvard University Press.

Gondolf, E. (1987). *Man against woman: What every woman needs to know about violent men*. Bradenton, Fla.: Human Services Institute.

Goodman, L. (1994, May 3). Spare the cane; teach the child. *Sarasota Herald-Tribune*, p. 10.

Goody, J. (1962). *Death, property, and the ancestors*. London: Tavistock.

Greenspan, M. (1983). *A new approach to women in therapy*. New York: McGraw-Hill.

Greven, P. (1990). *Spare the child: The religious roots of punishment and the psychological impact of physical abuse*. New York: Knopf.

Harbin, H. T., & Madden, D. J. (1979). Battered parents: A new syndrome. *American Journal of Psychiatry, 136*, 1288–1291.

Helfer, R., & Kempe, R. S. (1987). *The battered child* (4th ed.). Chicago: University of Chicago Press.

Herman, J. (1981). *Father-daughter incest*. Cambridge, Mass.: Harvard University Press.

Herman, J. (1992). *Trauma and recovery: The aftermath of violence*. New York: Basic Books.

Hilberman, E. (1980). Overview: The 'wife-beater's wife' reconsidered. *American Journal of Psychiatry, 137*, 1336–1347.

Hillman, D., & Solek-Tefft, J. (1988). *Spiders and flies: Help for parents and teachers of sexually abused children*. Lexington, Mass.: Lexington Books.

Hoff, L. A. (1990). *Battered women as survivors*. London: Routledge.

Hoff, L. A. (1992a). Battered women: Understanding, identification, and assessment—a psychosociocultural perspective (Part 1). *Journal of American Academy of Nurse Practitioners, 4*(4), 148–155.

Hoff, L. A. (1992b). Review essay: Wife beating in Micronesia. *ISLA: A Journal of Micronesian Studies, 1*(2), 199–221.

Hoff, L. A. (1993). Battered women: Intervention and prevention—a psychosociocultural perspective (Part 2). *Journal of American Academy of Nurse Practitioners, 5*(1), 34–39.

Hoff, L. A. (1995). *Violence issues: An interdisciplinary curriculum guide for health professionals.* Ottawa: Health Canada, Health Services Directorate.

Hoff, L. A. (1991). Human abuse and nursing's response. In P. Holden & J. Littlewood (Eds.), *Nursing and anthropology* (pp. 130–147). New York: Routledge.

Hoff, L. A., & Rosenbaum, L. (1994). A victimization assessment tool: Instrument development and clinical implications. *Journal of Advanced Nursing, 20,* 627–634.

Hoff, L. A., & Ross, M. (1993). *Curriculum guide for nursing: Violence against women and children.* Ottawa: University of Ottawa, Faculty of Health Sciences. French edition, 1994.

Hollenkamp, M., & Attala, J. (1986). Meeting health needs in a crisis shelter: A challenge to nurses in the community. *Journal of Community Health Nursing, 3*(4), 201–209.

Holmstrom, L. L., & Burgess, A. W. (1978). *The victim of rape: Institutional reaction.* New York: Wiley.

Hudson, M. F. (1986). Elder mistreatment: Current research. In K. A. Pillemer & R. S. Wolf (Eds.), *Elder abuse: Conflict in the family.* (pp. 125–166). Dover, Mass.: Auburn House.

Jackson, D. Z. (1994, September 7). Handguns in our homes put children at risk. *Boston Globe,* p. 13.

Jaffe, P., Wolfe, D., & Wilson, S. (1990). *Children of battered women.* Newbury Park, Calif.: Sage.

Jang, D., Lee, D., & Morello-Frosch, R. (1991). Domestic violence in the immigrant and refugee community: Responding to the needs of immigrant women. *Response to the Victimization of Women and Children, 13*(4), 2–7.

Jones, A. (1980). *Women who kill.* New York: Holt, Rinehart & Winston.

Judson, S. (Ed.). (1984). *A manual on nonviolence and children.* Philadelphia: New Society.

Kempe, H., & Helfer, R. E. (Eds.). (1980). *The battered child* (3rd ed.). Chicago: University of Chicago Press.

Kidd, R. F., & Chayet, E. F. (1984). Why do victims fail to report? The psychology of criminal victimization. *Journal of Social Issues, 40*(1), 39–50.

Kidder, L. H., Boell, J. L., & Moyer, M. M. (1983). Rights consciousness and victimization prevention: Personal defense and assertiveness training. *Journal of Social Issues, 39*(2), 155–170.

Korbin, J. E. (1987). Fatal child maltreatment. Paper presented at the Third National Conference on Family Violence, Durham, N.H.

Kurz, E. (1993). Physical assaults by husbands: A major social problem. In R. J. Gelles & D. R. Loseke (Eds.), *Current controversies on family violence* (pp. 88–103). Newbury Park, Calif.: Sage.

Lardner, G. (1993, May 28). 48 percent of rape cases dismissed, Senate panel finds. *Boston Globe,* p. 4.

Levinson, D. (1989). *Family violence in cross-cultural perspective.* Newbury Park, Calif.: Sage.

Levy, B. (1991). *Dating violence: Young women in danger.* Seattle: Seal Press.

Lobel, K. (Ed.). (1986). *Naming the violence: Speaking out about lesbian battering.* Denver, Colo.: National Coalition Against Domestic Violence.

Long, N. J., & Wilder, M. T. (1993). Massaging numb values LSI. *Journal of Emotional & Behavioral Problems, 2*(1), 35–40.

MacLean, M. (Ed.). (1995). *Abuse and neglect of older Canadians.* Toronto: Thompson Educational Publishing.

MacLeod, L. (1989). *Wife battering and the web of hope: Progress, dilemmas, and visions of prevention.* Ottawa: Health and Welfare Canada. National Clearinghouse on Family Violence.

Martin, D. (1976). *Battered wives.* San Francisco: Glide.

Mawby, R. I., & Walklate, S. (1994). *Critical victimology.* London: Sage.

McDonald, P. L., Hornick, J. P., Robertson, G. B., & Wallace, J. E. (1991). *Elder abuse and neglect in Canada*. Toronto: Butterworths.

McEvoy, A., & Erickson, E. (1994). *Abused children: The educator's guide to prevention and intervention*. Holmes Beach, Fla.: Learning Publications.

McLeod, D. (1994). Forgotten victims of abuse: Older women have no place to turn. *AARP Bulletin, 35*(8), 16–17.

Mirkin, M. P. (Ed.). (1994). *Women in context: Toward a feminist reconstruction of psychotherapy*. New York: Guilford.

Miller, J. B. (1986). *Toward a new psychology of women* (Rev. ed.). Boston: Beacon Press.

Mills, C. W. (1959). *The sociological imagination*. London: Oxford University Press.

Mones, P. (1993). Parricide: A window on child abuse. *Journal of Emotional and Behavioral Problems, 2*(1), 30–34.

Newberger, C. M., & Newberger, E. H. (1981). Prevention of child abuse: Theory, myth, practice. Presented at the meeting of the Society for Research in Child Development, Boston.

Newberger, E. (1980). New approaches needed to control child abuse. Presented before the Subcommittee on Select Education of the Committee on Education and Labor. Washington, D.C.: U.S. House of Representatives.

NiCarthy, G. (1989). *You can be free: An easy-to-read handbook for abused women*. Seattle: Seal Press.

Novello, A. C. (1992). From the Surgeon General: U.S. Public Health Service. *Journal of the American Medical Association, 267*(23), 3132.

Pillemer, K. A., & Wolf, D. W. (1986). *Elder abuse: Conflict in the family*. Massachusetts: Auburn House.

Pillemer, K., & Finkelhor, D. (1987). *The prevalence of elder abuse: A random survey*. Durham, N.H.: Family Violence Research Program.

Podnieks, E., & Pillemer, K. (1990). *National survey on abuse of the elderly in Canada. The Ryerson study*. Health and Welfare Canada. National Clearinghouse on Family Violence.

Powers, J., & Jaklitsch, B. (1989). *Understanding survivors of abuse: Stories of homeless and runaway adolescents*. Lexington, Mass. & Toronto: Lexington Books.

President's task force on victims of crime: Final report. (1982). Washington, D.C.: U.S. Government Printing Office.

Prothrow-Stith, D. (1986). Interdisciplinary interventions applicable to interpersonal violence and homicide in Black youth. In *Surgeon General's workshop on violence and public health: Report* (pp. 35–43). Washington, D.C.: Health Resources and Services Administration.

Pruschno, R., & Resch, N. (1989). Husbands and wives as caregivers: Antecedents of depression and burden. *The Journal of Gerontology, 29*, 159–162.

Renzetti, C. M. (1992). *Violent betrayal: Partner abuse in lesbian relationships*. Newbury Park, Calif.: Sage.

Ross, M. (1991). Spousal caregiving in later life: An objective and subjective career. *Health Care for Women International, 12*(1), 123–135.

Ross, M., & Hoff, L. A. (1994). Teaching nurses about abuse: A curriculum guide for clinical practice. *Canadian Nurse, 90*(6), 33–37.

Rubenstein, C. (1982). Real men don't earn less than their wives. *Psychology Today, 16*, 36–41.

Russell, D.E.H. (1982). *Rape in marriage*. New York: Collier Books.

Russell, D.E.H. (1986). *Secret trauma: Incest in the lives of girls and women*. New York: Basic Books.

Ryan, W. (1971). *Blaming the victim*. New York: Vintage Press.

Sadker, M. & Sadker, D. (1994). *Failing at fairness*. New York: Charles Scribner's Sons.

Sales, E., Baum, M., & Shore, B. (1984). Victim readjustment following assault. *Journal of Social Issues, 40*(1), 117–136.

Samaan, J. (1993). The challenge of street kids. *Spare Change, 2*(5), 16–17.

Schechter, S. (1982). *Women and male violence*. Boston: South End Press.

Segal, L. (1987). *Is the future female? Troubling thoughts on contemporary feminism.* London: Virago Press.

Shallat, L. (1993). Women, violence, and the world conference on human rights. *Women's Health Journal, 1,* 58–62.

Sommers, T., & Shields, L. (1987). *Women take care.* Gainesville, Fla.: Triad.

Stark, E. (1984). *The battering syndrome: Social knowledge, social therapy, and the abuse of women.* Unpublished doctoral dissertation, State University of New York, Binghamton.

Stark, E., Flitcraft, A., & Frazier, W. (1979). Medicine and patriarchal violence: The social construction of a "private" event. *International Journal of Health Services, 9,* 461–493.

Statistics Canada (November 18, 1993). The violence against women survey. *The Daily.* Ottawa.

Stephens, B. J. (1985). Suicidal women and their relationships with husbands, boyfriends, and lovers. *Suicide and Life-Threatening Behavior, 15*(2), 77–90.

Straus, M. A. (1993). Physical assaults by wives: A major social problem. In R. J. Gelles & D. R. Loseke (Eds.), *Current controversies on family violence* (pp. 67–87). Newbury Park, Calif.: Sage.

Straus, M. A., Gelles, R. J., & Steinmetz, S. K. (1980). *Behind closed doors: Violence in the American family.* New York: Anchor Books.

Sugg, N. K., & Inui, T. (1992). Primary care physicians' response to domestic violence: Opening Pandora's box. *Journal of the American Medical Association, 267*(23), 3157–3160.

Surgeon General's workshop on violence and public health: Report. (1986). Washington, D.C.: Health Resources and Services Administration.

Tilden, V. P., Schmidt, T. A., Limandri, B. J., Chiodo, G. T., Garland, M. J., & Loveless, P. A. (1994). Factors that influence clinicians' assessment and management of family violence. *American Journal of Public Health, 84*(4), 628–639.

VandeCreek, L., & Knapp, S. (1993). *Tarasoff and beyond: Legal and clinical considerations in the treatment of life-endangering patients* (Rev. ed.). Sarasota, Fla.: Professional Resource Press.

van der Kolk, B. A. (1987). *Psychological trauma.* Washington, D.C.: American Psychiatric Press.

Walker, H. M. (1993). Anti-social behavior in school. *Journal of Emotional and Behavioral Problems, 2*(1), 20–23.

Warshaw, C. (1989). Limitations of the medical model in the care of battered women. *Gender and Society, 3*(4), 506–517.

Warshaw, D. (1988). *I never called it rape.* New York: Harper & Row.

Wolfgang, M. E. (1986). Interpersonal violence and public health care: New directions, new challenges. In *Surgeon General's workshop on violence and public health: Report* (pp. 9–18). Washington, D.C.: Health Resources and Services Administration.

Yllo, K., & Bograd, M. (Eds.) (1987). *Feminist perspectives on wife abuse.* Newbury Park, Calif.: Sage.

CHAPTER NINE

THE VIOLENT PERSON: INDIVIDUAL AND SOCIOCULTURAL FACTORS

The theoretical overview in Chapter Eight introduced the concept of a continuum between violence against intimates and family members and the violence pervading the larger sociocultural milieu. For example, violence against female partners is no longer regarded as a private matter between the couple, but is now recognized as a major public health issue. One of the reasons for connecting what happens behind closed doors to the public domain is to avoid transferring the legacy of individual victim-blaming to the level of family-blaming. As noted in the last chapter, much personal misery can be traced to family dynamics, neglect, and patterns of harsh discipline or outright abuse and violence. But families do not exist in a social or cultural vacuum. In families, children absorb from their parents values that support aggression and violence as solutions to problems. The parents' behavior has been reinforced by policies and media celebrations that nourish—if they do not condone outright—aggression as an ideal in social life.

Aggression and Violence: A Contextual Versus Adversarial Approach

It has been a slogan of victims' rights organizations that victims deserve the same justice as their accusers and assailants. The last chapter amply supports this position. Yet, in addition to academic debates about "family" versus "feminist" research, there are polarizations, even within advocacy and feminist communities, that do not advance the common goal of reducing violence and caring for its victims. For example, women are portrayed *either* as victims *or* as having "made it" on equal terms with men. Of course, many women have made it, but the fact remains that millions of women worldwide are victimized and most of the assailants are men (PAHO, 1994; Yllo, 1993).

This chapter's focus on the perpetrators of violence—the crises of assailants and their sociocultural underpinnings— suggests that such arguments delay progress in reducing violence. Violence is a major public health problem as well as a criminal justice issue. An either-or position damages both victims/survivors and assailants at worst and constitutes empty polemics at best. Thus, it is not a question of whether we (1) *either* provide refuge and care for battered women *or* provide treatment programs for their batterers; (2) *either* hold parents accountable for the violent and abusive behavior of their children *or* offer parent effectiveness training and socioeconomic support to parents unduly burdened with the task of parenting; or (3) *either* teach inner-city youth anger-management skills *or* address the sociocultural and economic roots of their anger. Essentially, either-or debates are adversarial and reflect the power component of violence itself.

From the perspective of health and human service providers who deal with such crises, it is clear that a contextual *both-and* approach offers more than an either-or polarity. A long history of human service organizations reveals that when staff are divided along ideological and programmatic lines, *clients* are the ones who suffer the most severe consequences by falling through the cracks in a system. One group cannot do everything; a particular discipline or person cannot be all things to all survivors of abuse. But greater coordination could mend some of the serious systemic problems that can trigger crisis responses. And in the case of violence and victimization, the life-and-death consequences as well as the long-term health, financial, and social consequences are enormous in both human and financial terms.

Accordingly, assessment for the risk of assault and homicide is integral to a complete crisis assessment. When the indicators of dangerousness described in Table 9.1 and the assessment tool described in Chapter Three were introduced routinely in crisis and counseling clinics in western New York, staff were astounded at how many clients were entertaining violent fantasies. But crisis workers in that public mental health system also noted the clients' openness to receiving help in dealing with their anger and violent impulses. The next section discusses safety issues for police and crisis workers as well as criteria for such assessment, followed by elaboration of these themes with respect to two major categories of abusive and violent assailants: (1) the international increase in violence and antisocial behavior among young people, and (2) programs for men who batter their women partners.

Violence Against Police Officers, Health, Mental Health, and Crisis Workers

One of the first principles in crisis work is safety—for ourselves, our clients, significant others, and the general public. Violence as an occupational health hazard is only now gaining public attention (Levin, Hewitt, & Misner, 1992; Lipscomb & Love, 1992); police officers, health, mental health, and crisis workers make up a special category of victims. Among women who died as a result of workplace trauma, 41 percent were homicide victims (Jenkins, Layne, & Kisner, 1992). The killing of police officers is particularly demoralizing and frightening because it shows disrespect for the very people dedicated to ensuring public safety. The issue is compounded when workers are victims of violence but there is no certainty that a crime has been committed. This potentially dangerous situation in crisis work embroils us in the controversy introduced in Chapter Eight: the relationship between crime and mental illness (Daniels, 1978; Gove, 1975; Scheff, 1975; Szasz, 1974). Despite numerous debates on this topic, the distinctions between crime and mental illness overlap with relevance to life crises and our response to them; police and mental health professionals are often caught in the middle and become victims of violence. In many cases, their victimization could have been avoided (see Case Example: Robert, Chapter Four).

Why, then, is there an apparent increase in the number of crisis and other workers who are injured, killed, or threatened on the job? In considering this question, the focus is not on what to do if attacked, but on why known crisis intervention strategies are not used, or why they are ineffective. Research (Bard, 1972; Melick, Steadman, & Cocozza, 1979) suggests that three factors are related to this issue: (1) the lack of crisis intervention training, (2) the widespread absence of appropriate collaboration between police and mental health professionals, and (3) the social trend toward medicalization of life. The lack of general knowledge about danger assessment probably increases the hazard of workplace violence as well.

Crisis Intervention Training

Traditionally, nurses and psychiatric professionals have been taught that if they get hurt by mentally disturbed people it is probably because they missed cues to rising anxiety levels or they antagonized or otherwise dealt inappropriately with the disturbed person. Over the years, mental health professionals have worked to dispel the myth that all mental patients are dangerous; only a small percentage are. Psychiatric facilities usually have precise protocols for preventing and responding to violence among mental patients (Anders, 1977; Engel & Marsh, 1986; Morton, 1986). Police procedures are also precise and comprehensive. A basic principle in both disciplines is to avoid force and physical restraint except for protecting oneself and others. This interpretation is strongly supported by the research of Bard (1972) and his precedent-setting training for New York City police officers. The number of police injuries and deaths on the job were significantly reduced as a result of the application of crisis intervention techniques, especially in family disturbance calls. These techniques have been expanded to deal with terrorists through hostage negotiation strategies.

Details of hostage negotiation are beyond the scope of this book or the skills expected of an ordinary crisis worker. The highly sophisticated developments in this field, however, point to the importance of collaborative use of knowledge between police and behavioral science fields in responding to certain crises. Everyone who is even remotely involved with hostage situations— such as when a mentally ill relative holds a child hostage and threatens to commit murder and then suicide if a rescue is attempted—must recognize that offers by civilians to "handle him . . . because I know him better than anyone" can backfire and need thorough investigation. Even police officers chosen for hostage negotiation are carefully screened on several counts, including their professional success in handling general crisis situations. Everyone should also be familiar with ways to reduce the chances of injury or murder.

Besides their usefulness in standard criminal justice and police work, the criteria for assessing the degree of danger and the risk of assault apply in a number of situations:

1. In crisis, emergency, and forensic services
2. In the event the worker is threatened with violence or is being taken hostage
3. In all domestic disputes

The third situation in the list above would apply, for instance, when an abused woman is in imminent danger of being taken hostage or murdered. Such danger is heightened in relationships in which a man acts as though he "owns" his wife, as when he says, "If I can't have you, no one can." Most battered women are already aware of the danger they face, but for those who are not—for whatever reason—a crucial part of safety and crisis intervention planning for her includes a frank discussion of the potential for assault or homicide. While acknowledging that violent people can learn other ways, past violent behavior is still a powerful indicator of future behavior. And, as the triage questions in Exhibit 8.1 indicate, the abused woman's own potential for perpetrating assault following abuse must also be ascertained.

Assessing the Risk of Assault and Homicide

Crisis intervention training should include principles of assessment for risk of assault and homicide. As in the case of suicide risk assessment, there is no absolute prediction of homicide risk. The topic itself is highly controversial; Monahan (1981, p. 6), for example, cites three criticisms regarding prediction:

1. It is empirically impossible to predict violent behavior.
2. If such activity could be forecast and averted, it would, as a matter of policy, violate the civil liberties of those whose activity is predicted.

3. Even if accurate prediction were possible without violating civil liberties, psychiatrists and psychologists should decline to do it, since it is a social control activity at variance with their professional helping role.

Nevertheless, the clinical assessment of risk for assault and homicide is an inherent aspect of police officers' and health and crisis workers' jobs. And the average citizen is always calculating safety maneuvers when in known risk areas. This is not the same as making an official prediction of risk as part of the psychiatric or psychological examination of persons who are detained for crimes and who plead insanity (Halleck, 1987). While assessment of dangerousness by crisis workers is far from an exact science, it can be based on principles and data, not merely guesswork. Based on Monahan's (1981) research, these include:

1. *Statistics,* for example, men between the ages of eighteen and thirty-four commit a much higher percentage of violent crimes than older men or women of any age. Statistical indicators, however, should be viewed with the same caution as in suicide risk assessment (see Chapter Six).
2. *Personality factors,* including motivation, aggression, inhibition, and habit
3. *Situational factors,* such as availability of a weapon or behavior of the potential victim
4. *The interaction* between these variables

Toch (1969) claims that the interaction factor is a crucial one influencing violence. There are several stages in the interactional process. First, the potential victim is classified as an object or potential threat. Based on this classification, some action follows, after which the potential victim may make a self-protective move. Whether or not violence occurs depends on the interaction of such variables as the effectiveness of the victim's self-protection or the would-be attacker's interpretation of resistance as an "ego" threat demanding retaliation. This point is supported by Cooper (1976, p. 237), who states that the greatest threat to a potential victim is his or her dehumanization. Establishing a bond, therefore, between victim and terrorist is a persuasive argument for preventing an attack, although that strategy should not be relied on in all cases. This is the basis for a widely held principle in crisis intervention and hostage negotiation: *time* and keeping *communication* channels *open*—rather than precipitous action, taunts, or threats—are to the benefit of the negotiator and can save the lives of victims, terrorists, and suicidal persons.

Clearly, assessing danger is no simple matter, but lives can be saved by taking seriously the fact that only potentially dangerous people make threats of assault or homicide. Thorough training in crisis assessment and intervention is paramount, therefore, for professionals and others who work with disturbed or potentially violent people.

CASE EXAMPLE: MARTHA

Martha, age thirty-five, had filed for divorce on grounds of her husband's jealousy and abusive behavior. In the parking lot where she worked, he took her hostage and threatened to first kill her and then himself. As Martha's estranged husband, armed with a revolver, drove her across the state for several hours, Martha accommodated his desire to "talk," to the point that he trusted her when she asked to go to the ladies' room while they were in a restaurant. On her way to the rest room, she was able to whisper her plight to a waitress who quickly called the police. As she cowered beneath a stairwell, the police arrested her husband at the restaurant table. The time and communication principle that Martha so astutely applied most likely saved her life.

Police-Mental Health Collaboration

Crisis intervention alone is not enough to prevent violence. Another critical aspect of preventing victimization concerns collaboration between police and mental health professionals, especially when the boundaries of these institutions overlap (Baracos, 1974). The following case example illustrates the tragic results of failure in such collaboration.

CASE EXAMPLE: ARTHUR

A mentally disturbed man, Arthur, age sixty-one, was brought to a hospital emergency department by two police officers for psychiatric examination at the request of his wife. Arthur had a history of paranoid delusions and at this time was accusing his wife of infidelity, though he threatened no harm to her. Arthur's wife had committed him three times before when he refused to seek treatment. This time, as he was getting out of the car, Arthur grabbed the gun of one of the officers and shot him. The other officer in turn shot Arthur, who died instantly; the police officer died a few hours later. While Arthur had a history of mental disturbance, he had no lethal weapons at the time of the police investigation. His history of mental disturbance had never included violence, although he did get very angry each time his wife had him hospitalized.

This case suggests that if police officers had not been required to perform the tasks of mental health professionals—assessing danger and performing crisis intervention with an acutely disturbed mental patient—two deaths might have been avoided. As it was, the community in which this double tragedy occurred had no mobile crisis outreach capacity. The same situation prevails in other communities, to the point that "police are rapidly becoming the frontline mental health workers" (Taft, 1980). Many officers resent that—with justification, since mental health professionals are often unavailable to collaborate with police in cases such as Arthur's. If mobile crisis outreach teams are not available, police officers should have twenty-four–hour access to telephone consultation regarding mental patients.

Such arrangements between police and mental health professionals skilled in crisis intervention should exist in every community (Hoff & Wells, 1989). The need has become more urgent since the trend toward deinstitutionalization of mental patients, often with inadequate community support (Johnson, 1990). Mental patients are at great risk for all sorts of crises, often with no one available to help but police officers.

On the other hand, crisis intervention training for police should be routine. Some officers may resist such training, claiming that a police officer should spend more time preventing crime. However, 80 percent of an average officer's time is spent in service or domestic calls. Ignoring this reality is foolhardy and can cost officers' lives. Even if officers are not physically injured in hostage or other crisis situations, they and their families can suffer psychological trauma that may require weeks or months for recovery. Reactions similar to those of disaster victims are common (see Chapter Ten). Recognizing these reactions and the need for support, the FBI and police departments are making special services available to officers involved in shooting and other highly traumatic incidents.

Application of Assault and Homicide Risk-Assessment Criteria

Translated into everyday practice, the following criteria are helpful as guidelines to assess risk of assault or homicide:

- History of homicidal threats
- History of assault
- Current homicidal threats and plan
- Possession of lethal weapons
- Use or abuse of alcohol or other drugs
- Conflict in significant social relationships such as infidelity, threat of divorce, or labor-management disputes
- Threats of suicide following homicide

Assault and homicide risk assessment is illustrated in a variation of Arthur's case (see Table 9.1). This assessment is based on the risk criteria cited in the Comprehensive Mental Health Assessment tool presented in Chapter Three. Suppose that Arthur had been seen at home by two crisis outreach specialists and no guns were available. According to the criteria cited, Arthur was a low risk for assault or homicide, with a rating of 2 at most. His anxiety level increased as he was forcibly taken to a hospital; guns were available; the risk of homicide increased dramatically. It seems reasonable to suggest that both Arthur and the officer might be alive today if Arthur and his wife had had the advantage of skilled crisis assessment and intervention from mental health professionals, preferably in their home.

In Martha's case, the homicide risk was very high, 5 on the scale, while the necessity of collaboration with police was obvious since the husband was armed.

TABLE 9.1. LETHALITY ASSESSMENT SCALES: OTHER.

Key to Scale	Immediate Dangerousness to Others	Typical Indicators
1	No predictable risk of assault or homicide	No homicidal ideation, urges, or history of same; basically satisfactory support system, social drinker only
2	Low risk of assault or homicide	Has occasional assault or homicidal ideation (including paranoid ideas) with some urges to kill; no history of impulsive acts or homicidal attempts; occasional drinking bouts and angry verbal outbursts; basically satisfactory support system
3	Moderate risk of assault or homicide	Has frequent homicidal ideation and urges to kill but no specific plan; history of impulsive acting out and verbal outbursts while drinking and otherwise; stormy relationship with significant others with periodic high-tension arguments
4	High risk of homicide	Has homicidal plan; obtainable means; drinking history; frequent acting out against others, but no homicide attempts; stormy relationships and much verbal fighting with significant others, with occasional assaults
5	Very high risk of homicide	Has current high-lethal plan; available means; history of homicide attempts or impulsive acting out, plus feels a strong urge to control and "get even" with a significant other; history of drinking, also with possible high-lethal suicide risk

The Medicalization of Crime

It is true that the standards of crisis intervention training among health and mental health workers are far from being met. A minimum of forty hours of training for all frontline and specialty crisis workers (such as nurses, physicians, police, and mental health professionals) is recommended by the American Association of Suicidology, the national standard-setting body for comprehensive crisis services (Hoff & Miller, 1987; Hoff & Wells, 1989). Still, the level of exposure to risk is probably not much higher than it was ten or fifteen years ago, and in many instances workers have had some training in crisis intervention. Yet health and mental health professionals and others seem to be victims of violence in the course of their work more often than in the past. Why?

A health or mental health professional could be a paragon of perfection in crisis intervention practice and still be injured or killed on the job. Mental patients are probably no more violent than they were in the past, but nurses and others may be getting hurt more often by patients who should never have been admitted to a mental health facility in the first place. This assertion is based on overwhelming evidence that life is becoming increasingly medicalized. Nowhere are the consequences of medicalization potentially more dangerous than when this social trend is applied to violent behavior, for example, when a violent criminal is classified as mentally ill and assigned to medical rather than penal supervision. As Melick, Steadman, and Cocozza (1979, p. 235) state in their research in the state of New York, "The reason that a case does not reach trial [for criminal justice versus mental health dispositions] probably has as much to do with the strength of the prosecutor's case as it does with the mental state of the defendant." The medicalization of crime may also be related to overcrowded prisons and empty mental hospitals, conditions that have been created through the process of deinstitutionalization (Johnson, 1990). The availability of state-owned space in mental hospitals provides a coincidental but convenient argument for medicalizing criminal behavior. But apart from the public debate on this topic, practitioners in the crisis and mental health professions also should critically examine the trend to interpret life's problems in an "illness" framework (Hoff, 1993).

It is certainly true that some people who commit crimes are mentally deranged, thus entitling them to leniency before the law. Many insanity pleas, however, leave much room for doubt. Insanity is a legal, not a mental health, concept. Our difficulties in dealing with this issue in the United States are complicated by a criminal justice system that often denies a decent standard of treatment to criminals. The humanitarian impulse of most people is to spare even a violent person an experience that seems beyond the desserts of the crime. It is ironic, then, that the tendency to treat a person rather than hold him or her responsible for violent behavior exists in concert with the movement to assert the rights of mental patients (Capponi, 1992; Szasz, 1974). We cannot have it both ways. One cannot, on the one hand, exercise the freedom to reject treatment and hospitalization for behavioral disorders, and, on the other hand, plead temporary insanity when one fails to control violent impulses and commits a crime. The following cases illustrate this point, as well as the need for mental health professionals to examine their misplaced guilt feelings when they hold clients accountable for their behavior.

CASE EXAMPLE: CONNIE

Connie, age fifty-one, was being treated in a private psychiatric facility for a drinking problem and depression following a divorce. Mental status examination revealed that Connie was mentally competent and not suffering from delusions or other thought disorders, though she was very angry about her husband's decision to divorce her because of her drinking problem. Therefore, when Connie decided to check out of the residential treatment facility against medical advice, there was no basis for confining her

Case Example, cont.

involuntarily, according to any interpretation of the state's mental health laws. A discharge planning conference was held at which follow-up therapy sessions were arranged through a special program for alcoholic women. Connie failed to keep her counseling appointments. One week after leaving the psychiatric unit, Connie attempted to demolish her former husband's car by crashing her own car into it. She endangered the lives of other people by driving on sidewalks, where pedestrians successfully managed to escape her fury. Connie was arrested and taken to jail. Two mental health professionals involved with her case were called to testify. The defense attorney was incredulous that the mental health professionals did not plead with the judge to commit Connie to a mental health facility rather than to jail. The judge clearly seemed to prefer committing Connie to the psychiatric unit but was assured (against the protests of the defense attorney) that her mental status and physical capacity provided no basis on which to keep her from being a further menace to society.

CASE EXAMPLE: ERIC

Eric, age twenty-eight, was employed but distressed over interpersonal relationships on the job. He came to a group therapy session and shortly after the session began, got up and swung his clenched fist at one of the therapists. Then he swung at other clients while making threatening statements. Eric had apparently had something to drink, as the smell of alcohol was on his breath. But as he swung his fists at people, he seemed very controlled; he came just an inch or so from their noses. The therapists and other clients were unable to persuade Eric to stop his violent, threatening behavior, and therefore called the police. Eric was taken to the nearby jail. Meanwhile, the senior therapist—feeling overwhelmed with guilt about her client being in jail—reviewed the mental health laws to ascertain grounds for having Eric transferred from jail to a mental health facility. She reported the incident to the executive director (a psychiatrist) and explored with him the idea of having Eric committed for treatment. The psychiatrist replied, "Treated for what? Threatening you and the other clients?" The therapist revised some of her traditional ideas about "treating" people for violent behavior rather than holding them accountable for it.

These cases suggest that our response to crises of violence directed at helpers, like other crises of social origin, may help perpetuate the problem if larger social ramifications of the issue remain unaddressed. Obviously, this takes us well beyond the individual crisis worker's responsibility. Yet our safety in the work setting and our common humanity in a violent society demand such a two-pronged approach to this serious issue.

The Crisis of Youth Violence

Aggressive, antisocial, and violent behavior among children and adolescents is gaining international attention. In Scandinavian countries and England, for example, bullying and mobbing—usually mild, child-on-child aggression—can create terror in schools and has even been associated with suicide (Hoover & Juul, 1993). Perhaps because the overall rates of violence are higher, 80 to 90 percent of U.S. students (compared with 9 percent in Norway) felt they had been bullied during their school years (p. 27). Research on this issue in Europe traces such behavior to a combination of factors in the home (e.g., inconsistent discipline, abuse, alcohol), the school (more antisocial behavior in the worst schools), and the individual victims and perpetrators, underscoring this book's premise of the *interactional* character of aggression and its sequelae. Paralleling adult patterns, the majority of bullying and antisocial behavior is perpetrated by males against both males and females (Walker, 1993, p. 21; Hoover & Juul, 1993, p. 28). As Sadker and Sadker (1994) point out, however, families begin the process by raising boys according to the cultural ideal of being active, aggressive, and independent; schools inadvertently collude in rewarding their aggressiveness by "going the extra mile" with attention and resources for the nation's future male leaders, as destined by tradition (p. 198).

In the United States, behavioral specialists assert that antisocial behavior by children should be viewed as a national emergency. For example, in one North Carolina school, 35 percent of fifth-graders brought weapons to school, in effect creating police states within school buildings (Walker, 1993, pp. 22–23). Many of these children will be future school dropouts, batterers, and rapists. Given these cultural norms and the centuries-old domination of all major institutions by men reared to feel both entitled (Herman, 1981) and in charge (Dobash & Dobash, 1979), perhaps the most surprising thing is that there is not more violence. As a paradoxical commentary on the influence (or failure?) of the women's movement, many young girls and women use their newly found "freedom" to adopt the aggressive and violent norms of men, including arming themselves in the illusion of self-protection. While some men are discovering the pleasures and growth potential of assuming the parenting and nurturing roles traditionally dominated by women, some women choose violence. They have yet to learn from the plight of battered women that violence begets more serious violence (Hoff, 1990). Educators and youth workers Brendtro, Brokenleg, and Van Bockern (1990, pp. 6–7) trace the discouragement and alienation of youth at risk to four ecological hazards:

1. *Destructive relationships,* as experienced by the rejected or unclaimed child, hungry for love but unable to trust, expecting to be hurt again
2. *Climates of futility,* as encountered by the insecure youngster, crippled by feelings of inadequacy and a fear of failure
3. *Learned irresponsibility,* as seen in the youth whose sense of powerlessness may be masked by indifference or defiant, rebellious behavior
4. *Loss of purpose,* as portrayed by a generation of self-centered youth, desperately searching for meaning in a world of confusing values

In the United States, in view of such factors as racism, the powerful gun lobby, and the pauperization of mothers who are raising children alone in an inequitable labor market, not only must "teachers, parents, and peers" (Walker, 1993, p. 23) influence antisocial children, but policy makers, church leaders, and all who care about the future of humanity must look "upstream" to discover why children are lost to violence and despair (DuRant, et al., 1994; Holinger, et al., 1994; Way, 1993; West, 1994). As Marian Wright Edelman said following a recent survey commissioned by the Children's Defense Fund and the Black Community Crusade, "This poll confirms what black leaders already know—that we have a major black child crisis, the worst since slavery" (*Boston Globe*, 1994, p. 6).

In response to the crisis of youth violence that is primarily sociocultural in origin, will we invent yet another medicalized explanation like "urban stress syndrome" to excuse assailants and neglect victims? Or will we examine the urban environments we have created or allowed to fester as a plague that threatens the lives of all who dwell there? Jenkins and Bell (1992, p. 82) note, for example, that in a study of five hundred elementary school children, 24 percent had witnessed a murder. Many youthful offenders have had no support in healing from childhood trauma (Holinger, et al., 1994; Mendel, 1994). Will people make a connection between values (Eyre & Eyre, 1993), the proliferation of guns, and the shocking increase of children killing children—and others? Again, this is not an either-or dichotomy. Mitigating circumstances must be considered in judging individual cases, but excusing violent action does nothing to facilitate the growth and resiliency that distressed people are capable of when supported through crisis. While facing the enormous challenge of youth violence, it is crucial to remember that we are *influenced* by our past, not *determined* by it. Further, with social support, individuals who have endured almost unimaginable cruelty have lived to tell their stories of endurance and survival. Paul Mones, an attorney specializing in the defense of children who have killed their parents, notes that the most common trigger event before parricide is the child's despair after receiving no help when they finally report abuse to an adult (Mones, 1993, p. 32).

Crisis Prevention and Intervention Programs

Despite this grim picture, the tide may be turning; crisis intervention and anger management programs are being developed in many schools and special treatment settings for disturbed youth. Leona Eggert, for example, has developed a guide for teachers, school nurses, and others working with adolescents and young adults (Eggert, 1994). Fritz Redl developed "The Massaging Numb Values Life Space Interview" to help aggressive students—many with histories of abuse—who become overwhelmed with guilt and remorse about their destructive behavior (Long & Wilder, 1993). Holden and Powers (1993) describe a therapeutic crisis intervention program developed at Cornell University. The four phases in this model—Triggering, Escalation, Crisis, Recovery—correspond roughly to the phases of crisis development originally put forth by Caplan (see Chapter Two), with a particular focus on observing behavioral cues in young people. At the institutional or ecological level, Watson, et al. (1990) offer step-by-step guidelines to prevent and manage a range of school emergencies, including violence. Such ecological approaches include the active involvement of parents and the entire community to provide safety and a hopeful future for its most vulnerable citizens.

In their hope-inspiring book *Reclaiming Youth at Risk*, Brendtro, Brokenleg, and Van Bockern (1990) draw on values of a traditional Native society of North America, the Lakota Sioux, in their application of the medicine wheel with its four spokes depicting *Belonging, Mastery, Independence*, and *Generosity*. To many Native peoples, the number four has sacred meaning. They see the person standing in a circle—a symbol of life—surrounded by the four directions—the requisites for a child to feel whole, competent, and cherished as a member of the community.

The tradition in which the entire community assumes responsibility for its children is highlighted by a widely publicized case of tribal justice. Two seventeen-year-old boys of the Tlingit Nation in Alaska who were convicted of robbing and beating a man were turned over to their village by a judge in Washington state. Village elders meted out justice in the form of a year to eighteen-month exile on Alaska's uninhabited islands. The intent was for the boys to reflect on their behavior, observe the power of natural beauty, and emulate the basic skills taught by their elders—something offenders rarely learn in a locked cell. Holland (1994) shares similar hopeful themes among the people of Soweto, South Africa, who are trying to reclaim their heritage after the devastating effects of apartheid.

A central theme in these programs is that controlling, authoritarian responses by adults to aggressive behavior is part of the problem, not the solution. This is because much of youth violence springs from a history of abuse, neglect, and behaviors that *control* rather than nurture, direct, and foster growth through love and consistent nonviolent discipline. Many young people act out aggressively because they feel disempowered and alienated in a society that does not meet their needs. But as frightening as youth aggression and violence can be, it is crucial to remember that *violence begets violence* (Tierney, Dowd, & O'Kane, 1993). There are many models of effective intervention with troubled youth, and many professionals and others are skilled at using them. Outcome studies of programs such as skills training in anger management are not yet available, though preliminary results suggest that youthful participants respond positively to them (Jenkins & Bell, 1992, p. 79; Prothrow-Stith, 1986). Certainly, at-risk youth can learn and benefit from nonviolent responses to conflict situations. But if they see no hope of escape from racism and a neglected social milieu, their individual tactics to avoid violence may be very short-lived. The greater challenge, then, is in the *primary* prevention domain of changing the socioeconomic and other factors that severely shortchange young people, a nation's most precious resource (see Figure 8.1, Box 3).

Men Who Batter Women

Early work in the violence literature depicted wife battering as the norm in marriage and batterers as incorrigible, with character disorders or a problem with alcohol that excused them from accountability. Gondolf's (1985, 1987) research with violent men reveals four types of batterers: sociopathic, antisocial, chronic, and sporadic. Gondolf suggests that sociopathic batterers need continual restraint to stem their violence, while those with antisocial behaviors need a variety of co-ordinated interventions. In a controversial experimental study, Sherman and Berk (1984) found that arrest had the greatest impact on reducing recidivism (repeat battering) as compared with mediation and crisis intervention. Edleson and Tolman (1992, p. 132), citing later studies, note that community intervention such as the Minneapolis Intervention Project *combined* with criminal justice efforts may offer more protection to women. Similar findings have been reported in Canada, despite its aggressive arrest laws (MacLeod, 1989).

This view is supported by Klein's (1994) study of 664 men who were issued civil restraining orders by the Quincy, Massachusetts court. Reliance on such orders alone did not prevent more abuse, especially among younger, unmarried abusers with prior criminal records who also abused alcohol. Klein, chief probation officer of the Quincy Court, asserts, "These male batterers look like criminals, act like criminals, and re-abuse like criminals" (p. 111). The majority of men in this study who re-abused were not arrested, and if arrested were not sentenced to jail or probation supervision. Another finding with particular relevance for those who ask "Why doesn't she leave?" was that many of the victims had either divorced or physically separated from their abusers—suggesting how little control women have in preventing re-abuse (p. 113). Klein's study supports earlier critiques of the criminal justice system that has failed to treat domestic violence as criminal behavior. Newspaper accounts also reveal that restraining orders have not prevented the murders of women.

Programs for Violent Men

Moving beyond the debate about whether batterers should receive treatment or be arrested, the both-and approach discussed earlier should generally be the norm, even when the women who have been battered—especially those intent on salvaging their relationship and marriage—just want the violence to stop, by whatever means. To carry out that approach, the health and criminal justice aspects of domestic violence must be synchronized. There are two key facets of any program for men who batter, including diversion programs in which men are sentenced and then ordered to undergo treatment as an alternative to jail:

1. The need to assess and reassess their potential for further assault and/or homicide, as suggested in Table 9.1
2. The importance of holding the man *accountable* for his violent behavior, regardless of excuses such as that the woman's behavior "provoked" him to violence

These program elements imply regular contact with the woman who was abused and is possibly still at risk, particularly if she has filed a restraining order, and in instances when men present themes of jealousy, desperation, and ownership of their partner (Meloy, 1992).

Most programs for battering men are variations on an early model, Emerge, which men developed in Boston in response to battered women's advocates' requests that men assume responsibility for a batterers' program. Today in North America, most programs are modeled after the Domestic Violence Intervention Project developed by Ellen Pence and colleagues in Duluth, Minnesota. This and the Emerge model are informed primarily by feminist principles that define woman battering and sexual violence in terms of power and control (Adams, 1988; Kurz, 1993; Pence & Paymar, 1986; Yllo, 1993). In the Power and Control Wheel central to this model, eight spokes depict the ways in which men use violence to maintain power and control of women:

- Intimidation—smashing things, displaying weapons
- Emotional abuse—putting the woman down, making her think she is crazy
- Isolation—controlling what she does, where she goes
- Minimization of abuse—denying, blaming, making light of the abuse, saying she caused it
- Exploitation of children—using visitation to harass her
- Assertion of male privilege—treating her like a servant
- Economic abuse—giving her an allowance, taking her money
- Coercion and threats—threatening to leave or commit suicide

In most programs for men who batter, group counseling is the preferred mode (Edleson & Tolman, 1992), usually including other men who have been violent in the past but are no longer violent. This approach underscores the premise that violence is not inevitable but is learned and reinforced through parenting practices and its pervasiveness in the sociocultural milieu. Couples counseling and family systems approaches are highly controversial (Bograd, 1984), as they tend to obscure violence as the primary problem in the use of such terms as "transaction" and imply the counselor's "neutrality" in regard to criminal behavior. If couples counseling is used, safety, ownership of responsibility for violence, and a *prior* intention of reconciliation must first be established (Edleson & Tolman, 1992, pp. 88–107).

While programs for batterers and refuges for victims must be supported, these are only *secondary* and *tertiary* measures; essentially they are our reactive approaches to a problem that would be much less costly in financial and human terms if *primary prevention* were more valued and promoted, as discussed later in this chapter.

Crises of People Prosecuted for Violence

Many people believe that the perpetrators of crime have a clear advantage over their victims. Aside from the issue of accountability for violent behavior, we should remember that violent people or those who are apprehended for a crime, especially if they go to jail, are also in crisis—the parents who have beaten their child to death, the rapist, a woman batterer, an eighteen-year-old who goes to jail after his first offense of breaking and entering with intent to rob, the middle-class man who has sexually abused a child, the mother who loses custody of her children when she goes to prison for shoplifting and prostitution, and the murderer. In addition to the trauma of being arrested and incarcerated, the prisoner may experience extreme shame, desertion by family, or panic over homosexual advances. Or the prisoner may suffer from chronic mental illness. For mothers of young children, imprisonment may also result in permanent loss of custody of their children. With the increased number of women prisoners, space and other conditions are often more deplorable than they are in overcrowded men's prisons. Suicides are more likely in short-term detention facilities during the height of crisis when there is great uncertainty about one's fate; in long-term holding centers, they are often related to prison conditions.

Crisis Intervention with Assailants

All of the principles of crisis intervention apply to the violent person or to someone who is in prison for other reasons. The application of these principles to violent people can be summarized as follows:

1. *Keep communication lines open.* As long as a person is communicating, violence usually does not occur.
2. Facilitate communication between a disgruntled employee, for example, and the person against whom he or she is threatening violence.
3. Develop specific plans—*with* the dangerous person—for nonviolent expression of anger, such as time-out, jogging, punching a pillow, or calling a hotline.

4. Communicate by telephone or behind closed doors whenever possible when dealing with armed persons, especially until rapport is established and the person's anxiety subsides.

5. If dangerous weapons are involved, collaborate with police for their removal whenever possible; implement emergency procedures for appropriate application of force, such as calling security or police, mobilizing a team effort to warn fellow workers. Failure to work in teams can be life threatening (Anders, 1977).

6. Insist on administrative support and emergency back-up help.

7. Make hotline numbers and emergency call buttons readily available.

8. Examine social and institutional sources of violent behavior, for example, harsh authoritarian approaches to employee relations, which may trigger violence by a disgruntled worker; failure to help disturbed persons seek professional help as an alternative to violence; and rigid structures and rules for geriatric and psychiatric patients.

9. Warn potential victims of homicide, based on risk assessment and the principles of the Tarasoff case (see VandeCreek & Knapp, 1993).

10. Remember that a violent person who is also threatening suicide is a greater risk for homicide.

11. Follow-up: engage in social and political activity to prevent violence.

Several factors, however, may become obstacles to providing aid to these people in crisis: (1) the sense of contempt or loathing one may feel toward a criminal, (2) fear of the prisoner or other person threatening violence, and (3) the need to work within the physical and social constraints of the detention setting or workplace where one does not anticipate interaction with disturbed and/or violent persons. People working in these settings, therefore, must assess and deal with crises according to the circumstances of their particular situations. The works of Danto (1981); Groth and Birnbaum (1979); Halleck (1971); McGinnis (1993); and Tavris (1983) are particularly recommended.

Follow-Up Service

Specialists in criminal justice cite the problem of recidivism among people convicted of crimes. The ex-offender is stripped of status and community respect and often has been exposed to conditions that harden and embitter rather than rehabilitate. Considering the dire financial straits of the ex-prisoner—a situation that frequently was present before incarceration—along with his or her lack of job skills, discrimination in employment, and the absence of follow-up programs, it is not difficult to understand why crime becomes a career for some.

Advocates of prison reform and various church groups are working to bring about long-term change in the conditions that seem to breed rather than prevent crime. For the nonviolent offender (more than half the American prison population), alternatives to jail sentencing are being tried in many states—a penalty system used in Native communities and in Europe for years. These less costly and more effective options include: (1) community service, such as working in parks and public buildings; (2) restitution, a sanction that is particularly appealing because it takes into account the person most directly affected by the crime—the victim; (3) intermittent confinement, a strategy that spares total disruption of work and family; and (4) intensive probation, that is, no more than twenty-five persons per officer. These humane approaches should be weighed against the thousands of dollars spent each year to keep a person in prison.

The Families of Prisoners

Inmates and ex-offenders are not alone in their distress. Historically, their families—especially children—are also neglected. While there are generally fewer women than men in prison, at least a quarter of a million U.S. children have mothers who are incarcerated. Families not only lose a spouse, parent, or child to prison, but may also lose a source of income and status in the community. Poverty, loneliness, and boredom are just a few of the problems faced by these families. Those who attempt to sustain relationships find that prison regulations (such as body searches of visitors and lack of privacy) or societal pressure and personal circumstances thwart their efforts. Children of imprisoned parents feel sadness, anxiety, guilt, and anger. If a divorce occurs during or following imprisonment, the post-release problems of the ex-offender are increased.

To address the crises of prisoners' families, more self-help groups such as Families and Friends of Prisoners in Dorchester, Massachusetts are needed. This group provides moral support, counseling, information, and inexpensive transportation to state and federal prisons. A similar group, Aid to Incarcerated Mothers (AIM), focuses on the special needs of mothers and children. A mother speaking about the services of this group wrote:

> When I first came to prison, I didn't want my children to have to see their mother in such a place. I didn't want them to have to go through the search, and transportation was a problem. I wanted desperately to see my children but was afraid of the impression the prison might have on them. After talking with AIM, a lot of my fears were put to rest. . . . I can't explain the feeling I had when I went to the visiting room and saw my son and daughter, after not seeing them for two months. Seeing my children has put my mind at ease and made my time a little easier to deal with. . . . Ladies, your children love and care about you as much as you love and care about them. They want to know that you are OK just as much as you want to know they are OK. AIM is people who care about you and want to help you keep that bond between mother and children. So, let them help you as they have helped me (AIM, 1982).

Primary Prevention of Crime and Antisocial Behavior

Chapter One presented a general picture of primary prevention as it pertains to life crises, emphasizing the public health and communitywide action necessary if we are to *prevent* stressful events and situations from escalating into full-blown crises. Here, this approach is explicated with particular reference to crises of both victims and perpetrators of violence and antisocial behavior. Clearly, as long as loopholes exist in the criminal justice system's response to battering, refuges are no less than life-saving for many women. Similarly, residential treatment programs for out-of-control youth are necessary. But the very fact that an entire system of *residential* programs for battered women have been established speaks to the tendency, especially in the United States, toward *reactive* rather than *preventive* approaches. History reveals that all societies establish rules for how to treat deviant members.

Criminal justice system loopholes and refuges for victims suggest an alternative approach. Instead of forcing victims to live like fugitives, with the additional burden of single parenting, what if *perpetrators* were required to leave and receive counseling in alternative housing as an incentive to stop their violent behavior? Perhaps when the cultural milieu and would-be offenders are saturated with the message of zero tolerance for violence—in the next generation, we hope—the present refuges for victims might be retrofitted for perpetrators instead (Hoff, 1990).

But how do we get to that point? We certainly will not get there without the communitywide endeavors generally intrinsic to the primary approach to health care. Such measures have already been suggested in the section on youth violence; more strategies follow.

Personal and Social-Psychological Strategies

When sincerely addressing the issue, individuals may become overwhelmed by the pervasiveness of violence and withdraw out of a sense of helplessness, self-protection, or both. It is important therefore to focus on selected actions and obtainable goals. These may include:

1. Adopting nonviolent language in everyday social interaction
2. Using nonviolent ways of disciplining children; attending parent effectiveness training groups to assist with difficult child-rearing challenges
3. Attending self-defense courses as a means of bolstering self-confidence and providing a substitute for arming oneself; avoiding violence as a response to violence
4. Reading about and attending continuing education courses on nonviolent conflict resolution in personal relationships

5. Avoiding sex-role stereotyping in child rearing and other interactions with children
6. Organizing neighborhood patrols and systematic ways of watching out for one another

Sociopolitical Strategies

These strategies are most successful when combined with personal and social-psychological approaches on the premise that people need grounding in information and self-confidence in order to stand firm against obstacles in the political arena. Among the most obvious are:

1. *Educating the public through schools, community organizations, and churches.* How many people who have attended church, synagogue, or mosque, for example, have heard a sermon condemning violence against women and children or have sponsored programs to explicitly address such issues? Probably not many have done so. Abused people often turn to clergy for help, and many religious leaders are now responding to the unique opportunity they have in preventing violence (Fortune & Hertze, 1987).
2. *Contacting legislators and organizing for change in laws that may be outdated or otherwise do not address the issues local people confront.* In the United States, this includes addressing the powerful gun lobby.
3. *Using advocacy and systematic organizing around racial and economic justice,* including equality in educational opportunities.

Professional Strategies

In the United States, the Surgeon General's Report (1986) recommended that all licensed professionals be required to study and pass examination questions in violence prevention and the treatment of various victims of violence. As a complement to this public policy statement, individual professionals can exert leadership and advocacy within their own groups for curriculum and in-service program development to systematically address this topic. At present, such educational endeavors are incidental at best (Hoff & Ross, 1995; Tilden, et al., 1994). In Canada, the federal government has published a document entitled *Violence Issues: An Interdisciplinary Curriculum Guide for Health Professionals,* that covers education about violence prevention and service for victims and assailants (Hoff, 1995). This document is addressed to the following disciplines: dentistry, medicine, nursing, occupational therapy, pharmacy, physical therapy, psychology (clinical), and social work. Similar programs have been developed for criminal justice professionals in North America and other countries.

The vast knowledge already available to professionals must be combined with personal strategies in order to:

- Widely disseminate new knowledge about this poignant topic to the public
- Change the values and attitudes that have served as fertile soil for nurturing violent and antisocial behavior
- Effect broad policy and functioning of social institutions through the political process necessary to bring about needed change

Summary

The crisis of increasing violence, especially among the young, is gaining international attention, while more and more health professionals and educators are joining grassroots community groups to address the crisis. Since children and youth are a nation's most precious resource, few crises command more urgent attention, not only for the sake of the assailants and their victims but for the future of a nation. Sociopolitical responses must be joined with assistance to the individuals and families affected by violence.

References

Adams, D. (1988). A profeminist analysis of treatment models of men who batter. In K. Yllo & M. Bograd (Eds.), *Feminist perspectives on wife abuse* (pp. 176–199). Beverly Hills: Sage.

AIM: Aid to Incarcerated Mothers (1982). *Newsletter,* p. 2. Boston.

Anders, R. L. (1977). When a patient becomes violent. *American Journal of Nursing, 77,* 1144–1148.

Baracos, H. A. (1974). Iatrogenic and preventive intervention in police-family crisis situations. *International Journal of Social Psychiatry, 20,* 113–121.

Bard, M. (1972). *Police, family crisis intervention, and conflict management: An action research analysis.* Washington, D.C.: U.S. Department of Justice.

Bograd, M. (1984). Family systems approaches to wife battering: A feminist critique. *American Journal of Orthopsychiatry, 54*(4), 558–568.

Brendtro, L. K., Brokenleg, M., & Van Bockern, S. (1990). *Reclaiming youth at risk: Our hope for the future.* Bloomington, Ind.: National Educational Service.

Capponi, P. (1992). *Upstairs in the crazy house.* Toronto: Penguin.

Charney, R. (1993). Teaching children nonviolence. *Journal of Emotional and Behavioral Problems, 2*(1), 46–48.

Cooper, H.H.A. (1976). The terrorist and the victim. *Victimology, 1,* 229–239.

Cotten, N. U., Resnick, J., Browne, D. C., Martin, S. L., McCarraher, D. R., & Woods, J. (1994). Aggression and fighting behavior among African-American adolescents: Individual and family factors. *American Journal of Public Health, 84*(4), 618–622.

Daniels, A. K. (1978). The social construction of military psychiatric diagnosis. In J. G. Manis & B. N. Meltzer (Eds.), *Symbolic interaction* (3rd ed.) (pp. 380–392). Boston: Allyn & Bacon.

Danto, B. (1981). *Crisis behind bars: The suicidal inmate.* Warren, Mich.: Dale.

Dobash, R. P., & Dobash, R. E. (1979). *Violence against wives: A case against the patriarchy.* New York: Free Press.

DuRant, R. H., Cadenhead, C., Pendergast, R. A., Slavens, G., and Linder, C. W. (1994). Factors associated with the use of violence among urban black adolescents. *American Journal of Public Health, 84*(4), 612–617.

Edleman, M. W. (1994, May 27). Poll finds pervasive fear in blacks over violence and their children. *Boston Globe,* p. 6.

Edleson, J. L., & Tolman, R. M. (1992). *Intervention for men who batter: An ecological approach.* Newbury Park, London, New Delhi: Sage.

Eggert, L. L. (1994). *Anger management for youth: Stemming aggression and violence.* Bloomington, Ind.: National Educational Service.

Engel, F., & Marsh, S. (1986). Helping the employee victim of violence in hospitals. *Hospital and Community Psychiatry, 37*(2), 159–162.

Eyre, L., & Eyre, R. (1993). *Teaching your children values.* New York: Simon & Schuster.

Fortune, M. & Hertze, J. (1987). A commentary on religious issues in family violence. In M. Pellauer, B. Chester, & J. Boyajian (Eds.), *Sexual assault and abuse: A handbook for clergy and religious professionals* (pp. 67–83). New York: Harper & Row.

Gondolf, E. (1985). *Men who batter: An integrated approach for stopping wife abuse.* Holmes Beach, Fla.: Learning Publications.

Gondolf, E., & Russell, D. (1986). The case against anger control treatment programs for batterers. *Response, 9*(3), 2–5.

Gondolf, E. (1987). *Research on men who batter.* Bradenton, Fla.: Human Services Institute.

Gove, W. (1975). *The labeling of deviance.* New York: Wiley.

Groth, A. N., & Birnbaum, H. J. (1979). *Men who rape: Psychology of the offender.* New York: Plenum.

Halleck, S. L. (1971). *The politics of therapy.* New York: Science House.

Halleck, S. L. (1987). *The mentally disordered offender.* Washington, D.C.: American Psychiatric Press.

Herman, J. (1981). *Father-daughter incest.* Cambridge: Harvard University Press.

Hoff, L. A. (1990). *Battered women as survivors.* London: Routledge.

Hoff, L. A. (1993). Review essay: Health policy and the plight of the mentally ill. *Psychiatry, 56*(4), 400–419.

Hoff, L. A. (1995). *Violence issues: An interdisciplinary curriculum guide for health professionals.* Ottawa: Health Canada, Health Services Directorate.

Hoff, L. A., & Miller, N. (1987). *Programs for people in crisis: A guide for educators, administrators, and clinical trainers.* Boston: Northeastern University Custom Book Program.

Hoff, L. A., & Ross, M. (1995). Violence content in nursing curricula: Strategic issues and implementation. *Journal of Advanced Nursing, 21,* 137–142.

Hoff, L. A., & Wells, J. O. (Eds.). (1989). *Certification standards manual* (3rd ed.). Denver: American Association of Suicidology.

Holden, M. J., & Powers, J. L. (1993). Therapeutic crisis intervention. *Journal of Emotional and Behavioral Problems, 2*(1), 49–52.

Holinger, P. C., Offer, D., Barter, J. T., & Bell, C. T. (1994). *Suicide and homicide among adolescents.* New York: Guilford.

Holland, H. (1994). *Born in Soweto.* London: Penguin.

Hoover, J. H., & Juul, K. (1993). Bullying in Europe and the United States. *Journal of Emotional and Behavioral Problems, 2*(1), 25–29.

Jenkins, E. J., & Bell, C. C. (1992). Adolescent violence: Can it be curbed? *Adolescent Medicine: State of the Art Reviews, 3*(1), 71–86.

Jenkins, L., Layne, L. A., & Kisner, S. M. (1992). Homicide in the workplace: The U.S. experience, 1980–1988. *American Association of Occupational Health Nursing Journal, 40*(5), 215–218.

Johnson, A. B. (1990). *Out of bedlam: The truth about deinstitutionalization.* New York: Basic Books.

Klein, A. (1994). Re-abuse in a population of court-restrained male batterers after two years: Development of a predictive model. Unpublished doctoral dissertation, Northeastern University (Law, Policy, and Society Program), Boston.

Kurz, D. (1993). Physical assaults by husbands: A major social problem. In R. J. Gelles & D. R. Loseke (Eds.), *Current controversies on family violence* (pp. 88–103). Newbury Park: Sage.

Levin, P. F., Hewitt, J. B., & Misner, S. T. (1992). Female workplace homicides: An integrative research review. *American Association of Occupational Health Nursing Journal, 40*(5), 229–236.

Lipscomb, J. A., & Love, C. C. (1992). Violence toward health care workers: An emerging occupational hazard. *American Association of Occupational Health Nursing Journal, 40*(5), 219–228.

Long, N. J., & Wilder, M. T. (1993). From rage to responsibility: A massaging numb values LSI. *Journal of Emotional and Behavioral Problems, 2*(1), 35–40.

MacLeod, L. (1989). *Wife battering and the web of hope: Progress, dilemmas, and visions of prevention.* Ottawa: Health and Welfare Canada. National Clearinghouse on Family Violence.

McGinnis, C. (1993). *Lifeline: A training manual.* Boston: Suffolk County Jail.

Melick, M. E., Steadman, H. J., & Cocozza, J. J. (1979). The medicalization of criminal behavior among mental patients. *Journal of Health and Social Behavior, 20*, 228–237.

Meloy, R. (1992). *Violent attachments.* Northvale, N.J.: Jason Aronson.

Mendel, M. P. (1994). *The male survivor.* Newbury Park: Sage.

Monahan, J. (1981). *Predicting violent behavior: An assessment of clinical techniques.* Beverly Hills: Sage.

Mones, P. (1993). Parricide: A window on child abuse. *Journal of Emotional and Behavioral Problems, 2*(1), 30–34.

Morton, P. G. (1986). Managing assaultive patients. *American Journal of Nursing, 86*(10), 114–116.

Pan American Health Organization (PAHO) (1994, November 16 & 17). *Inter-American Conference on Society, Violence, and Health.* Washington, D.C.: Author.

Pence, E., & Paymar, M. (1986). *Power and control: Tactics of men who batter.* Duluth: Minnesota Program Development.

Prothrow-Stith, D. (1986). Interdisciplinary interventions applicable to prevention of interpersonal violence and homicide in black youth. In *Surgeon General's workshop on violence and public health: Report* (pp. 35–43). Washington, D.C.: Health Resources and Services Administration.

Report: Surgeon General's workshop on violence and public health. (1986). Washington, D.C.: U.S. Department of Health and Human Services.

Sadker, M., & Sadker, D. (1994). *Failing at fairness.* New York: Charles Scribner's Sons.

Scheff, T. J. (Ed.). (1975). *Labeling madness.* Englewood Cliffs, N.J.: Prentice-Hall.

Sherman, L. W., & Berk, R. A. (1984). The specific deterrent effects of arrest for domestic assault. *American Sociological Review, 49*(4), 261–272.

Straus, M. A. (1993). Physical assaults by wives: A major social problem. In R. J. Gelles & D. R. Loseke (Eds.), *Current controversies on family violence* (pp. 65–87). Newbury Park, Calif.: Sage.

Szasz, T. S. (1974). *The myth of mental illness* (Rev. ed.). New York: Harper & Row, Perennial Library.

Taft, P. B. (1980). Dealing with mental patients. *Police Magazine*, 20–27.

Tarasoff v. the Regents of the University of California. (1976). 551P. 2d 334. Also in 131 California Reporter 14. Supreme Court of California.

Tavris, C. (1983). *Anatomy of anger.* New York: Simon & Schuster.

Tierney, J., Dowd, T., & O'Kane, S. (1993). Empowering aggressive youth to change. *Journal of Emotional and Behavioral Problems, 2*(1), 41–45.

Tilden, V., Schmidt, T. A., Limandri, B. J., Chiodo, G. T., Garland, M. J., and Loveless, P. A. (1994). Factors that influence clinicians' assessment and management of family violence. *American Journal of Public Health, 84*(4), 628–633.

Toch, H. (1969). *Violent men.* Chicago: Aldine.

Walker, H. M. (1993). Anti-social behavior in school. *Journal of Emotional and Behavioral Problems, 2*(1), 20–24.

Watson, R. S., Poda, J. H., Miller, C. T., Rice, E. S., & West, G. (1990). *Containing crisis: A guide to managing school emergencies.* Bloomington, Ind.: National Educational Service.

VandeCreek, L., & Knapp, S. (1993). *Tarasoff and beyond: Legal and clinical considerations in the treatment of life-endangering patients.* (Rev. ed.). Sarasota, Fla.: Professional Resource Press.

Way, D. W. (1993). I just have a half heart. *Journal of Emotional and Behavioral Problems, 2*(1), 4–5.

West, C. (1994). *Race matters.* New York: Vintage Books.

Yllo, K. (1993). Through a feminist lens: Gender, power, and violence. In R. J. Gelles & D. R. Loseke (Eds.), *Current controversies on family violence* (pp. 47–62). Newbury Park, Calif.: Sage.

CHAPTER TEN

VIOLENCE AND CRISIS FROM DISASTER

The natural world is both a nurturing home and a source of potential destruction. The sun warms us. The beauty of foliage, sea coasts, forests, plains, and mountains satisfies our aesthetic needs and inspires us to write, sing, and love one another. Yet these same elements have the capacity to destroy us if we do not protect ourselves from nature's violent forces. For example, we must build shelters to prevent freezing to death in a snowstorm. We are also in danger if we misuse or destroy nature's resources, for example, by uncontrolled burning of coal which causes acid rain and destroys lakes and the creatures that live in them.

As human beings, we can see and respond to the differences and connections between natural elements and ourselves. Our ability to rationally construct our social and material world allows us to contain the forces of nature for our own protection. The natural world yields much of what we need for survival; yet the victims of fires, floods, tornados, tidal waves, earthquakes, and snowstorms provide ample evidence of nature's destructive potential in spite of great technological attempts to decipher nature's mysteries and direct them for human ends.

> "I saw deaths, devastation, agony, and misery of a magnitude I have never seen before. . . . The bodies were decomposed and the stench was unbearable."

> "Our people have learned to resist difficulties and consider the national disaster to be a divine test."

> "In some places, whole streets are gone. Entire buildings are just piles of rubble. . . . Many of the victims are school children."

Dulal Biswas had given thanks that his five-year-old daughter Shanti was safe with her grandparents. A few days later, on his way to get her, Dulal stumbled upon a child's body on the bank of the Pasur River. He peered in disbelief at the bloated, decomposing body. Then he screamed, beat his chest, and cried, "Shanti, my little doll, Shanti." Biswas's wife had died a year earlier of cholera, and Shanti was his only child. As he related his story to the Red Crescent Society worker, he was almost incoherent with grief.

"I [an AIDS patient] have wanted to die so badly. . . . It took a 7.0 earthquake to make me rudely aware that I didn't want to die half as badly as I thought I did."

"Some of our guys were crawling on their stomachs through the lower section of the freeway. There was a space of only eighteen inches. People were alive. The workers said they could hear them, but they couldn't get to them. I know those people didn't make it through the night."

"There are no dead to mourn. There can be no funerals. The passengers have simply vanished."

"This is a village of people buried alive."

These are a few of the reactions of victims and survivors of the volcanic eruption in Columbia in 1985, floods in the midwestern United States in 1993, the cyclone in Bangladesh in 1991, the San Francisco Bay Area earthquake in 1989, and the Armenian earthquake in 1988. Internationally, similar disasters have occurred in Manila, Los Angeles, Iran, South Carolina, and Egypt. The number of dead, injured, and homeless from these disasters is staggering, for example: 138,000 dead from a Bangladesh hurricane; 20 dead from Hurricane Andrew; 100,000 dead and a half-million homeless in Armenia; 40,000 dead in Iran; more than 200 dead and injured in San Francisco. In the worst natural disaster in Colombia's history, the 1985 eruption of a volcano in Armero killed more than 22,000 people, with another 20,000 injured or left homeless. The 1985 earthquake and its aftershocks in Mexico City left 10,000 dead, more thousands homeless, and millions of pesos worth of damage.

Human Potential for Catastrophic Violence

However, nature's potential for violence seems small beside the destructive possibilities for disaster caused by human beings. In Bhopal, India, a gas leak at a chemical plant killed 2,000 people and disabled tens of thousands more. Besides the 300 dead and 10,000 evacuated from the Chernobyl nuclear accident in the former Soviet Union, radioactive fallout affected people and animals thousands of miles away, while illness and death from this accident are still being counted. Sur-

vivors of a fire in a North Carolina chicken plant that had violated safety regulations—doors were locked; there were no sprinklers or fire alarms—are still
haunted by victims' screams a year later. Similarly, survivors of the underground
gold mine explosion near Yellowknife in the Northwest Territories, Canada, cite
the tragedy as proof of the need for reform of labor-management relations. Also,
the famines in Ethiopia, Mozambique, and Somalia, although apparently "natural," can be traced to human origins (Wijkman & Timberlake, 1984). By most
accounts, the inferno that killed at least eighty people in Waco, Texas, could have
been avoided. "Ethnic cleansing" and tribal wars in the former Yugoslavia and
Rwanda are the most recent man-made disasters creating incalculable misery and
loss of life; the systematic slaughter of people in Rwanda is being compared to the
Nazi Holocaust in the war crimes category. "Environmental racism," a reference to placing toxic waste dumps in communities where ethnic minority groups
live and in poor countries, surely takes its toll.

Human potential for both good and evil seems limited only by the technology we create. For example, a child can be saved through a liver transplant; amputated hands can be replaced; energy from the sun can be collected and stored;
but technology also made it possible for the Nazis to perform inhuman experiments on Jews and others in concentration camps and for most of the population
of Hiroshima and Nagasaki to be destroyed by atomic bombs. While many enjoy
the benefits of scientific knowledge, others suffer. For example:

Ask Those Who Really Know

Ask the Victims of Love Canal why they need immediate permanent relocation, and why some will refuse to leave their motel rooms once funds are
cut off.

Ask the innocent victims of corporate profits.

The reasons are simple. We cannot lead a normal life, we:

Cannot go in our basements because of contamination from Love Canal.

Cannot eat anything from our gardens because of soil contamination.

Cannot allow our children to play in our yards because of contaminated
soils.

Cannot have our children attend school in the area—two have been
closed due to Love Canal contamination.

Cannot breathe the outside air—because of air contamination we are
now in hotels.

Cannot become Pregnant—miscarriage rate is state defined: 45 percent.
Homeowners' survey: 75 percent.

Cannot have normal children—because of 56 percent risk of birth
defects.

Cannot sell our homes. Love Canal was not mentioned in our deeds; who wants a contaminated house?

Cannot get a VA or FHA loan in Love Canal; even the government is reluctant.

Cannot have friends or relatives visit us on holidays; they're scared it's unsafe.

Cannot have our Pregnant daughters, or our grandchildren visit: it's unsafe for them.

We need your support and your help to end the suffering of men, women, and especially children of Love Canal. We have lost our constitutional rights of life, liberty and the pursuit of happiness. Justice for all but not Love Canal Victims. We cannot live at Love Canal—we cannot leave Love Canal (Gibbs, 1982).

The disastrous effects of violence from natural and human sources can be described in both personal and social terms. Although people are now moving back to Love Canal, this highly publicized disaster holds lessons for other communities still struggling against toxic waste. How do people respond to disasters of natural origin, as compared with those of human origin? Why are disasters of human origin, such as Love Canal and Hiroshima, not usually viewed as a form of violence? What can individuals and groups do to reduce our vulnerability to disasters from natural and human sources? Our answers to these questions could affect:

• What happens to disaster victims
• The quality of our everyday lives
• The quality of life on earth we can realistically anticipate
• Whether or not we ultimately destroy ourselves and our planet

Natural and Accidental Disaster: Prevention and Aid

One can only guess at the extent to which a disaster such as a flood, fire, or earthquake affects the people who experience it. The depth of the tragedy is private and immeasurable. Although the negative consequences of disaster are not always clear, some research suggests that survivors suffer long-term stress (Baum, Fleming, & Singer, 1983; Erikson, 1994). Preventive measures and help for survivors are therefore of great importance. What do we need to know about disaster and its victims in order to help? The nature of a disaster affects the victims' response. A disaster usually occurs rapidly and is therefore completely unexpected and shocking. The following account (Glasheen & Crowley, 1993, p. 11) portrays vividly the depth of loss and destruction of life and property that resulted from the Mississippi flood.

> She's a friendly, look-you-in-the-eye kind of woman who has been through a lot but prefers not to talk about it. But today, showing visitors the wreckage of her home of 37 years, Dorothy Flowers, 70, struggles for her composure.
>
> "That building up there—it doesn't belong here. It floated in here. That refrigerator over there? It's not mine—or any of my neighbors'." She steps into her house, now knee deep in black mud, confiding, "I'm scared to death of snakes."
>
> She's been out of her home since April, when flood waters stood four feet deep in her one-story frame house. In the midst of cleaning up after the spring flood, the river rose again—up and over the roof.
>
> Flowers has lost a lot to the Mississippi. Her husband died while they were living temporarily in a mobile home after the '79 flood, his death, she believes, hastened by stress. Her only child, Randy, died in the flood of '83, at 18 years old, his truck swallowed up by water. She talks about other losses, many tied to the river landscapes around which she has spent her life. "Valmeyer, Illinois—that town is gone. That's where I was born. Kaskaskia Island is gone—that's where I spent every summer. That's where my grandparents lived all their lives. Now it is gone."
>
> She rummages around her yard, looking for familiar sights. "I had 10 roses there," she says. Vandals have knocked over her birdbath. "Now that's uncalled for," she says, stricken. She walks around the yard, pointing. "I planted a garden before the first flood. Then I planted a garden again. I had window boxes up there—they were loaded with geraniums."
>
> She stops and looks around. "I don't want to come back," she says finally. "I don't want to go through another flood. But I can't just walk away. My friends are all here," she says wistfully. "Oh, this was a beautiful community. If anybody couldn't cut the grass because they were sick or something, why somebody else would cut it for them. Everybody shared everything with everybody."
>
> The authorities want Flowers to raise her house over the flood level—to the roof line. "I don't have that kind of money," she says. "I can't just give [the property] away for nothing. And I'm too old to pay $100,000 for a house someplace. But I've got nothing to come home to."

Fortunately, tragedies like this happen rarely—or perhaps not at all—to most people. Most of our expectations of disaster are formed in the abstract. This lack of experience, along with the suddenness and unexpectedness with which most disasters strike, greatly reduces the opportunity for escape and for effective problem solving.

Technological and Political Factors Affecting Aid to Victims

Rescue operations and assistance with physical necessities occur in disaster-stricken communities throughout the world. Foreign countries and the International Red Cross assist in such relief work: millions of dollars in aid were sent to Armenia, Iran, Colombia, and Mexico following their devastating disasters. Also, a country's ability to respond is related to the amount and quality of its resources, technological developments, and the bureaucratic functioning of its government.

The uncontrolled forces of nature may not seem to differentiate between rich and poor, north and south, or between white people and those of color. But the effects of these forces differ. Widespread flooding in the United States, for example, is less frequent and results in fewer lost lives than it did years ago because the resources and technology needed for good prevention programs—building dams, for example—are available. But a poor country like India still has difficulty preventing massive floods that take thousands of lives. A poor nation also has fewer government resources for assisting survivors. Similarly, fires of the proportion of the Cocoanut Grove disaster, which claimed 492 lives in Boston in 1942, are rare today because political action has enforced building safety regulations. Federal aviation policy has likewise been tightened to prevent jetliner crashes due to faulty technology or the nonenforcement of safety codes. However, news accounts of disaster worldwide repeatedly emphasize the difference between rich and poor countries' access to resources for preventing, or at least warning of, impending disaster. Presidents of poor countries often plead for technical assistance to warn people of impending disaster so they can take measures to avoid injury.

Consider, for example, the contrast in flood damage and compensation in a rich nation, the United States, and a poor nation, Bangladesh. As Fauzia A. Ahmed, South Asia coordinator of Oxfam America, wrote:

Hurricane Andrew claimed 20 lives. Last year, a hurricane with no name struck Bangladesh, killing 138,000 people. Both hurricanes had winds of 140 miles per hour. But why was one hurricane approximately 7,000 times more lethal? The answer is poverty. Bangladesh has 300 shelters for hurricanes. It needs 5,000, which could be built for less than the cost of one C-17 military cargo aircraft.

When Hurricane Andrew came to Miami, it found a ghost town. Most people had fled to shelters. In Bangladesh, hundreds of thousands of people tried to run as a huge wall of water advanced on them. Abdul, a survivor, told me, "My two children could not run fast enough. The wave caught up with them and they died. The roar of the sea was so great I could not even hear their cries for help."

There was also tremendous psychological devastation. In Miami, a businessman died of a heart attack after seeing his business reduced to rubble. In

Bangladesh, mothers were forced to choose which children to save. They will somehow have to go on living with the consequences of this choice. "I had four children," one mother told me. "But I only have two hands. With one hand I grasped a tree and held my six-month-old baby with the other. I had to watch my three other children drown because I could not save them."

In Florida, there was insurance for homeowners. The Federal Emergency Management Agency dispensed money for the cleanup. In Bangladesh, there was no compensation for people who lost their livestock—which was often the sum total of all their worldly possessions.

Bangladesh is a nation where there are more riverways than dirt tracks and more dirt tracks than paved roads. In good times, fishermen live off the water. In hurricanes, the water drags them to their death. The overall lack of quality roads makes it impossible for relief supplies to reach people in remote areas.

In Florida, the warning system and evacuation plan worked. Bangladesh's 80 percent illiteracy rate makes it difficult for many citizens to understand storm warnings. In Bangladesh, illiteracy runs highest among women. The majority of the dead in the hurricane with no name were women.

Despite all this, people were resilient and struggled to help one another. Women talked of searching for food and finding some rice buried in the sand. A thirteen-year-old boy found his father's body and gave him proper burial rites. He felt proud that he was able to do his duty toward his father. The media did not report this. In Florida, pictures were shown on TV of neighbors helping each other. Reporters interviewed survivors, asking them how they hoped to return to normal lives. But in Bangladesh, the media showed only dead bodies and masses of dark-skinned people begging for food. Fourteen million people were made homeless, but the media left them as nameless as the hurricane.

This sort of coverage led to absurd queries. Why do these stupid people live in a disaster prone area? Aren't there too many people in Bangladesh already? Nobody is asking why forty-four million people crowd into hurricane prone counties from Texas to Maine.

The truth is, death like this does not have to be inevitable in the developing world. What is more important: one C-17 airplane, or enough shelters to keep 138,000 people from floating away [Ahmed, 1992, p. 15]?

Material, financial, and human resources, then, play an important part in preventing disasters from natural or accidental causes. These economic, political, and technological conditions highlight the continued need for international programs of aid and cooperation in the distribution and use of natural and human resources. Bureaucratic and political rivalries can result in further tragedy and loss of life. Technology and effective political organizations are central to controlling nature and aiding disaster victims. Social and behavioral sciences also have contributed to the reduction in human error and accidental disaster through, for example, research on perception and reaction times of pilots and air traffic controllers.

Psychological and Other Factors

In the psychological realm, confronting the unhealthy mechanism of denial is central to preventing victimization by natural disaster. Because a natural disaster is a dreaded experience, most people deny that it could happen to them, even when they live in high-risk areas for floods, tornados, or earthquakes. People use denial as a means to go on living normal lives while under more or less constant threat of disaster. Escape and problem solving are also affected by the extent of a person's denial. Jerry Jefferson in Wilkes-Barre, Pennsylvania ignored the flood warnings and convinced his wife that they should go to bed as usual because, he said, "it will never get so high that we'll have to move." His wife Ann was unconvinced and kept watch on the rising water during the night. Each new warning from Ann left Jerry unconvinced that the flood could really hit them. When the water reached the second floor of their house, Jerry finally gave up his denial. Fortunately, this couple was rescued and did not lose their lives. But Francis King, also of Wilkes-Barre, refused to leave his home despite all warnings. Eventually, he clung to a telephone pole and was rescued by helicopter. Others may be in special circumstances that prevent them from hearing the warnings.

CASE EXAMPLE: MARTIN AND EVELYN SCHONER

Martin Schoner, age seventy, and his wife Evelyn, age sixty-eight, had lived all their lives in a valley neighborhood. The Schoners had both been retired for several years; Martin had been a men's clothing merchant and Evelyn a nurse. They enjoyed the activities of their retirement years, including occasionally baby-sitting their five grandchildren. They and their two children exchanged visits frequently.

The evening before the flood, Martin was admitted to the hospital for chest and stomach discomfort. When Evelyn left her husband at the hospital that evening, they still did not know his diagnosis nor did they have any suspicion that disaster was imminent. Meanwhile, numerous flood warnings were being broadcast by radio and televi-

sion. Evelyn, however, heard none of these. She went to bed as usual, only to be awakened at 5 A.M. by a telephone call from a friend advising her of the flood and the need to leave her house quickly. She immediately packed a bag and drove to her friend's house. A few hours later, she heard on the radio that houses in her neighborhood were filled with water up to the second floor. She was unable to reach her husband; the hospital was also flooded and the patients had been evacuated. Both Martin and Evelyn were beside themselves with fear and worry, for each had no idea of the whereabouts of the other.

One of Evelyn's special concerns was Martin's medical condition. She still did not know whether or not his symptoms signaled

Case Example, cont.

heart trouble. As it turned out, Martin's symptoms were from food poisoning. He had been moved to a local college that was converted into a temporary shelter; seriously ill patients were in another hospital. Martin, however, was so upset and worried about his wife that rescue workers finally sent a hospital chaplain to talk with him. Martin said afterward that he found it a tremendous relief to pour out his worry to a sympathetic listener who helped him through a good cry without embarrassment or shame. Evelyn had no way of knowing these facts because public communication networks were not operating.

Two days later, Evelyn finally learned from a friend that Martin was at the college emergency shelter. Evelyn went to pick him up; they stayed for a few days at a friend's house before returning to their neighborhood to assess the damage. When they returned, they were grief-stricken over the loss of their possessions and the destruction of the home they had treasured. Evelyn was particularly upset. She kept repeating, "If only I had known that this was going to happen, I would have moved at least some of our precious things upstairs or packed them up to take with me."

Martin and Evelyn, with the help of their friends, decided to stay in the neighborhoodand rebuild their home with the help of federal aid. In the aftermath of the crisis, Martin gained a new lease on life despite the tragedy. He no longer had empty hours in his days; he single-handedly took on the job of repairing the flood damage and refinishing the house. He became a source of support and encouragement for others in the neighborhood. But Evelyn felt the flood left an indelible mark on her. She seemed unable to stop grieving over the loss they had suffered. Evelyn said, "If only our minister hadn't been out of town at the time, I would have had someone to talk to when it happened." Martin and Evelyn did not know that specially trained crisis counselors were available to survivors of the disaster. This highlights the fact that communication in a disaster-stricken community is often inadequate.

Martin, Evelyn, and their neighbors live in fear of another flood; they have no assurance that adequate precautionary measures have been taken to prevent a recurrence. They decided, however, to take a chance and live their last years in the neighborhood they love, with the resolution that, should another flood occur, they will move away once and for all.

It is difficult for anyone who has not experienced a flood to imagine that heavy rain alone can produce enough water to break a dam and flood a whole city. People are used to associating certain results with certain causes. When cause and effect are unfamiliar, denial is likely.

Preventive Intervention

It is impossible to prepare for the crisis of disaster the way one can prepare for transition states such as parenthood, retirement, or death. However, we can act on a communitywide basis before disaster strikes. This is particularly important in communities at high risk for natural disasters. Such preparation is a form of psychological immunization. There are several things a community can do to prepare for possible disaster:

1. Make public service announcements during spring rains or tornado seasons urging people not to ignore disaster warnings.
2. Broadcast educational programs on television dramatizing techniques for crowd control and for helping people who are panic stricken or in shock.
3. Review public safety codes to assure adequate protection against fire in public gathering places such as restaurants, theaters, and hospitals.
4. Make public service announcements urging people to take first-aid courses with local Red Cross and fire departments.
5. Broadcast educational programs on radio and television to acquaint people with social agencies and crisis services available to them in the event of disaster.
6. Initiate a program of crisis intervention training for mental health and social service workers as an addition to their traditional skills.
7. Institute an upgraded program of disaster preparation by medical, health, and welfare facilities, including mechanisms for community coordination of disaster rescue services. In communities with an excellent medical disaster plan, survivors had adequate medical and health care during and after floods.
8. Develop plans for support of disaster relief workers who themselves usually are shocked and numbed from the experience. For example, workers assigned to recover human remains from an airplane wreckage (typically emergency medical and firefighting personnel) can tolerate only a few hours at a time confronting the horror. They need time-out and an opportunity to process what they have witnessed with a crisis or mental health counselor.

These preparations will not prevent the devastating effects of a disaster, but they may reduce the impact of the trauma and help people live through the experience with less physical, social, and emotional damage than they might otherwise suffer.

Individual Responses to Disaster

Reactions to the stress and trauma of a disaster are not unlike reactions to transition states such as migration or loss of a loved one through death. They also resemble responses to victimization by crime (see Chapter Eight). Tyhurst (1951, 1957a, 1957b) has identified three overlapping phases in disaster reaction. These are similar to the four phases noted by Caplan (see Chapter Two) in the development of a crisis state:

1. *Impact:* In this period, the person is hit with the reality of what is happening. In catastrophic events, the impact period lasts from a few minutes to one or two hours. The concern of disaster victims during the impact phase is with the

immediate present. An automatic stimulus-response reaction occurs, with the catas-trophe as stimulus. Victims are struck later with wonder that they were able to carry on as well as they did, especially if they finally break down under the full emotional impact of the experience. During the impact phase, individual reac-tions to the disaster fall into three main groups:

a. Ten to twenty-five percent of the victims remain calm and do not fall apart. Instead, they assess the situation, develop a plan of action, and carry it through.
b. Seventy-five percent of the victims are shocked and confused. They are un-able to express any particular feeling or emotion. The usual physical signs of fear are present: sweating, rapid heart beat, upset stomach, and trembling. This is considered the "normal" reaction to a disaster.
c. Another ten to twenty-five percent become hysterical or confused or are par-alyzed with fear. These victims may sit and stare into space or may run around wildly. The behavior of this group is of most concern for rescue workers and crisis counselors who may be on the scene during emergency operations.

Evelyn Schoner, caught in the Wilkes-Barre flood because she did not hear the warnings, had the first type of reaction during the impact phase. When she fi-nally received the warning telephone call, she packed her bag and drove to safety. She had no difficulty doing this, even though she ordinarily depended heavily on her husband when in distress, and he was in the hospital. Evelyn stated: "It re-ally only hit me afterward . . . that everything I treasured was lost. I just had to drive away and leave everything behind. You don't know what that's like—saving precious things all your life, then all of a sudden they're gone—even the photo-graphs of our family." There are no studies that identify or predict which people will fall into the last group of reactors to disaster. However, prediction criteria (see Chapter Three) indicate that the following types of people are particularly vul-nerable to crisis or emotional disturbance following acute stress from a disaster:

• The elderly who have few physical resources and a reduced capacity to adapt to rapid change
• Those who already are coping with stress in self-destructive or unhealthy ways such as taking solace in alcohol
• Those who are alone and friendless and who lack physical and social resources they can rely on in an emergency

During the San Fernando Valley earthquake, mental health staff at the Los Angeles County–Olive View Medical Center observed that some acutely disturbed mental patients reacted more rationally than usual during the acute phase of the quake. For example, they helped to rescue fellow patients (Koegler & Hicks, 1972). In Rapid City, South Dakota, seventy-one-year-old Gertrude Lux stood for five hours in shoulder-deep water balancing her disabled granddaughter Vicki on a foam mattress floating in the room where they were trapped. In Armero, Colombia, rescue workers dug with their bare hands and bailed out water with tin cans to save a thirteen-year-old girl trapped beneath a cement slab. These incidents reveal the commonly observed heroism and humanity of disaster victims despite personal pain and loss. People rise dramatically to the occasion and mobilize resources to help themselves and others.

2. *Recoil:* During this phase, there is at least a temporary suspension of the initial stresses of the disaster. Lives are no longer in immediate danger, although other stresses such as cold or pain from injury may continue. Along the Mississippi, more floods followed the first one, and aftershocks follow earthquakes. During the recoil phase, survivors are typically en route to friends' homes, or they have found shelter in community facilities set up for the emergency. They may look around for someone to be with. They want to be taken care of—to receive a cup of coffee or a blanket. Chilled survivors of an earthquake, for example, huddle in makeshift camps and tent cities, lighting fires to keep warm. The disaster experience leaves some survivors with a childlike dependency and need to be with others. At this phase, survivors gradually become aware of the full impact of what they have been through. Both women and men may break down and weep. Survivors have their first chance to share the experience with others. Their attention is focused on the immediate past and how they managed to survive. This phase has the greatest implication for crisis workers helping the survivors.

3. *Post-trauma:* During this period, survivors become fully aware of the losses they have sustained during the impact phase: loss of home, financial security, personal belongings, and particularly, loved ones who may have died in the disaster. In this phase, much depends on a person's age and general condition. As Jane Cantor, a Wilkes-Barre survivor put it, "A disaster can bring out the best and the worst in a person." Those who are too old to start over again find their loss of home and possessions particularly devastating. Older people who prize the reminders of their children and earlier life feel robbed of what they have worked for all their lives. Anger and frustration follow. If loved ones have died in the disaster, grief and mourning predominate. Murphy (1986, p. 339) cites studies of bereavement suggesting that the recovery period varies from several months to several years and is subjectively defined. Murphy found that among survivors who lost a loved one in a close relationship to the Mt. St. Helen's volcanic eruption, bereavement was intense and prolonged, especially if they perceived the disaster as preventable. Some survivors of the Rapid City flood felt overwhelming guilt over the death of loved ones: "Why me? Why was I spared and not she?" Many survivors describe the horror of listening to screams, of watching people being swept past them to their deaths, and of being helpless to save them. Lifton and Olson (1976) have described this reaction as "death guilt." Survivors somehow feel responsible for the death of their relatives or others they were unable to save. They cannot quite forgive themselves for living, for having been spared. At the same time, they may feel relief at not being among the dead. This, in turn, leaves them feeling guiltier.

During this third phase, survivors may have psychotic episodes, reactive depressions, anxiety reactions, and dreams in which they relive the catastrophic experience. Some agencies report increased numbers of hospital admissions for emotional disturbances following disaster. Staff of the Child Guidance Center in San Fernando Valley counseled hundreds of parents and children following the earthquake. Children typically were afraid to be alone and afraid to go to sleep in their own beds. Bennet (1970), in his study of survivors of the 1968 floods in Bristol, England, found that twelve months after the disaster the health of flooded people was worse than the general health of those not in the flood and that the likelihood of older people dying within twelve months was increased. Lifton and Olson (1976) report that when survivors perceive a disaster as a reflection of human callousness—rather than an act of God or nature—the psychological effects are more severe and long-lasting.

This post-traumatic phase may last for the rest of a person's life, depending on his or her predisaster state, the extent of loss, the help available during the disaster, and whether the disaster was natural or from human origins (Richman, 1993). Evelyn Schoner said, "I don't think I'll ever be the same. I just can't get over it. . . . I live in constant fear that there might be another flood. . . . There's just no guarantee that there won't be another one."

A small group of disaster survivors gives up. These people remain despondent and hopeless for the rest of their lives (Farberow, 1967). Most survivors, however, gather together and reconstruct their lives, their homes, and their community. While a number of people in flood-prone areas move to higher elevations, many others rebuild their homes on the same location, even though there is no guarantee against further flooding. This is particularly true for older people who find it too costly to start over and who want to keep the comfort of a familiar neighborhood, even though they have lost everything else.

Rescue and crisis workers have the most influence during the impact and recoil phases (Joseph, et al., 1993), while mental health workers play a key role during the post-traumatic phase. As noted throughout this book, crisis intervention—available at the right time and in the right place—is the most effective means of preventing later psychiatric disturbances. As Evelyn Schoner said: "If only I would have had someone to talk to when it happened." The availability of crisis assistance to individuals, however, is intricately tied to the community response to disaster.

Community Responses to Disaster

The most immediate social consequence of a disaster is the disruption of normal social patterns on which all community members depend (Tyhurst, 1957a). The community suffers a social paralysis. People are separated from family and friends and spontaneously form other groups out of the need to be with others.

When disaster strikes, large numbers of people are cut off from public services and resources that they count on for survival. These can include water—one of the first resources to go in the event of a flood—electricity, and heat. People scramble for shelter, food, and water. Traffic controls are out, so accidents increase. In flooded areas, many people fall in the slippery mud and break limbs, thus placing more demands on hospital staff. Often, hospitals are flooded out, and all patients must be transferred to other facilities. Schools and many businesses close, creating further strain and chaos in homes and emergency shelters.

Disaster can bring out the worst in people. Some take advantage of the disorder to loot and steal; some business owners take advantage of the occasion to profit from others' misfortune by inflating the prices of necessary supplies.

Since normal communication networks are either destroyed or are very limited, rumors abound and panic and chaos increase. Communication problems and physical distance also make information about relief benefits difficult to disseminate. This causes resentment among those who feel they did not receive a fair share of the benefits. Residents who are not even on the scene of the disaster can be affected by media generalizations and sensationalistic reports.

The Schoners in Wilkes-Barre observed that the flood was instrumental in bringing the people of their neighborhood closer together. Professional evaluators observed the same phenomenon (Zusman, Joss, & Newman, 1973). During the impact period of a disaster, there is greater cohesion among community members; later, people focus on their individual concerns. People must rely on each other for help and support during a disaster in a way that was not necessary before, as was illustrated in Rapid City. During the flood, a group of professionals were attending a conference on death and dying. A call was put out to the conference participants to assist families in identifying members who had died. The helpers reported that many friends had already turned out to help the bereaved families.

During the impact and recoil stages of a disaster, community control usually passes from elected government officials to professionals who direct health, welfare, mental health, and public order agencies. This occurs out of necessity, because of the reactions cited above. Elected officials have the important function of soliciting assistance for the community from state, federal, and sometimes international resources. The community's priorities are rapidly defined by professional leaders, and an emergency health and social service system is quickly established. This emergency network focuses on:

- Preservation of life and health: rescue activities, inoculations, treatment of the injured
- Conservation and distribution of resources: organization of emergency shelters, distribution of supplies such as water, food, and blankets
- Conservation of public order: police surveillance to prevent looting and accidents arising out of the chaos and the scramble for remaining resources

- Maintenance of morale: dispatching mental health, welfare, and pastoral coun-selors to assist the panic stricken and bereaved during the acute crisis phase

Material, social, and psychological services should be available for as long as they are needed.

In summary, a community's response to disaster is poignantly revealed in the following description by Kizzier (1972) of Rapid City, and is repeated many times over in communities.

> With all of this help from private, city, county, state, and federal funds and with the compassion and support offered from an entire nation, Rapid City is restor-ing and rebuilding with a new appreciation for life. It has pulled together for a purpose before, but never before has it become a pulsating, throbbing being as it is now, in the aftermath of a flood.
>
> Not one person has been untouched by the drama of recovery. Through the silent heartache and compassion, we again remember what it is like to be pa-tient with each other. There is a need for the comfort of physical contact as we greet each survivor with a thankful hug.
>
> We are more aware of the things we take for granted like the utility companies, bridges, and the National Guard. We now look at the police with new respect, feel thankful for the closeness of the air force base and vow never again to pass the ringing Christmas bells of the Salvation Army without dropping in a coin.
>
> We empty our food closets and our clothes closets in an attempt to lend a hand to someone who was left with nothing. We shake our heads in dismay as the big scoops move in on the destruction to clear away the mess.
>
> We go to the citywide memorial service on Sunday, feeling sad and empty and discouraged after being threatened by another torrent of rain the night before. We see people there who have lost far more than we have, bearing their burden with surprising spirit. We want to cry with all the pent-up emotion, but we are being told that we must overcome our grief, rejoice, and sing and carry on with life. And so we will, just like everyone around us will, because people need to laugh or they will break. We come from the memorial service feeling renewed and we try laughing and it makes us feel warm inside and a little lightheaded.

Factors Affecting Recovery of Survivors

Tyhurst (1957a) notes that the nature and severity of reactions to disaster and the process of recovery are influenced by several factors:

1. *The element of surprise:* If and when warnings are given, they should be fol-lowed by instructions in what to do. Warnings followed by long silences and no

action plan can heighten anxiety and lead to the commonly observed denial of some residents that a disaster is imminent.

2. *Separation of family members:* Children are particularly vulnerable to damaging psychological effects if separated from their families during the acute period of a disaster (Blanford & Levine, 1972; Durkin, et al., 1993; Zeidner, Klingman, & Itskowitz, 1993). Therefore, families should be evacuated as a unit whenever possible.

3. *Outside help:* Reasonable recovery from a disaster requires aid from unaffected areas. Since military forces have the organization, discipline, and equipment necessary for dealing with a disaster, their instruction should include assisting civilians during disaster.

4. *Leadership:* As in any crisis situation, a disaster demands that someone have the ability to make decisions and give direction. The police, the military, and physicians have leadership potential during a disaster. Their training should include preparation to exercise this potential appropriately.

5. *Communication:* Since failures in communication give rise to rumors, it is essential that a communication network and public information centers be established and maintained as a high priority in disaster work. Much impulsive and irrational behavior can be prevented by the reassurance and direction that a good communication network provides.

6. *Measures directed toward reorientation:* Communication lays the foundation for the reidentification of individuals in family and social groups. A basic step of reorientation is the registration of survivors so that they can once again feel like members of society. This also provides a way for relatives and friends to find each other.

7. *Evacuation:* In any disaster, there is a spontaneous mass movement to leave the stricken area. Planned evacuation will prevent the panic that results when people find their escape blocked or delayed. Failure to attend to the psychological and social problems of evacuation can result in serious social and interpersonal problems.

Resources for Psychological Assistance

Although federal aid for reconstruction has been available to communities stricken with disaster for many years, there was no comparable aid for victims' psychological needs until 1972. At that time, the National Institute of Mental Health (NIMH) was prepared organizationally to provide disaster victims with emotional first-aid services, that is, crisis intervention. As a result of this change, communities in the United States receive financial aid to assist in offering crisis services to disaster victims (Okura, 1975). The significance of this policy is twofold. First, it demonstrates the need for outside mental health assistance in times of disaster to supplement local resources. Local mental health workers may be disaster victims themselves and temporarily unable to help others in distress. Second, it confirms that the ability of people to help others in crisis is strongly influenced by their prior skill or training in crisis intervention.

In most communities, the special federal aid for crisis intervention supplements crisis services offered by other groups. For example, Jewish Social Services from New York deployed social workers to Wilkes-Barre to assist disaster victims (Birnbaum, Coplon, & Scharff, 1973). Catholic, Mennonite, and various protestant denominations traditionally offer help to disaster-stricken communities.

It is probably impossible to have an oversupply of crisis intervention services for people struck by a disaster. Gordon (1976) notes that community mental health agencies must have prior crisis intervention skills in order to mobilize the resources necessary when a disaster occurs. Health and mental health workers, along with other community caretakers, must know how to put these crisis intervention skills to use when a disaster strikes. Since there is little or no time to prepare for the disaster, there is no time to prepare as a crisis worker once a disaster is imminent. Workers must be ready to apply their knowledge, attitudes, and skills in crisis intervention.

In spite of much progress in this area, more long-term planning is needed to better meet the psychological needs of disaster victims, many of whom suffer from severe shock. The National Organization for Victim Assistance (NOVA) recognizes this need through services offered by its Crisis Response Team.

Help During Impact, Recoil, and Post-Trauma Phases

The helping process during disaster takes on distinctive characteristics during the disaster's impact, recoil, and post-trauma phases. Table 10.1 illustrates the kind of help needed and who is best suited to offer it during the three phases of a disaster. The table also suggests the possible outcomes for disaster victims if help is not available in each of the three phases.

Crisis Intervention and Follow-Up Service

The basic principles of crisis management should be applied on behalf of disaster victims. During and after a disaster, people need an opportunity to:

- Talk out the experience and express their feelings of fear, panic, loss, and grief
- Become fully aware and accepting of what has happened to them
- Resume activity and begin reconstructing their lives with the social, physical, and emotional resources available

To assist victims through the crisis, the crisis worker should:

- Listen with concern and sympathy; ease the way for the victims to tell their tragic story, weep, and express feelings of anger, loss, frustration, and despair

TABLE 10.1. ASSISTANCE DURING THREE PHASES
OF NATURAL DISASTER.

	Help Needed	Help Provided by	Possible Outcome if Help Unavailable
Phase I: Impact	Information on source and degree of danger	Communication network: radio, TV, public address system	Physical injury or death
	Escape and rescue from immediate source of danger	Community rescue resources: police and fire departments, Red Cross, National Guard	
Phase II: Recoil	Shelter, food, drink, clothing, medical care	Red Cross	Physical injury
		Salvation Army	Delayed grief reactions
		Voluntary agencies such as colleges to be converted to mass shelters	Later emotional or mental disturbance
		Local health and welfare agencies	
		Mental health and social service agencies skilled in crisis intervention	
		Pastoral counselors	
		State and federal assistance for all of the above services	
Phase III: Post-trauma	Physical reconstruction	State and federal resources for physical reconstruction	Financial hardship
	Social reestablishment	Social welfare agencies	Social instability
	Psychological support concerning aftereffects of the event itself; bereavement counseling concerning loss of loved ones, home, and personal property	Crisis and mental health services	Long-lasting mental, emotional, or physical health problems
		Pastoral counselors	

- Help the survivors accept the reality of what has happened a little bit at a time—perhaps by staying with them during the initial stages of shock and denial, accompanying them to the scene of the tragedy, and supporting them when they are faced with the full impact of their loss
- Assist victims in making contact with relatives, friends, and other resources needed to begin the process of social and physical reconstruction—perhaps by making telephone calls to locate relatives, accompanying people to apply for financial aid, and giving information about social and mental health agencies for follow-up services

In group settings where large numbers are housed and offered emergency care, those who are panic stricken should be separated from the rest and given individual attention to avoid the contagion of panic reactions. Assigning these people simple, physical tasks will move them in the direction of constructive action. Any action that helps victims feel valued as individuals is important at this time. Yet, in spite of massive efforts to help survivors of disaster, it seems almost impossible to prevent life-long emotional scarring among the people who live through the experience. Crisis and bereavement counseling can at least reduce some negative effects and should be available to all victims.

One lesson learned in Wilkes-Barre's Project Outreach was the necessity of actively seeking out those in need of crisis counseling (Zusman, Joss, & Newman, 1973). Crisis workers became acquainted with residents on a block-by-block basis and were thereby able to assess needs and make crisis services available to people who otherwise might not have used them.

No local community can possibly meet all of the physical, social, and emotional needs of its residents who are disaster victims. The Wilkes-Barre experiment of providing federal funds for crisis services as well as for physical reconstruction sets a precedent for assisting communities that are struck by disaster in the future. This will be necessary even when local mental health, welfare, and health workers are better trained in crisis intervention. In most disasters, the need is too great for the local community to act alone, especially since some of its own human service workers (police officers, nurses, clergy, and counselors) will themselves be among the disaster victims (Laube, 1973).

In summary, individual responses and the needs of natural disaster victims— as in other crisis situations—vary according to psychological, economic, and social circumstances. Natural disaster victims seem to have something in common for coping with this kind of crisis: they interpret these tragedies as acts of God, or fate, or bad luck—and thus beyond anyone's control. Accounting for an event from a common viewpoint is an important aspect of constructive crisis coping at the cognitive level. Emotional coping can then occur through grief work and can be followed by behavioral responses to rebuild lives. The victims' interpretation of these crises as "natural" and beyond their control is the basis for the hope felt by survivors of natural disasters in spite of enormous suffering. It is the reason they can rise from the rubble and begin a new life; it lets them move beyond the emotional pain and gain new strength from the experience. This element of disaster response and recovery constitutes the greatest distinction between natural disasters and those occurring from human indifference, neglect, or design.

Disasters from Human Origins

The world knows about the atomic bombs dropped in Japan, the Nazi Holocaust, and the destruction of Love Canal. War and environmental pollution are planned disasters that bring about physical, social, and emotional destruction of immeasurable proportions. Some survivors of Hiroshima describe the horror:

> People who were laying there and dying and screaming and yelling for help and the people who were burned were hollering, "I'm so hot, please help me, please kill me" and things like that and . . . it was terrible (Mary).

> We had a hospital near our place and many, many hundreds of injured people came to the hospital and there weren't too many adequate medical supplies and there were some doctors there, some nurses there, but they didn't have enough medicine to take care of all the people. And these people were thirsty and hurt and dying and all night long I could hear them calling, "mother, mother," and it sounded to me like ghosts calling out in the middle of the night (Mitsuo).

> In the Japanese tradition, you're supposed to look for your family. I walked for three weeks, every single day, looking for my grandparents and my brother. It was a feeling of real loneliness and looking at the devastation of the whole city wondering why God left me here alone. You know, why didn't he take me too. At the time, yeah, I did want to go too. I felt they should have . . . I should have gone too instead of being left alone (Florence). (*Survivors,* 1982, pp. 4–6; WGBH Educational Foundation, 1982.)

On August 6, 1945, the first atomic bomb was dropped on Hiroshima. Three days later, Nagasaki was bombed. Six days later, World War II was over. Over 80 percent of the people within one kilometer of the explosion died instantly or soon afterward. By December 1945, the number of dead in Hiroshima and Nagasaki was over 200,000. By 1950, another 140,000 people had died from the continuing effects of radiation exposure; since then, 100,000 more people have died from radiation-related cancer. Before and during the same war, millions of Jews, gypsies, homosexuals, mentally retarded people, and others viewed as undesirable by the Nazis were systematically exterminated in what many consider the most horrible crime in the history of the world.

When Japanese-American victims of the atomic bomb declared themselves as survivors, insurance companies withdrew their health and life insurance policies, and employers discriminated against them. Nightmares, flashbacks, and fear for themselves and their children are common today among these survivors. Over ten years ago, they formed the Committee of Atomic Bomb Survivors in the United States to gain medical benefits from the U.S. government—to no avail; several bills introduced in Congress have failed to pass. Vietnam War veterans did finally succeed in gaining veterans' benefits for health damage they claim resulted from exposure to the defoliant Agent Orange, damage affecting at least 250,000 U.S. families. For many Vietnam veterans, America's most unpopular war still rages; many still feel that the loss of life and limb—accepted as necessary in earlier wars—was not justified in a war that should never have been fought. Veterans of the Gulf War (Desert Storm) have had a much shorter struggle. They have been given compensation for damages they believe to have resulted from exposure to as-yet-unidentified agents during warfare, based on testimony in Congress from sick veterans and their advocates.

In Buffalo Creek, West Virginia, a mining corporation carelessly dumped coal waste, which formed artificial dams that eventually broke and caused dozens of deaths. Buffalo Creek residents knew that the dam was considered dangerous and that the mining corporation had neglected to correct the problem (Lifton & Olson, 1976). When loved ones, homes, and the natural environment were destroyed, survivors concluded that the mining company regarded them as less than human. In fact, one of the excuses offered by the company for not correcting their dangerous waste disposal method was that fish would be harmed by alternative methods. The survivors' feelings of devaluation were confirmed by their knowledge of the coal company's proposal of hasty and inadequate financial settlements. The physical damage to the community was never repaired, either by the company or through outside assistance. Residents are constantly reminded of the disaster.

Unlike the Rapid City community described earlier, Buffalo Creek survivors did not respond to the disaster with community rejuvenation born out of the tragedy. Lifton and Olson (1976) attribute this tremendously different response to the disaster's human (rather than natural) origin. Even though the mining company was forced to pay 13.5 million dollars in a psychic damage suit, Buffalo Creek residents seem to feel that they and their community will never be healed. Considering genetic, health, and material damage such as that suffered by Love Canal residents, monetary compensation becomes practically meaningless. Money cannot repair such losses. *Prevention* of and *learning* from such tragic neglect seem the only reasonable responses.

Reactions of Buffalo Creek and Love Canal survivors are similar to those observed among survivors, including children, of Hiroshima, the Nazi Holocaust, and other wars (Apfel & Simon, forthcoming; Lifton, 1967). Lifton and Olson (1976) state, "As the source of stress shifts from indiscriminate violence by nature to the discriminate oppression by man, the damage to human personality becomes less remediable." Survivors of planned disaster—including war—feel that their humanity has been violated. Their psyches are bombarded to such a degree that their capacity for recovery is often permanently damaged.

In a related category are victims and survivors of technological disaster, an increasing occurrence worldwide as people demand more goods and energy, technical errors occur, and more toxic wastes are produced (Baum, Fleming, & Singer, 1983). The most outstanding international examples are the Bhopal, Chernobyl, and Challenger space shuttle disasters. At least seven thousand people died in the Bhopal industrial calamity; ten years later, a half-million survivors have yet to receive compensation, while the plant officials charged with manslaughter have not been brought to trial (Ganguly, 1994, p. 7). On a less dramatic scale are the increasing numbers of people exposed to occupational hazards, as evidenced by increasing rates of infertility, especially among low-paid workers (predominately women of color) in the least protected environments. For example, two women in Silicon Valley, California developed an immune deficiency syndrome traceable to their exposure to toxic chemicals in the presumably "clean" computer chip industry (Spake, 1986). Central to the emotional recovery of persons exposed to such events are the concepts of "meaning" and "control." As discussed in Chapter Two, emotional recovery seems to require that traumatized people be able to incorporate events into their meaning system and to maintain at least some perception of control. If a situation seems beyond one's control, self-blame may be used as a way to cope with the event (Baum, Fleming, & Singer, 1983, p. 134).

Thus, if the origin of trauma or prolonged distress is external, that is, if people are exposed to occupational hazards or are victims of disasters traced to negligence, it is important that victims attribute responsibility to its true sources rather than to themselves. Interpreting a person's anger and demand for compensation as a "dependency conflict" or in other psychopathological terms is a form of blaming the victim (Schottenfeld & Cullen, 1985, p. 1126). Instead, such traumatized people should be linked to self-help and advocacy groups through which they might channel their anger into constructive action for necessary change—in this case, improved safety standards on the job (Chavkin, 1984)—or social change regarding toxic waste (Grossfeld, 1993; Hoff & McNutt, 1994) (see Figure 8.1, Box 3, right circle). This is not to say that prior psychopathologies do not play a role in some injury claims, but these should not be used to obscure the fact that injurious exposure reduces some people to joblessness, ill health, and poverty (Schottenfeld & Cullen, 1985, p. 1126).

Many of these ideas are now being examined in studies of "post-traumatic stress disorder" (PTSD), a controversial concept describing a chronic condition that may occur years after an original trauma experienced outside the normal range of life events, such as during a war or in a concentration camp (Davidson, et al., 1985; McCarroll, et al., 1993; Peterson, Prout, & Schwarz, 1991). Although PTSD has some features common to depression, panic disorder, and alcoholism, its increasing prevalence underscores the importance of crisis intervention for all traumatized people in addition to renewed efforts to prevent trauma in the first place.

Maintaining or regaining health (salutogenesis) and avoiding illness is a greater challenge when the crisis originates from sociocultural sources—in this case, disasters of human origin. This is because the emotional healing process requires, among other things, that people answer this question for themselves: Why did this happen to me? If the answer is, "It was fate," "It was God's will," or "That's life; some bad things just happen," people are able to recover and rebuild their lives, especially with social support. But if the answer can be traced to prejudice; neglect or hatred of individuals, groups, or a corporation (as in environmental pollution); ethnic cleansing; or to any other human origin, the persons affected must receive a message of caring and compensation to counteract the devastating effects of such malevolent actions. Otherwise, a person's sense of coherence, including comprehensibility, meaningfulness, and manageability (Antonovsky, 1987, pp. 17–19) is shaken; they tend to absorb the blame and devaluation implied by others' neglect or outright damage. This process is similar to the downward spiral to depression and possible morbidity discussed in Chapter Two (Figure 2.2), which can occur when victims of violence are blamed for their plight.

Follow-Up and Prevention

Vietnam veterans are still trying to rebuild their lives after a generation of being made scapegoats for a nation's guilt and shame about a war they were not personally responsible for starting. Holocaust survivors have formed awareness groups as resources for support and the preservation of history. Atomic bomb survivors say their sacrifice was worthwhile if only the bomb is never used again. First Nations people are fighting for their cultural survival as well as against the destruction of the environment, which they view as a crime against the harmony that should exist between nature and human beings (Mousseau, 1989). Lois Gibbs (1982) has told about the Love Canal tragedy; her story moved a nation to awareness of similar hazards in numerous other communities. Not unlike the parent survivors of teenage suicide, these survivors are trying to find meaning in their suffering by sharing the pain and tragedy of their lives to benefit others. The survivors of human malice, greed, and prejudice tell us something about ourselves, our world, and the way we relate to each other and the environment.

Yet, more than 100 years after the American Civil War, a half century after the Holocaust, and twenty-five years after the Vietnam War, we still have:

- Racially motivated violence and institutionalized racism across the United States, which seems to be increasing in recent years
- Crimes with apparent anti-Semitic and other ethnic, religious, and political motives from Boston to Ireland, Bosnia, Haiti, Rwanda, and the Middle East
- A systematic attempt to declare the Holocaust a "myth" that never happened
- Repeated famines in African countries that can be traced to war and to the widening gap between haves and have-nots of the world (Wijkman & Timberlake, 1984)
- An international nuclear capacity for destruction more than one million times the power of the atomic bomb dropped on Hiroshima

To meet the challenges of these potentially destructive forces, there are now national and international debates about nuclear proliferation, regional wars, and arms trade that are unparalleled in the history of the human race in their importance to our ultimate survival. But the social, political, religious, and psychological ramifications of national and international crises and chronic problems are complex, controversial, and passionately debated. People are deeply divided, for example, in their views about:

- Whether or how "ethnic cleansing" should be stopped
- What the division of government spending should be between "guns and butter"
- Whether the environmental crisis is as serious as some claim

These issues will probably be argued for a long time. Nevertheless, the following facts remain:

- Many crises can be traced to social, economic, and political factors of local and global origins.
- Children are pressing their teachers for answers about crime and environmental threat.
- Fear about nuclear power and environmental pollution have increased since the Chernobyl disaster.
- Effective crisis intervention cannot be practiced without considering the sociocultural context of the crisis.

It is imperative that individual crises be understood in terms of their public meaning (Mills, 1959). Public issues should be debated and acted on, not abstractly, but in terms of their impact on each of us—you, me, our families and friends, and others. Not only is there a dynamic interplay between public and private life, but in both realms our sensitivity to others' perceptions and value systems regarding controversial issues can foster cooperation and prevent conflict.

Each person's unique perception of traumatic events is central to understanding and resolving a crisis. Without communication, we cannot understand another's interpretation of an event or issue, and we may become a hindrance to constructive crisis resolution. In fact, two compelling reasons to practice crisis intervention are the reward and stimulation of discovering the uniqueness of others and the satisfaction of helping people in crisis discover their own capacities for solving problems. Communication is central to such discovery. The differences in interpretations of personal, social, and political problems are as diverse as community members themselves. Unquestionably, communication is the key to uncovering these interpretations and thus understanding and helping people in crisis. A person tells his or her traumatic experience through emotional display, behavior, and verbal communication—Hansell's (1976) "crisis plumage." If we do not listen and respond with caring and support, or if there is no one to tell the story to, the chances of a constructive crisis outcome are diminished.

This is also true at the social and political level or when large groups of people are in crisis. Victims of disasters of human origin, like victims of crime, often have a hard time finding people to listen to them. Friends or crisis counselors may listen, but as noted in earlier chapters, these individual responses are not enough if the crisis did not originate from individual circumstances or if the whole community is affected. Social and political action are pivotal to a positive crisis outcome if the *origin* of the crisis is social and political.

No matter how public and widespread the calamity, we should remember that society is made up of individuals with particular interpretations of events—with distinct shades in their "crisis plumage." These individuals are more real than the casualty figures reported on the evening news make them seem.

- Richard, a Vietnam War veteran with recurrent nightmares, is someone's husband, father, son, and brother. He is forty-eight years old and lives on Locust Street in a town of 45,000.
- Shigeko is an atomic bomb survivor who has had twenty-six operations on her face and lips and is glad that she is alive and that her eight-year-old son is not ashamed of her appearance.
- Diane is a woman from Love Canal who has had multiple miscarriages.
- Bobby is a little boy from Love Canal who has nightmares about what chemicals look like. He imagines "a thing" attacking him.
- Jane, age five, lives near a hazardous waste site and has toxic hepatitis.

These people and many others like them tend to get lost in statements of "statistically significant" incidences (of cancer, deformed children, or other medical problems), scientific jargon, and "investigative procedures" for determining whether corrective action is in order. This process of generalizing does not seem to apply to real people. The abstractness, along with the grossness of the figures—10,000,000 victims of the Holocaust; nearly 500,000 dead from atomic bomb blasts—contribute to denial and psychic numbing for the average person. The numbers, the destruction, and the sheer horror are unimaginable for most of us. To defend ourselves against the terror, we deny and try to convince ourselves that there is nothing we personally can do about these global issues.

Although the Cold War is officially over, there are still stockpiles of nuclear arms sufficient to destroy the planet several times over, even as the United Nations Security Council debates how to deal with one regional crisis after another in which thousands of innocent civilians (many of them children) are slaughtered or wounded by warring factions. As Apfel and Simon (1994, p. 72) note, "If we decide it is the responsibility of the enemy's leadership to take care of its own children, then we can more easily go ahead with our bombing program. If we decide children anywhere in the world are also our children, we can less easily bomb. We distance ourselves and say that children who are far away are not our children, and if they suffer it is because their leaders and their parents are irresponsible." In the spirit of violence prevention and Ruddick's (1989) thesis regarding "maternal practice," it is reasonable to suggest that if men and women shared equally in the everyday tasks of caring for children and learned the conflict resolution tactics demanded by nonviolent parenting, they would insist that more resources be spent to promote peace and conserve lives and resources than are presently spent on war and destruction (Goodman & Hoff, 1990).

Denial and scientific objectification of actual and potential disaster victims are similar to the process discussed in the last chapter: (1) dehumanizing victims and enemies; and (2) maintaining distance from the object of criminal terrorism so that ordinary human compassion and other feelings do not interfere with the ultimate purposes of terrorism and war. From a safe distance, it is relatively easy to think of our enemies as less than human and therefore worthy of destruction. As in our attitudes toward the homeless, deinstitutionalized mental patients, and unwed mothers, our enemies are distant; they belong to groups and are the responsibility of the state or church. When they are thus objectified, we do not have to think of them as someone's sister, father, mother, or friend.

Our worst enemies are people like ourselves: they eat, sleep, make love, bear children, feel pain, fear, and anger, communicate with one another, bury their dead, and eventually die. Statistics and machines will never be a substitute for human interaction, just as rating scales can *aid* but not *displace* clinical judgment in evaluating individual suicide risk. As Albert Einstein said, "Peace cannot be kept by force. It can only be achieved by understanding."

In a particular crisis situation, if we do not *communicate*, for example, with a suicidal person, we will not understand why death is preferable to life for that individual and therefore may be ineffective in preventing suicide. If we take the time to *talk* with and *listen* to a person in crisis, we are less likely to suggest or prescribe a drug as a crisis response. Similarly, at the national and international levels, if we keep communication open and foster political strategies to handle crises, there is less likelihood of resorting to mechanical and chemical approaches to problem solving. Human communication, then, not only distinguishes us from the animal kingdom, it is central to our survival—as individuals and as a world community.

Nevertheless, our ethnocentrism is often so strong, and greed and power motives are often so disguised, that the average person may find it difficult to think of disasters occurring from human design as a form of violence. Victims of disasters and traumas of human origin, however, feel violated. They have experienced directly the destruction of their health, their children, their homes, their sense of security, their hopes for the future, and their sense of wholeness and worth in the human community.

In many ways, the poignant testimonies and tragic lives of the victims of ethnic, class, and political conflicts speak for themselves. Still, two of the most painful aspects of their crises are that they feel ignored and often cannot receive even material compensation for their enormous losses. They feel denied. If we have not listened, or if we have been silent when we should have spoken, convinced that we have nothing to say about public issues, perhaps we should reexamine what Nobel Peace Prize recipient Albert Schweitzer said in 1954: "Whether we secure a lasting peace will depend upon the direction taken by individuals—and, therefore, by the nations whom those individuals collectively compose." Survival is too serious to be confined to partisan politics, the government, or liberal versus conservative debates. Every citizen—and certainly crisis workers—should be informed on the critical issues confronting the human race (see, Ekins, 1992; Foell & Nenneman, 1986; Hoff & McNutt, 1994). It is time for crisis workers to confront denial and to understand its implications for prevention and for the response to victims. Therapist "neutrality" is a concept that will not do in cases of crisis originating in sociocultural and political sources.

When confronted with the enormity and horror of disaster from human sources, denial is understandable. Most of us feel helpless and powerless. But, in fact, we are not. The opinions of officials and professionals are not necessarily wiser or more life-saving than those of ordinary citizens. Lois Gibbs (1982) documents this point and illustrates the urgency of our attention to the threat of disaster from human sources. In describing why she wrote *Love Canal—My Story,* she emphasizes the fact that, as an average citizen with limited education and almost no funds, she was able to fight city hall and the White House and win!

Murray Levine, a community psychologist, wrote, in his introduction to Gibbs's story (Gibbs, 1982, pp. xii–xviii), reasons why the story should be told; he also illustrated crisis and preventive responses to a disaster of human origins:

1. Lois Gibbs is in many respects a typical American woman: a mother of two children and a housewife. In response to crisis and challenge, she courageously "transcended herself and became far more than she had been."
2. Her story informs us of the relationship between citizens and their government, and shows that the government's decisions about a problem are not necessarily in the interests of ordinary people whose lives are threatened by these decisions.
3. Lois Gibbs's story is one of "inner meanings and feelings of humans," a story that "provides a necessary and powerful antidote to the moral illness of those cynics and their professional robots who speak the inhuman language of benefit-cost ratios, who speak of the threat of congenital deformities or cancers as acceptable risks."

In conclusion, the differences between disasters of natural and human origin are striking: the uncontrolled, violent forces of nature (fire, water, wind, and temperature)—destructive as they are—are minuscule in comparison to disasters from human sources. The possible crisis outcomes for the victims are also markedly different, with enormous implications for prevention. Ironically, through technology and public health planning, much has been done to harness some of the destructive potential of nature. Natural disaster-control technology and resources for aid to victims should now be shared more widely in disaster-prone areas of the world. Concerning disaster from human sources, however, we have been much less successful in directing and controlling conflict and indifference toward the health and welfare of others. This is unfortunate but not hopeless. Violence is not inevitable (Lifton, 1993); it results from our choices, action, and inaction.

In the discussion of understanding people in crisis in Chapter Two, emphasis was placed on the examination of crisis origins. In the case of disasters of human origin, such an examination inevitably leads us into the most pressing social, political, and economic questions facing humankind. After hearing the voices of survivors of nuclear bombs, of the downwind fallout in Utah, of Love Canal, of the concentration camps, or of still another war, the crisis worker may well begin to question the social and political choices that led to these disasters. The broad view suggested by these questions is important for the crisis worker to develop, in tandem with individualized crisis intervention strategies. Without it, he or she may begin to perceive the task of helping victims of man-made disasters as an exercise in futility. Frustration, loss of effectiveness, and burnout may replace the understanding, sensitivity, and problem-solving ability that the crisis worker should bring to this task.

Summary

Disaster is experienced as a crisis unlike any other a person will ever live through. Victims may face a threat to their lives, may lose loved ones, homes, and personal belongings in a single stroke. Many spend the rest of their lives mourning these tragic losses and trying to rebuild their homes and lives. Rescue services, crisis intervention, and follow-up care for physical, emotional, and social rehabilitation are necessary for all survivors. While financial aid for physical restoration and rehabilitation has been available for years, crisis counseling services are a newer phenomenon on the disaster scene. Communities will be better equipped to handle the emotional crisis related to the disaster experience when health and social service workers, as well as other caretakers, are prepared in advance with skills in crisis management. The urgency of preventing disasters of human origin is self-evident.

References

Ahmed, F. E. (1992, September 1). The Bangladesh hurricane had no name. *Boston Globe*, p. 15.

Antonovsky, A. (1987). *Unraveling the mystery of health.* San Francisco: Jossey-Bass.

Apfel, R. J., & Simon, B. (1994, February 13). Children in the cross-fire. *Boston Globe*, pp. 69, 72.

Apfel, R. J., & Simon, B. (Eds.) (forthcoming). *Minefields in the heart: Mental life of children of war and communal violence.* New Haven, Conn.: Yale University Press.

Baum, A., Fleming, R., & Singer, J. E. (1983). Coping with victimization by technological disaster. *Journal of Social Issues, 39*(2), 117–138.

Bennet, G. (1970). Bristol floods. Controlled survey of effects on health in local community disaster. *British Medical Journal, 3,* 454–458.

Birnbaum, F., Coplon, J., & Scharff, R. (1973). Crisis intervention after a natural disaster. *Social Casework, 54,* 545–551.

Blanford, H., & Levine, J. (1972). Crisis intervention in an earthquake. *Social Work, 17,* 16–19.

Chavkin, W. (Ed.). (1984). *Double exposure: Women's health hazards on the job and at home.* New York: Monthly Review Press.

Davidson, J., Swartz, M., Storck, M., Krishman, R. R., & Hammett, E. (1985). A diagnostic and family study of post-traumatic stress disorder. *American Journal of Psychiatry, 142*(1), 90–93.

Durkin, M. S., Khan, N., Davidson, L. L., Zaman, S. S., & Stein, Z. A. (1993). The effects of a natural disaster on child behavior: Evidence for post-traumatic stress. *American Journal of Public Health, 83*(11), 1549–1553.

Ekins, P. (1992). *A new world order: Grassroots movements for global change.* New York: Routledge.

Erikson, K. (1994). *A new species of trouble.* New York: W.W. Norton.

Foell, E., & Nenneman, R. (1986). *How peace came to the world.* Boston: MIT Press.

Farberow, N. L. (1967). Crisis, disaster, and suicide: Theory and therapy. In E. S. Shneidman (Ed.). *Essays in self-destruction.* New York: Science House.

Ganguly, D. (1994, December 4). Anger in India ten years after Bhopal. *Boston Globe,* p. 7.

Gibbs, L. (1982). *Love Canal: My story.* Albany: State University of New York Press.

Glasheen, L., & Crowley, L. (1993, December). Facing a difficult situation, impossible choices. Washington, D.C.: *AARP Bulletin, 34* (11), 11.

Goodman, L. M., & Hoff, L. A. (1990). *Omnicide.* New York: Praeger.

Gordon, N. (1976). Disaster, research, training, service. Workshop presented at American Association of Suicidology Ninth Annual Meeting, Los Angeles, Calif.

Grossfeld, S. (1993, March 28). The exhausted earth: Life in the poison zones. *Boston Sunday Globe,* pp. 1, 24–27.

Hansell, N. (1976). *The person in distress.* New York: Human Sciences Press.

Hoff, L. A. (1995). *Violence education: An interdisciplinary curriculum guide for health professionals.* Ottawa: Health Canada. Health Services Directorate.

Hoff, M. D., & McNutt, J. G. (Eds.). (1994). *The global environmental crisis.* Aldershot, England: Avebury.

Joseph, S., Yule, W., Williams, R., & Andrews, B. (1993). Crisis support in the aftermath of disaster. *British Journal of Clinical Psychology, 32*(Part 2), 177–185.

Keck, B. (1991, March). War—A public health disaster! *The Nation's Health,* p. 2.

Kizzier, D. (1972). *The Rapid City flood.* Lubbock, Tex.: C.F. Boone.

Koegler, R. R., & Hicks, S. M. (1972). The destruction of a medical center by earthquake. *California Medicine, 116,* 63–67.

Laube, J. (1973). Psychological reactions of nurses in disaster. *Nursing Research, 22,* 343–347.

Lifton, R. J. (1982). Interview for national public television documentary. *Survivors.* Boston: WGBH Educational Foundation.

Lifton, R. J. (1967). *Life in death.* New York: Simon & Schuster.

Lifton, R. J. (1993). *The protean self: Human resilience in an age of fragmentation.* New York: Basic Books.

Lifton, R. J., & Olson, E. (1976). The human meaning of total disaster: The Buffalo Creek experience. *Psychiatry, 39,* 1–18.

McCarroll, J. E., Ursano, R. J., & Fullerton, C. S. (1993). Symptoms of post-traumatic stress disorder following recovery of war dead. *American Journal of Psychiatry, 150*(12), 1875–1877.

Mills, C. W. (1959). *The sociological imagination.* London: Oxford University Press.

Mousseau, M. (1989). *The medicine wheel approach to dealing with family violence.* Canada: West Region Child and Family Services.

Murphy, S. A. (1986). Status of natural disaster victims' health and recovery 1 and 3 years later. *Research in Nursing and Health, 9,* 331–340.

Okura, K. P. (1975). Mobilizing in response to a major disaster. *Community Mental Health Journal, 11,* 136–144.

Peterson, K. C., Prout, M. F., & Schwarz, R. A. (1991). *Post-traumatic stress disorder: A clinician's guide.* New York: Plenum.

Richman, N. (1993). After the flood. *American Journal of Public Health, 83*(11), 1522–1523.

Ruddick, S. (1989). *Maternal thinking: Toward a politics of peace.* Boston: Beacon Press.

Schottenfeld, R. S., & Cullen, M. R. (1985). Occupation-induced post-traumatic stress disorders. *American Journal of Psychiatry, 142*(2), 198–202. See also "Reply" in Letters to the Editor, *142*(9), 35–42, 93–95.

Spake, A. (1986). A new American nightmare? *Ms., 14*(9), 1125.

Survivors (1982). Boston: WGBH Educational Foundation.

Tyhurst, J. S. (1951). Individual reactions to community disaster. *American Journal of Psychiatry, 107,* 764–769.

Tyhurst, J. S. (1957a). Psychological and social aspects of civilian disaster. *Canadian Medical Association Journal, 76,* 385–393.

Tyhurst, J. S. (1957b). The role of transition states—including disaster—in mental illness. Symposium on preventive and social psychiatry. Washington, D.C.: Walter Reed Army Institute of Research and the National Research Council.

Wijkman, A., & Timberlake, L. (1984). *Natural disaster: Acts of God or acts of man?* London & Washington, D.C.: International Institute for Environment and Development.

Zeidner, M., Klingman, A., & Itskowitz, R. (1993). Children's affective reactions and coping under threat of missile attack: A semiprojective assessment procedure. *Journal of Personality Assessment, 60*(3), 433–457.

Zusman, J., Joss, R. H., & Newman, P. J. (1973). *Final report: Project Outreach.* Buffalo: Community Mental Health Research and Development Corporation.

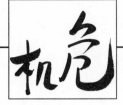

PART THREE

CRISES RELATED TO SITUATIONAL AND TRANSITION STATES

Hazardous life events—both anticipated and unanticipated—are traditionally defined as transitional and situational state crises (see Crisis Paradigm). In presenting these crises, the first three chapters of Part Three address the theme of passage: from health to illness, from employed to unemployed status, from one residence to another, from adolescence to adulthood, as well as other changes in status and role throughout life. Chapter Thirteen highlights rites of passage during life crises, including the final crisis for all—passage from life to death—and suggests ways we can help ourselves and others through this last developmental task. The concluding chapter illustrates situational, transitional, and sociocultural aspects of AIDS, one of the most devastating crises of the twentieth century.

CHAPTER ELEVEN

THREATS TO HEALTH STATUS AND SELF-IMAGE

Many have said that if their health is intact, they can endure almost anything else. This is because a change in health status is not only hazardous in itself and potentially life-threatening, but poor health status leaves one more vulnerable than otherwise to hazardous events. To avoid a crisis state, all of us need to have:

- A sense of physical and emotional well-being
- An image of self that flows from general well-being and acceptance of one's physical attributes
- Some control in everyday life functions and the activities of daily living

These aspects of life are acutely threatened by illness, accidents, surgery, physical or mental handicap, and the uncontrolled use of alcohol and other drugs. Several of our basic needs are in jeopardy when events that are hazardous to health occur. A full crisis experience can be avoided if the threatened person is supported by family, friends, and health workers and receives necessary treatment regardless of financial status. Self-defeating outcomes such as suicide, assault or homicide, mental illness, and depression can also be avoided if appropriate treatment and emotional support are available when threats to health status occur (see Figure 11.1, Crisis Paradigm).

People in emotional crisis related to illness, injury, surgery, or handicap rarely come to the attention of crisis specialists or mental health workers in the acute crisis stage. Mental health workers often see people *after* a crisis episode when they may have become dependent on alcohol or other drugs, lapsed into depression,

FIGURE 11.1. CRISIS PARADIGM.

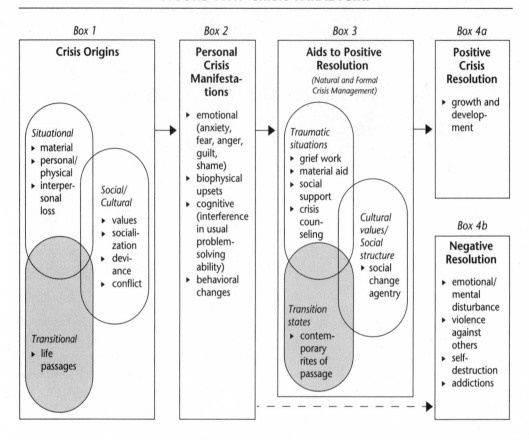

Box 1   *Box 2*   *Box 3*   *Box 4a*

Crisis Origins

Personal Crisis Manifestations

Aids to Positive Resolution
(Natural and Formal Crisis Management)

Positive Crisis Resolution
- growth and development

Situational
- material
- personal/ physical
- interpersonal loss

Social/ Cultural
- values
- socialization
- deviance
- conflict

- emotional (anxiety, fear, anger, guilt, shame)
- biophysical upsets
- cognitive (interference in usual problem-solving ability)
- behavioral changes

Traumatic situations
- grief work
- material aid
- social support
- crisis counseling

Cultural values/ Social structure
- social change agentry

Box 4b

Negative Resolution
- emotional/ mental disturbance
- violence against others
- self-destruction
- addictions

Transitional
- life passages

Transition states
- contemporary rites of passage

or experienced other emotional disturbance. This pattern underscores the pivotal role of general health workers such as physicians and nurses in the crisis assessment and management process, especially at various entry points to the health care system. In addition, many frontline workers such as police, rescue teams, firefighters, and Traveler's Aid caseworkers are the first to confront a person injured or in emotional shock from an accident, violent attack, or fire.

Centuries ago, Hippocrates said that it is more important to "know the man who has the disease than the disease the man has." More recent research, along with the human potential movement, documents the intrinsic relationship between mind, body, and spirit (Benson & Klipper, 1976; Borysenko, 1987; Chopra, 1993). The congressional document, *Action for Mental Health* (1961) and federal legislation have led to pioneering efforts in the community mental health movement in the United States, including national survey data documenting the fact that many distressed people *first* visit physicians or clergy, *not* mental health professionals.

These data underscore a premise of this book, that the crisis response is a *nor-*

mal, not pathological, life experience. Yet, crisis assessment and intervention in general health care practice is by no means routine. As Sugg and Inui (1992) report, physicians are afraid of opening Pandora's box by inquiring about the possibility of abuse. Similarly, Moore and Schwartz (1993) report that emergency nurses may not be delivering the psychosocial support they believe they are. On the other hand, many health and frontline workers are already doing crisis intervention but may lack self-confidence because they have no formal training in the field. They often need reinforcement and confirmation from crisis specialists for work they are doing with distressed people (Adamowski, et al., 1993).

This chapter addresses the crisis management process as applied in *general* health care situations when a person is in a status change from health to illness or from physical intactness to handicap. The strategies apply in doctors' offices; emergency, intensive care, and other hospital departments; primary care settings such as prenatal clinics—in virtually all health and human service settings, including long-term care facilities. Points discussed here assume the underpinnings of general assessment and intervention strategies and life-threatening situations addressed elsewhere in this book.

Crisis Care in Primary Health Care Settings

Since the essential features of formal crisis intervention have not changed much since the era when it was deemed a mere Band-Aid, we have a paradoxical situation. On the one hand, mental health care and crisis intervention are being increasingly cited in health reform policy statements (e.g., Fiedler & Wight, 1989; *Putting People First,* 1993). On the other hand, a mind-body split is still evident as many general health practitioners hesitate to deal with emotional issues, citing either discomfort with them or lack of time. Understandably, most nonpsychiatric physicians and nurses do not think of themselves as psychotherapists, yet the psychosocial facet of treatment and care is a given whether the primary health problem is physical or emotional. And therein may lie insight into the paradox. As discussed in Chapter One, while crisis intervention shares certain techniques with psychotherapy and may have *therapeutic* outcomes if aptly applied, it is not psychotherapy. The social construction of crisis intervention as therapy within a decade of having discounted it as a Band-Aid may partially explain the continued reluctance of general health practitioners to incorporate the model into routine health care practice. The medicalization of crisis intervention is one facet of the tradition, especially in North America where equating "health" care with "medical" care is common (Rachlis & Kushner, 1994; Smith, 1994). There is a need to reclaim the primary prevention model espoused by Caplan (1964) and recast crisis intervention within the public health model, rather than the medical model (Feingold, 1994; Navarro, 1994).

The increasing emphasis on primary care in the face of worldwide recession and escalation of health care costs, underscores the inclusion of crisis intervention as an essential element of comprehensive health care. As Figure 1.2 in Chapter One illustrates, prevention (including through crisis intervention) is less costly than treatment, especially in residential facilities. On the other hand, crisis approaches must not be used as *financially expedient* substitutes for the longer-term care and rehabilitation which some problems require (Hoff, 1993; Johnson, 1990). In many of these primary care situations, crisis assessment, social support, and/or a referral to a peer group as discussed in Chapter Five (e.g., for people with diabetes or cancer) will do. For example, one woman said that her physical and emotional recovery after a mastectomy might have been much more precarious if a nurse had not comforted her when she broke down crying the first time she looked in the mirror. This was the beginning of her grief work around the loss of her breast. It was facilitated by a surgical nurse who was not a psychotherapist; the nurse simply understood and responded to the crisis dimensions of the woman's transition in health status and, potentially, her self-image.

Hazards to Physical and Emotional Health

Physical illnesses or accidents are often the beginning of a series of problems for an individual as well as for his or her family (Lindemann, 1979; Werner-Beland, 1980). If struck by a potentially fatal illness such as cancer, the person may experience the same sense of dread and loss that death itself implies. A person's self-image is also threatened by physical deformity resulting from a mastectomy, amputation of an arm or leg, scars from an accident or extensive burns, AIDS (see Chapter Fourteen), or genital herpes. If injury and illness result from a disaster of human origins, crisis resolution that avoids despair, revenge, or violence is especially challenging. People with sexually transmitted diseases (STDs) such as herpes II are also particularly crisis prone. For example, shame, revulsion, ignorance, and fear about such diseases can precipitate marriage breakups, suicidal tendencies, social isolation, self-loathing, and depression. And if a person realizes that STD may be a forerunner of AIDS and was caused by having unprotected sex, the potential for crisis is increased. This is also true when HIV is transmitted through rape.

In addition to facing the illness or accident itself, the person acutely or chronically ill often faces another crisis: institutionalization in a hospital or nursing home. As noted in Chapter Three, hospital admission in itself may precipitate a crisis (Polak, 1967). Hospitals and other institutions can be considered as subcultures in which the longest-term occupants—the staff—know the procedures and rules that prevent chaos and help them do their jobs. The sick person however, especially one who has never been hospitalized, may experience culture shock—a condition that can occur when the comfort of familiar things is missing. Because the staff of these institutions become enculturated to their work environment, they often forget that a hospital admission is a "blip on the screen" of the sick person's normal, everyday existence.

Without support, in the "foreign" institutional environment a person's usually successful response to life's ups and downs may be weakened. In extreme cases, a person in culture shock feels too surprised and too numbed by a new culture's unfamiliarity to proceed with the successful management of everyday life tasks. Add in the fear of the unknown regarding the outcome of treatments, and it is easy to understand why some patients lash out at staff in what may appear to be unreasonable outbursts, or manifest other classic signs of culture shock or crisis. Even in long-term care placements, attention to these crisis manifestations, especially upon admission, can avoid much pain for both client and staff. Complicating this scenario is the potential crisis response of a patient who feels unready for discharge. In this era of cost containment and concern about dependency issues, timely discharge may seem cost-efficient. But premature discharge does not save money and may eventually cost more through readmission or extreme responses such as suicide (Hoff, 1993).

In some instances, people's illnesses and the crisis of hospitalization are complicated further by negligence, mishandling, or unethical medical practice. Millman (1978) discusses the systematic cover-up of iatrogenic illness and death (that is, caused by the health care provider). In addition to the original illness, the patient (or survivor) must contend with personal damage (or death) inflicted by the people he or she trusted. Despite progress in the women's health movement, some women are still dying prematurely from illnesses that were dismissed as manifestations of their "neurotic personalities" (Ehrenreich & English, 1979). In one 1993 case, a forty-three-year-old woman died of ovarian cancer within a year of diagnosis after spending six months trying to persuade her physician to take her symptoms seriously. When he finally examined her, she already had nine metastatic sites.

Patients and families, however, are not the only ones in crisis around these issues. Nursing and medical colleagues face the moral dilemma of collusion in cover-up of negligence. If lawsuits occur, a new series of crises may unfold: joblessness, financial loss, and damage to professional status.

A related issue concerns unnecessary surgery. A historic account of surgery (Dally, 1992) documents experimentation on women and black slaves. While unnecessary elective surgery is under scrutiny for ethical and cost-containment reasons, cosmetic surgery such as breast implants continue despite highly controversial results such as disfigurement and immune system breakdown. Without the profits to be made and the cultural component of women's general concern (and sometimes obsession) with body image, some of the crises related to these health issues might be avoided. Among those surgeries with the highest nonconfirmed rates—those in which the second opinion did not support the initial recommendation—are breast surgery, hysterectomy (removal of the uterus), and, in men, removal of the prostate gland. Women have the majority of unnecessary operations and also receive 50 percent more prescription drugs than men (Boston Women's Health Book Collective, 1992). This practice is especially significant in view of women's emotional and physical assets: on average, women in industrialized societies live seven years longer than men and are assumed worldwide to be the emotional and social caretakers of society. But they have unequal access to care. These facts are linked to the political economy of medicine and to cultural values about women that portray women as less valuable than men and, when sick, in need of medical intervention and control (Becktell, 1994; Ehrenreich, 1978; Ehrenreich & English, 1979; Lugina, 1994).

The issue of unnecessary surgery is particularly poignant in the case of breast surgery. Despite continued controversy over ethical violations in some clinical trials, these randomized trials reveal that radical mastectomy for breast cancer is no more effective than other forms of treatment. The first experimental research supporting this finding was carried out in England and Scandinavia, where surgeons' fees are significantly lower than they are in the United States. Considering the cultural symbolism of the female breast, it is not difficult to imagine the loss of a breast as the occasion for acute crisis, in addition to the crisis over the threat to life from cancer. Preparing a woman for a mastectomy and explaining alternative treatments can help her live through this crisis (Bredenburg, 1991; Jamison, Wellisch, & Pasnaw, 1978; Penman, et al., 1987). Offering support through self-help referrals after surgery is equally important. Yet in one New England state, the legislature had to pass a law requiring physicians to make nonsurgical options known to women with breast cancer. Increasingly, women who have had mastectomies are referred to self-help groups such as Reach for Recovery, who offer emotional support during this crisis-prone period. However, in communities where physician control prevails, advocacy is needed to ensure such referrals. As the rates of breast cancer steadily grow and research begins to examine possible environmental causes such as contamination of the food chain by pesticides, it is important to link this personal traumatic event with broader social concerns.

Men having surgery on sex organs also need communication and accurate information. Although radical surgery (prostatectomy) has increased dramatically in recent years, there is no proof that this surgery saves lives, while there is evidence of incontinence and impotence following the operation. Nurses are in especially strategic positions to encourage male patients to communicate their feelings regarding this sensitive issue and to assist them in making informed decisions about surgery (Gammon, 1993). The crisis for men having such surgery is heavily tinged by the threat to male potency and self-image that is signaled by cancer or surgery affecting sex organs. The hazards of such a diagnosis are compounded because males have been socialized not to cry or to express feelings readily. While there were only a handful of prostate cancer support groups until recently, nearly 300 such groups exist now, according to the American Foundation for Urologic Disease, which has helped organize them. Some physicians recommend that men begin routine screening for prostate cancer at age fifty, although the issue is still controversial. Education, as well as communication with the man's sex partner, are important (Shipes & Lehr, 1982). Besides crisis prevention and management, post-traumatic stress disorder can also be prevented by timely support during medical and surgical care (Shalev, et al., 1993).

The physician plays a pivotal role in such crisis situations. Alex, for example, was upset with the news that his wife intended to divorce him. When his physician diagnosed his cancer of the testicle, he was even more distressed. The physician simply told him to check into the county hospital's psychiatric unit thirty miles away if he continued to feel upset. Instead, Alex went home, told his wife what the physician had said, and shot himself in his front yard.

Alex had been discussing the impending divorce with a crisis counselor who lived in Alex's community; the physician also practiced there. Even if the physician had no time to listen to Alex, he should have made a local referral. This case illustrates how local crisis specialty services may go unused if effective linkages with health and other frontline professionals are lacking (Hoff, 1983; Hoff & Miller, 1987).

If illness, surgery, and hospitalization are occasions of crisis for most adults, they are even more so for children and their parents (Kruger, 1992). Research has revealed the traumatic effects of hospitalization on children, and a new organization has emerged: Association for the Care of Children in Hospitals. Professionals with special training in child development now work in Child Life Departments of many hospitals. They arrange preadmission tours and listen to children's questions and worries:

- Sam, age four, has been told by his doctor that a hole will have to be made in his stomach to make him well again. Because the doctor neglected to mention that the hole will also be stitched up again, Sam worries that "the things inside me will fall out."
- Cindy, age nine, sees an intravenous bottle and tubes being wheeled to her bedside. She had once seen the same apparatus attached to her cousin Jeffrey, who later died. As the needle is being inserted, she wonders if she is as sick as Jeffrey was.
- Ken, a junior high school football player, is confined to a traction frame. Unable to dress or wash himself each morning, he suffers acute embarrassment in front of the nurses.

If a child is going to the hospital, Child Life workers offer the following advice to parents:

1. Accept the fact of the hospitalization.
2. Be honest with your child.
3. Prepare yourself; for example, find out about procedures.

4. Prepare your child, for example, through preadmission get-acquainted tours.
5. Whenever possible, stay with your child.

In addition to these general health care situations, frontline health workers need to increase their vigilance on behalf of victims whose first contact after injury is a health care professional or emergency medical technician (Hoff & Rosenbaum, 1994; Surgeon General's Report, 1986).

Crisis Response of People in Health Status Transition

To better understand the crisis responses of those who are ill and/or hospitalized, some questions must be addressed, such as, How do sick and hospitalized people feel? How do they perceive their illness and its relationship to their beliefs and lifestyle? How do they behave in the "sick role" (Brody, 1988)? The person whose physical integrity, self-image, and social freedom are threatened or actually damaged by these hazards to health shows many of the usual signs of a crisis state (see Figure 11.1 and Chapter Three).

1. *Biophysical response:* Besides the pain and discomfort from the disease or injury itself, the person losing health and bodily integrity suffers many of the biophysical symptoms experienced after the loss of a loved one (see "Loss, Change, and Grief Work" in Chapter Four). For example, Parkes (1975) compares the "phantom limb" experience to the "phantom husband" of widows, noting the influence of connections between psychological factors and the nervous system.

2. *Feelings:* After an amputation or a diagnosis such as heart disease, AIDS, herpes II, diabetes, or cancer, people respond with a variety of feelings:

- Shock and anger: "Why me?"
- Helplessness and hopelessness in regard to future normal functioning: "What's left for me now?"
- Shame about the obvious scar, handicap, or reduced physical ability, and about dependence on others: "What will my husband think?"
- Anxiety about the welfare of spouse or children who depend on them: "How will they manage at home without me?"
- Sense of loss of bodily integrity and loss of goals the person hoped to achieve before the illness or accident: "I don't think I'll ever feel right again."
- Doubt of acceptance by others: "No one will want to be around me this way."
- Fear of death, which may have been narrowly escaped in an accident or which now must be faced in the case of cancer: "It was almost the end," or "This is the end."
- Fear that one's sex life is over: "Am I condemned to lead a celibate life now?"

3. *Thoughts and perceptions:* The fears raised by a serious illness, accident, or operation usually color the person's perception of the event itself—the understanding of the event, and how it will affect the future. For example, a young woman

with diabetes assumed that she would be cut off from her cocktail party circuit, which she felt was necessary in her high, executive position. She lacked knowledge about how social obligations might be synchronized with diabetes.

A person with heart disease may foresee spending the future as an invalid; the reality is that he or she must only change the manner and range of performance. The woman with a mastectomy may perceive that all men will reject her because of the deformity; in reality only some men would do so. A woman who does not have a secure relationship with a man before a mastectomy may experience rejection; we can help such a woman consider the value of a relationship with a man who accepts her only for her body. Women with stable relationships are seldom rejected by their husbands or lovers following a mastectomy.

4. *Behavior:* The behavior of people who are ill or suffering from the physical effects of an accident or surgery is altered by several factors. First, hospitalization enforces a routine of dependency, which may be necessary when people are weak, but the routine also keeps the hospital running according to established rules of hierarchy. This hierarchy has little or nothing to do with patient welfare. In fact, rigidity in the hierarchy often defeats the purpose for which hospitals exist: quality care of patients (Schain, 1980).

The environment of an intensive care unit—the tubes, lights, and electrical gadgets—is a constant reminder to the patient and family members of proximity to death (Kleeman, 1989; Kuenzi & Fenton, 1975). Furthermore, a patient's fears, anger, and lack of knowledge about illness, hospital routines, and expectations can elicit the worst behavior from a person who is otherwise cooperative and likable. The rules and regulations governing visitors to these settings present a further hazard to people already in a difficult situation (Fuller & Foster, 1982).

To understand and respond appropriately to the emotional, perceptual, and behavioral responses of people to illness, pain, and hospitalization, we must be sensitive to cultural differences. The role of culture and value systems in the development of and response to crisis was discussed in the first four chapters; the cultural component becomes even more important in the face of illness, pain, and hospitalization. For example, Zborowski's (1952) classical study of Jewish, Italian, Irish, and other Americans revealed that: (1) similar reactions to pain by different ethnocultural groups do not necessarily reflect similar attitudes to pain; (2) similar reactive patterns may have different functions in various cultures. For instance, Jews' responses to pain elicit worry and concern, whereas Italians' elicit sympathy. Standard texts on health, illness, and healing in cross-cultural perspective offer further discussion of this topic (Conrad & Kern, 1990; Foster & Anderson, 1978; Galanti, 1991; James, Stall, & Gifford, 1986; Landy, 1977; McElroy & Townsend, 1985; Spector, 1991).

Nurses, physicians, social workers, chaplains, and others familiar with common signs of patients in crisis can do much to relieve unnecessary stress and harmful outcomes of the hospital experience. The patient in crisis needs an opportunity to

- Express the feelings related to his or her condition
- Gain an understanding of the illness, what it means in terms of one's values, what limitations it imposes, and what to expect in the future.
- Have the staff understand his or her behavior, how it relates to the person's feelings and perception of the illness, and how the behavior is related to the attitudes and behavior of the entire staff

CASE EXAMPLE—CRISIS MANAGEMENT: MICHAEL AND MARIA FRENCH

Michael French, age fifty-five, had suffered from prostate cancer for several years. During the past year, he was forced to retire from his supervisory job in a factory. The cancer spread to his bladder and colon, causing continuous pain as well as urinary control problems. Michael became very depressed and highly dependent on his wife, Maria, age fifty-one. Stress for both of them increased. Michael began to suspect Maria of infidelity.

Maria was scheduled to go to the hospital for a hysterectomy for fibroids of the uterus, but repeatedly cancelled the surgery. Her husband always protested her leaving and, at the last minute, she would cancel. Finally, her doctor pressed her to go through with the operation. Since Maria did not look

sick to Michael, he felt she was abandoning him unnecessarily. Along with the ordinary fears of anyone facing a major operation, Maria was very worried about her husband's condition when she went to the hospital. However, she was too embarrassed by Michael's accusations of infidelity to discuss her fears with the nurses or with her doctor.

While in the hospital, Maria received a message from a friend that Michael was threatening to kill her when she came home. He had dismissed their tenants without notice and changed the locks on the doors. The friend, who was afraid of Michael in this state, also called a local community health nurse who, in turn, called a nearby crisis clinic. The nurse had been making biweekly visits to supervise Michael's medication.

Crisis management took the following form:

1. The crisis counselor called Maria in the hospital to talk about her concerns and to determine whether Michael had any history of violence or whether guns were available. Michael's accusations of infidelity—which, according to Maria, were unfounded—may have been related to his concern about his forced dependency and to feelings of inadequacy, since he had cancer of the sex gland (Shipes & Lehr, 1982).

2. The crisis counselor called Michael and let him know that he (the counselor), Maria, and the neighbors were all concerned about him. Michael accepted an appointment for a home visit by the counselor within the next few hours. He expressed his fears that people were trying to take advantage of him during his wife's absence. This was his stated reason for dismissing the tenants and changing the locks. Further exploration revealed that he felt inadequate to handle household matters and the tenants' everyday requests that Maria usually managed (Maxwell, 1982).

3. Michael agreed to the counselor's recommendation for a medical-psychiatric-neurological check-up to determine whether his cancer might have spread to his brain. The counselor explained that brain tumors can contribute to acute emotional upsets such as Michael was experiencing.

4. Since Michael had no independent means of visiting Maria in the hospital, the counselor arranged for such a visit. The counselor also scheduled a joint counseling session between Michael and Maria after they had had a chance to visit. This session revealed that Michael and Maria each had serious concerns about the welfare of the other. In their two telephone conversations during Maria's stay in the hospital, Michael and Maria had been unable to express their fears and concern. The joint counseling session was the highlight in successful resolution of their crisis. Michael's threat to kill Maria was a once-in-a-lifetime occurrence triggered by his unexpressed anger at her for leaving him and the troubles he experienced during her absence.

5. When Maria returned from the hospital, a joint session was held at the Frenches' home including the two of them, the community health nurse, and the friend who had made the original calls (see "Social and Group Process in Crisis Intervention" in Chapter Five). This conference had several positive results: (a) it calmed the neighbor's fears for Michael; (b) it broadened everyone's understanding of the reactions people can have to the stress of illness and hospitalizations; (c) the community health nurse agreed to enlist further home health services to relieve Maria's increasingly demanding role of nurse to her husband (Skorupka & Bohnet, 1982); and finally, (d) Michael and Maria agreed to several additional counseling sessions to explore ways in which Michael's excessive dependency on his wife could be reduced. Michael and Maria had never discussed openly the feelings they both had about Michael's progressive cancer (Pruchno & Potashnik, 1989; Sontag, 1978). In future sessions, the Frenches dealt with ways they could resume social contacts with their children and friends, whom they had cut off almost completely.

Preventive Intervention

This case history reveals at least three earlier points at which crisis intervention should have been available to the Frenches:

1. At the time Michael received his diagnosis of cancer
2. When Michael was forced to retire
3. Each time Maria delayed her operation, as well as at the point of Maria's hospitalization

In each of these instances, nurses and physicians were in key positions to help the Frenches through the hazardous events of Michael's illness and Maria's operation. Sessions with the crisis counselor confirmed the fact that the Frenches, like many other people facing illness, received little or no attention regarding the fears and social ramifications of their illnesses and hospitalization.

When Maria expressed to the community nurse her original concern about Michael's early retirement, the nurse might have extended her ten-minute visits to a half hour, thus allowing time for Maria to express her concerns. For example, the nurse might have said, "Maria, you seem really concerned about your husband being home all the time. Can we talk about what's bothering you?" Or the nurse might have made a mental health referral after observing Michael's increasing depression.

The gynecologist attending to Maria's health problems might have explored the reason for her repeated cancellations of the scheduled surgery, saying, "Mrs. French, you've cancelled the surgery appointment three times now. There must be some serious reason for this, as you know that the operation is necessary. Let's talk about what's at the bottom of this." Such a conversation might have led to a social service referral.

The nurse attending Maria before her operation—as well as the community health nurse visiting the home—might have picked up on Maria's concerns about the effect of her absence on Michael. Such a response requires listening skills and awareness of psychological cues given by people in distress.

CASE EXAMPLE: INTERVIEW WITH MARIA

Nurse: Mrs. French, you've been terribly quiet, and you seem tense. You said before that you're not particularly worried about the operation, but I wonder if something else is bothering you.

Maria: Well, I wish my husband were here, but I know he can't be.

Nurse: Can you tell me more about that?

Maria: He's got cancer and isn't supposed to drive. . . . I hated leaving him by himself.

Nurse: How about talking with him by phone?

Maria: I've done that, but all we talk about is the weather and things that don't matter—I'm afraid if I tell him how worried I am about him, he'll think I'm putting him down.

Nurse: Mrs. French, I understand what you're saying. A lot of people feel that way. But you know there's really no substitute for telling people honestly how we feel, especially those close to us.

Maria: Maybe you're right. . . . I could try, but I'd want to be really careful about what I say. There's been a lot of tension between us lately.

Nurse: Why don't you start by letting him know that you wish he could be here with you and that you hope things are OK with him at home. (Pause) You said there's been a lot of tension—do you have anyone you can talk to about the things that are bothering you?

Maria: No, not really.

The nurse might then explain the hospital resources, such as social services or pastoral care—ways of helping Maria explore the problem further.

In this brief interaction about a hazardous event such as surgery, the nurse has (a) helped Maria express her fears openly, (b) conveyed her own understanding of Maria's fears, (c) helped Maria put her fears about not communicating with her husband in a more realistic perspective, (d) offered direct assistance in putting Maria in touch with the person most important to her at this time, and (e) made available the resources for obtaining counseling service if Maria so desires.

This type of intervention should be made available to everyone who has a serious illness or who experiences the traumatic effects of an operation, burns, or an accident. Putting people in touch with self-help groups, as discussed in Chapter Five, is another important means of reducing the hazards of illness and hospitalization. Such groups exist for nearly every kind of illness or operation a person can have: heart disease, leukemia, diabetes, mastectomy, amputation, and others. Many hospitals also hold teaching and discussion groups among patients while they are still in the hospital. This is an excellent forum in which people can air their feelings with others who have similar problems, gain a better understanding of an illness or operation and how it will affect their lives, and establish contacts with people who may provide lasting social support in the future.

Crisis Intervention in Mental Institutions, Transitional Housing, and Hostels

As noted in Chapters Two and Three, admission to a psychiatric facility is a sign that crises have not been constructively resolved at various points along the way (Polak, 1967). Whenever possible, crisis hostels and other alternatives to psychiatric hospitalization should be used if a person cannot be helped in the home environment (Polak, 1976). Although mental hospitals are intended to relieve acute breakdowns or stress situations, they—like general hospitals—create another kind of crisis.

CASE EXAMPLE: ANGELA

Angela, age eighteen, highly suicidal, upset, and dependent on her family, was brought to a private mental hospital by her mother on the advice of a psychiatrist whom the mother had called a few hours earlier. Angela and her mother arrived at the hospital at 3:00 P.M. The admitting nurse stayed with them until 3:30 P.M. when she was sched- uled to go off duty. Angela was just beginning to calm down but became very upset again when the nurse left. The nurses were unable to reach the physician to obtain an order for tranquilizing medication. Meanwhile, visiting hours ended, and Angela's mother was asked to leave. At this point, Angela became even more upset. The nurse on

Case Example, cont.

the evening shift was unable to quiet or con-   controllable, and she was placed in a high-
sole her. With still no order for tranquilizing   security room as she became more suicidal.
medication, Angela's behavior became un-

In this case, the rules and regulations of the hospital and the absence of a call system to obtain doctors' orders for emergency medication clearly contributed to Angela's crisis state, which reached the point of panic. Richardson's (1987) study of in-patients' perceptions of the seclusion-room experience revealed that in 58 percent of the cases, patients experienced negative interaction with the staff before being secluded; 50 percent said that seclusion protected them; 58 percent perceived seclusion as a form of punishment, and 50 percent said that a different approach would have averted the need for seclusion.

In general, the same principles of crisis management discussed in earlier chapters apply in mental institutions and residential settings. The worker should (a) help people express their feelings; (b) help them understand their situation and develop new ways of problem solving; and (c) help them reestablish themselves with family and community resources. The staff in residential facilities should examine their programs and routines to determine whether people become even more upset than they were originally as a result of the rules, thus defeating the purpose of the residential program (Kavanagh, 1988).

For example, most psychiatric facilities routinely search patients on admission for dangerous articles, contraband, and anything that might be used as a weapon. Considering the number of dangerous people now admitted to psychiatric centers instead of prisons and the frequency of attacks on staff (see Chapter Nine), such searches seem reasonable. They should not, however, be done without a full explanation to the patient as to the reasons. A person's psychotic condition does not preclude the prospect of experiencing culture shock, or eliminate the need for respect and personal integrity, including for those committed involuntarily to a mental institution (Anders, 1977; Farberow, 1981).

Physical and Mental Handicap

Becoming a parent can be a crisis, even if everything occurs as expected. The birth of a handicapped child, however, presents a serious threat to the parents' image of themselves as successful parents. Frequently, the parent asks: "What did I do wrong? What have I done to deserve this?" Parents conclude mistakenly that something they did or failed to do is responsible for their child's handicapped condition.

Because of the strength of the parent-child bond, the child's physical or mental handicap is, in a sense, the parent's handicap as well (Childs, 1985). The intergenerational and family aspects of handicap suggest that initial and successive crisis points related to birth and the continued care of a handicapped person extend well beyond childhood. The degree of handicap and the level of parental expectation of a normal child are key factors influencing the likelihood of crisis for concerned parents. Handicaps vary greatly. Down's syndrome is a mental deficiency with distinctive physical signs: slanting, deep-set eyes that are close together and often crossed; flattened nose; loose muscles; thick, stubby hands; and short stature. Hydrocephalus is characterized by an enlarged head containing excessive fluid. In addition to Down's syndrome and hydrocephalus, the range of handicaps varies from gross deformity to minor physical deformity, to developmental disabilities that surface later, such as a learning disability or hypothyroidism.

Initial Crisis Point

In many cases, birth defects are obvious immediately after birth. Sometimes, however, the handicap is not noticed until the child is obviously lagging in normal development. Whenever the handicap becomes known to the parents, the usual response includes anger, disbelief, a sense of failure, numbness, fear for the child's welfare, guilt, and an acute sense of loss—loss of a normal child, loss of a sense of success as parents. The parents' initial reactions of disbelief and denial are sometimes compounded unnecessarily by medical personnel who withhold the truth from them. Seventy to eighty percent of mentally retarded children also have physical disabilities, but parents should not be encouraged to believe that when these physical conditions are remedied, the mental condition will be cured as well.

CASE EXAMPLE: ANNA

Edward and Jane took their six-year-old daughter, Anna, for kindergarten evaluation. They were told bluntly that she required special education. They were shocked by the news. No psychological or social services had been made available to these parents. Edward and Jane had tried to ignore their daughter's obvious differences from other children and had not questioned their physician, who was noncommittal. Finally, the grandparents and a sister convinced them to seek guidance from the local Association for Retarded Children.

A child's physical or mental handicap can be a source of crisis for a parent even before the child is born. When medical tests reveal a fetal handicap, parents face the decision of whether or not to abort the fetus. An infant born with devastating brain damage can now be kept alive through advanced medical technology. Like the spouses and children of the dying elderly, parents are caught in the middle of passionate public debates on life and death issues such as whether it is morally justifiable to sustain physical life by extraordinary means when brain death is certain (Lynn & Childress, 1991; Solomon, et al., 1993). Parents of unborn children who are certain to die now face another moral dilemma: whether to carry the infant to term in order to donate healthy organs to other infants. Sensitive health care workers will make themselves available to parents who need to work through these dilemmas.

Successive Crisis Points

Parents of children who are developmentally disabled or otherwise handicapped can experience crisis at many different times, the most common of which are:

- When the child is born
- When the child enters school and does not succeed in a normal classroom
- When the child develops behavior problems peculiar to his or her handicap
- When the child becomes an adult and requires the same care as a child
- When the child becomes an intolerable burden and parents lack the resources to care for him or her
- When it is necessary to institutionalize the child
- When institutionalization is indicated and parents cannot go through with it out of misplaced guilt and a sense of total responsibility
- When the child is rejected by society and parents are reminded once again of their failure to perform as expected

The classic signs of crisis are easily identified in most parents of handicapped children:

1. *Feelings:* They deny their feelings and may displace their anger onto doctors, nurses, or each other. They feel helpless about what to do. Essentially, they feel they have lost a child as well as their role as successful parents.
2. *Thoughts:* Expectations for the child are often distorted. The parents' problem-solving ability is weakened; they lack a realistic perception of themselves as parents and sometimes expect the impossible. In short, they deny reality.
3. *Behavior:* Sometimes parental denial takes the form of refusing help. Sometimes help is not readily available, or parents are unable to seek out and use available help without active intervention from others.

The following case illustrates these signs of crisis and the manner in which a maternal health nurse successfully intervened.

CASE EXAMPLE: MONA ANDERSON

Mona Anderson, age thirty-one, had been married for ten years when she finally became pregnant after many years of wanting a child. Her baby girl was born with Down's

Case Example, cont.

syndrome. When Mona was tactfully informed of this by the physician and nurse in the presence of her husband, she became hysterical. Initially, she refused to look at the baby. Whenever the nurse attempted to talk with her about the baby's condition, she denied that she could have given birth to a defective child. The nurse allowed her this period of denial, but gradually and consistently informed her of the reality of her child's condition. During this time, her husband was also very supportive. Neither he nor the nurse insisted that she see the baby before she was ready. When she felt ready and the nurse brought the baby in, Mona broke down, crying, "All I wanted was a normal baby—I didn't expect a genius." Mona continued to grieve over her loss of a normal child. Gradually, she was able to talk with the nurse about her hopes for her child, her

sense of loss, and what she could and could not expect of her baby girl. While the nurse could not answer all of Mona's or her husband's questions, she referred them to a children's institute for genetic counseling. They were also given the name and number of a self-help group of parents of children with Down's syndrome.

The nurse was also helpful to other members of Mona's family who were drawn into the crisis. Mona's sister had had a baby two months previously. She concluded, wrongly, that she could not come to visit Mona with her normal baby because such a visit would only remind Mona again of her "abnormal" baby. The nurse counseled the family members against staying away, as it would only support Mona's denial of the reality of her child's condition.

The nurse, in the course of her usual work in a maternity ward, practiced successful crisis intervention by supporting Mona through her denial and mourning periods, offering factual information about the reality of Down's syndrome, and actively linking Mona to her family as well as to outside resources who could continue to help in the future. Because hospital stays after delivery now average only twenty-four to forty-eight hours, a visiting nurse would also be a key figure in a situation like Mona's. An important source of continued help for these families is the availability of respite care (Ptacek, 1982). Other crises associated with birth and parenthood are discussed in Chapter Thirteen.

Besides crises around parenting a handicapped child, any person—child or adult—with a handicap is more vulnerable than others to additional stressors, trauma, and potential crises. For example, physical limitations may prevent one from self-protection in cases of domestic dispute, rape, or robbery; lack of access to public transportation and buildings affect one's mobility, financial security, and other requisites for a healthy self-image. The alienation and feelings of powerlessness associated with such stressors can also lead to unhealthy coping such as excessive drinking (Seeman & Seeman, 1992). Recent federal legislation in the United States has facilitated addressing some of these issues affecting the health, crisis vulnerability, and general welfare of people with disabilities.

Substance Abuse and Other Chronic Problems

Alcoholism and drug and food abuse are not crises in themselves. A common view of these problems is that they are diseases; another view is that they are possible outcomes of crisis. In either case, the person who abuses alcohol, other drugs, or food is engaging in a chronic form of self-destructive behavior (see Figure 11.1 and Chapter Six). The abuse of food by excess eating is sometimes accompanied by bulimia: compulsive gorging followed by self-induced vomiting to avoid weight gain. This is related to excess dieting, which may result in anorexia nervosa, a life-threatening condition of severe weight loss. Since eating disorders are most common among young women, they are increasingly linked to female identity issues and the pressure on young women to conform to traditional images of women's roles and body size (Chernin, 1985).[1] Crises arising from these chronic problems can bring about lasting change in the tendency to abuse food. It can be assumed that when people were in crisis at earlier points in their lives, they lacked the social support and personal strength to resolve the crisis in a more constructive manner. People abusing food, drugs, and alcohol commonly avoid getting help for their problem until another crisis occurs as a result of the addiction itself. Frequently, a crisis takes the form of a family fight, eviction from an apartment, loss of a job, or trouble with the law. Depending on the attitude and skill of helpers at such times, later crises can be the occasion of a turning point.

CASE EXAMPLE: ANITA

Anita was abused physically and verbally by her husband for years. Her way of coping with the abuse was by overeating to the point that she gained more than 100 pounds. When her husband threatened her life, she finally left the violent marriage and sought refuge in a shelter for battered women. This crisis was a turning point that led Anita to seek help for her compulsive overeating in Overeaters Anonymous, a peer support group similar to Alcoholics Anonymous.

Chronic Self-Destructive Behavior and Crisis Intervention

The opportunity to change a self-destructive lifestyle is often missed. This is due, in part, to the lack of appropriate long-term treatment facilities and, in part, to the negative attitudes some hospital and clinic staff members hold toward self-destructive people. Careful application of crisis intervention techniques can greatly reduce the sense of defeat experienced by client and staff alike. Crisis principles that apply especially to the drug-, alcohol-, or food-dependent person include:

[1]For detailed information on eating disorders, contact MEDA/ABC (Massachusetts Eating Disorder Association/Anorexia Bulimia Care), 1162 Beacon Street, Brookline, MA 02146; telephone (617) 738–6332; fax (617) 738–7470.

1. Crisis represents a turning point, in this case, a turning away from drugs or food as a means of coping with stress. For example, intravenous drug users are at high risk for AIDS and therefore are offered clean needles, in a nonjudgmental manner, to reduce the risk of transmitting HIV. Users might reach a turning point in their lives through this constructive interaction with health and social service workers.

2. In crisis intervention, we avoid doing things *for* rather than *with* people. Proposed solutions to problems are mutually agreed on by client and staff person. The substance-dependent person will often act helpless and try to get staff to do things for him or her unnecessarily, thus increasing dependency even more. While expressing concern, staff should avoid falling into this rescue trap.

3. Basic social attachments that have been disrupted must be reinstated or a substitute found to help avoid further crises and more self-destructive behavior. Usually, people who abuse drugs, alcohol, and food are more isolated than most.

4. For all of these reasons, the principles and techniques of social network intervention (see Chapter Five) are particularly helpful in assisting the person in repeated crisis because of chronic underlying problems. While other approaches often yield little progress, clinicians skilled in network techniques point to impressive results (Garrison, 1974; Hansell, 1976; Polak, 1971).

Failure to observe these points leads to greater dependency of the client and increasing frustration of the staff. These crisis management techniques should be practiced in hospitals, transition facilities, doctors' offices, and by police and rescue services—wherever the food- or chemical-dependent person is in crisis. The use of these techniques would be a first step for many persons toward a life free of these harmful addictions.

CASE EXAMPLE: EMMA JEFFERSON

Emma Jefferson, age forty-two, had been drinking heavily for about fifteen years. When she was thirty-five, her husband divorced her after repeated pleading that she do something about her drinking problem. He also obtained custody of their two children. Emma was sufficiently shocked by this turn of events that she gave up drinking, joined Alcoholics Anonymous (AA), remarried at age thirty-seven, and had another child at age thirty-eight. She had hurried into her second marriage, the chief motive being that she wanted another child.

A year later, Emma began drinking again and was threatened with divorce by her second husband. Emma made superficial attempts to stop drinking and began substituting Valium when she had episodes of anxiety and depression. Her second husband divorced her six months later. This time, Emma retained custody of her child, though it was a close fight.

Emma took a job, was fired, went on welfare assistance, and began spending a lot of time in bars. On the urging of a friend, Emma finally decided to seek help for her

Case Example, cont.

alcohol and Valium dependency. She gave up drinking but continued a heavy use of Valium, sometimes taking as many as six 5-mg. tablets a day. Emma was inconsistent in carrying out plans to reorganize her life to include less dependence on drugs and more constructive social outlets.

One day, a neighbor reported to the Child Protection Agency that she believed Emma was neglecting her child and should be investigated. The child-welfare worker learned that Emma indeed had few social contacts outside the bars and occasionally left her two-year-old child unattended. Emma was allowed to maintain temporary custody of her child with regular home visits by a case worker to supervise her parenting activity. The threat of loss of her third child was apparently a sufficient crisis to act as a turning point for Emma. The case worker urged Emma to seek continued help with her problems from her counselor. Emma finally gave up her dependency on Valium, developed a more satisfying social life, and returned to work. She also made plans for another marriage, this time being more selective in her choice of a partner and less desperately dependent on a man for security.

The crisis of losing her children as a result of chronic dependence on alcohol and drugs, led Emma to give up her self-destructive lifestyle. Two divorces resulting from her drug dependency were not enough to make her change. In fact, Emma did not seek available counseling on either of these occasions. She said she was ashamed to ask for help and in any case did not think she could afford it.

Other people abusing drugs and alcohol seek help and make changes after serious financial or job failures, threats of imprisonment, or brushes with death such as DTs (delirium tremens, a sign of advanced alcoholism), bleeding ulcers, liver damage, or near-fatal suicide attempts.

Emma's case illustrates the damaging effects of alcoholism on children. According to the National Institute on Alcoholism and Alcohol Abuse, an estimated 26,000,000 American minors living at home have at least one alcoholic parent. Besides the daily stresses and crises experienced by these children, many become alcohol-dependent themselves. College students in the United States engage in binge drinking at alarming rates. The increasing availability of crisis services and follow-up treatment programs should result in earlier choices toward growth rather than self-destruction for substance-dependent people. Also, there are increasing numbers of self-help groups for adult children of alcoholics that can be contacted through local AA branches.

Influence of Societal Attitudes

The values of a given society naturally affect the use of drugs in that society. In the United States, many attitudes toward drug use are contradictory. For example, a drug such as marijuana is often regarded as dangerous, while many consider the excessive use of alcohol to be acceptable. A stable, law-abiding citizen can be censored or convicted for the use of marijuana, but if the same person chose to use alcohol, there would be no legal restrictions.

If alcohol is consumed privately with no damage to others, there are no sanctions against its use, even if excessive. Yet those who use alcohol chronically often suffer eventual liver or brain damage. A legal crisis can occur for the user of alcohol only if he or she excessively indulges in public and then damages others or others' property, as in the case of reckless driving. For the drunken person's innocent victims, however, it is different. U.S. society's implicit support of alcohol abuse is illustrated by the looseness of laws punishing drunken drivers. For the most part, alcoholism has been decriminalized, and the concept of alcoholism as a disease is now widely accepted. However, whether or not alcoholism is a disease, the combination of drinking and driving takes an enormous social toll. The loss and crises of drunk driving victims and their families are the focus of a concerted effort to stop what has been called a national slaughter on U.S. highways resulting from the abuse of alcohol.

The user of other drugs can experience a crisis simply by the purchase or possession of a substance like marijuana. In the United States, a few states have changed the drug possession laws in this regard, but the use of drugs other than alcohol is still predominately a political issue. Little effort is made to distinguish between the *user* and the *abuser* of drugs. Many crises, such as arrest and imprisonment of people using illegal drugs, occur by design of the social system. The most serious drug abuse problems receive the least attention. The most widespread and dangerous abuse problems today are alcoholism and the overuse or misuse of prescribed drugs, both of which are legal.

The story of Ruth illustrates further the complex interplay between chronic problems and acute crises: beatings as a child, feelings of rejection, a troubled marriage, suicide attempts, depression, death of a husband by suicide, and alcohol dependence (see "Stress, Crisis, and Illness" in Chapter Two). It also highlights how crisis intervention (in contrast to something like electric shock "treatment") can be the occasion for a turning point in a chronically troubled life.

CASE EXAMPLE: RUTH

I called the Crisis Center because I was afraid I'd attempt to take my life again. All my suicide attempts stemmed from feeling rejected, especially by my father. He picked on me and favored my older sister. I couldn't do anything right. Once I stole some money from my mother's purse so I could buy a gift for my friend (now I think I was trying to buy friendship). My father beat me so that my hands were bleeding; then he made me show my hands to my mother. My mother cried when he beat me, but I guess she was afraid to stop him. When my father was dying, he asked me to forgive him.

I dropped out of school after tenth grade and got a job in a stockroom and later worked as a bookkeeper. I got married when I was nineteen. Our first five years were beautiful. We had three boys. I loved my husband very much and waited on

Case Example, cont.

him hand and foot. We bought a home, and he helped finish it. During the second five years, he started changing and got involved with another woman. My family and everyone knew, but I kept denying it. Then he left for about four months. I made a suicide attempt by turning on all the gas. I didn't really want to die, I just wanted him to stop seeing the other woman and come back to me. He came to pick me up at the hospital, and two weeks later I went over to his girlfriend's house and beat her up. I could have gotten in trouble with the law for that, but she didn't press charges.

After that, we tried to patch things up for about four months, but it didn't work. Then I started seeing other men. We had lots of arguments. I threatened divorce and he threatened to kill himself, but I didn't believe him.

One night he sat in his car and wouldn't come in to go to bed when I asked him. At 7:00 A.M. my oldest son reported finding Dad dead in his car. I thought it was my fault. Even today I tend to blame myself. His parents also blamed me. My father was still alive then, and he and my mother stood by me. After my husband's death, I made another suicide attempt. I was in and out of the hospital several times and received a lot

of shock treatment. Nothing seemed to help in those days.

Three years after my first husband's death, I remarried. We argued and fought and again I felt rejected. When I was afraid of taking an overdose of aspirin, I called the Crisis Center and was referred to the local crisis and counseling center near my home. I can't say enough good things about how my counselor, Jim, helped me. After all those years of being in and out of hospitals, having shock treatments, and making several suicide attempts, I'm so glad I finally found the help I needed long ago.

I don't think I'd ever attempt suicide again. I still struggle with the problem of feeling rejected, which I think is the worst thing in the world to go through. But I can cope a lot better now and I'm not half as bad about condemning myself as I used to be. He keeps reminding me that I've done these things for myself, but I have a hard time giving myself credit for anything.

Even though I feel I'm on the horizon of something much better, I still have my down days and have to watch that I don't drink too much. But I don't think I'd ever let myself get as down and out as I've been in the past. I've seen that real help is available when I need it.

Rescue Workers, Nurses, Physicians, and Social Workers in Acute-Care Settings

Crisis situations demanding response are as diverse as the people experiencing them. Health practitioners have numerous opportunities to assist people in crisis because of threats to health, life, and self-image from illness, accidents, and related problems. All human service workers have a responsibility to assist people in crisis, but health care personnel in emergency and acute-care settings are in a particularly strategic position to influence the outcome of high-risk crisis situations. The nature of emergency and acute-care settings, with a focus on life-saving procedures, precludes the opportunity to assist a person to complete resolution of an emotional crisis originating from threats to health and life. If life is at stake, no one would place the expression of feelings, however intense these may be, before life-saving measures.

Yet, because of the tense atmosphere of emergency medical scenes, it is important to remember that emotional needs do not disappear when physical needs take on life and death importance. Both physical and emotional needs must be met. An appropriate attitude and a sensitivity to the emotional needs of victims and survivors must accompany necessary life-saving procedures, and a team approach accomplishes this best; the strain on nurses, physicians, and emergency medical technicians would be enormous without teamwork. Staff burnout in these settings is often very high in any case, and the lack of teamwork and staff support, inappropriate placement of personnel in high-risk work, or lack of training in crisis intervention frequently contribute to such burnout (Fullerton, et al., 1992; Hoff & Miller, 1987; McCarroll, et al., 1993). Not everyone is suited for crisis work, but

---

CASE EXAMPLE: RESCUE TEAM

No matter how long we work in the rescue business, there are still scenes we never get used to. One of the hardest is the death of a child. Lately, it seems we've had so many calls for children—an eight-year-old killed on the expressway, a ten-year-old hit by a car. My heart really goes out to the parents. I'm a parent too, and it hurts to witness these tragedies.

One of the saddest things happened last night. We were called to the foster home of a child who had originally been abandoned. She died of liver cirrhosis in spite of the foster mother's efforts to make up for years of neglect. It's very sad to watch a child die; I thought about it all day.

Another scene that haunts me is the man we found yesterday in the driveway of the hospital when we pulled in with our ambulance. He was just standing there with tears rolling down his cheeks. We asked the hospital guards and EMTs (emergency medical technicians) what was wrong. They said they didn't know and just laughed. We had to go out on another call right away. Now I can't get the man out of my mind; maybe I'll still call the hospital.

There seem to be a lot of overdose cases at our local college. Sometimes the other students interfere and even the residence counselor won't give us the information we need because of fear of getting someone in trouble. If residence counselors were trained better, they could help us a lot in this kind of emergency.

Another frequent call is to the scene where a death has already taken place. One call that I remember well was for an elderly woman who had died of cancer. She had taken a bath and told her daughter to leave her alone, that she wanted to go to sleep. The daughter thought her mother was still alive when she called. From what the daughter said, it seems this lady knew her time was up and prepared herself to die. Often, the dying seem to be thinking more of those left than of themselves.

Rescue work is exciting, but there's only so much we can do. In most cases, it's up to the hospital emergency staff to pick up where we leave off. Sometimes that doesn't happen, I'm afraid, and that's really sad.

those who are should not feel burned out or develop callous attitudes toward people in life-threatening situations. Acute-care nurses, for example, need the time and opportunity to air their feelings about the person who is comatose for days from a drug overdose. When the patient comes through the critical stage and survival seems certain, many nurses find it difficult to communicate empathetically with such a person.

In cases of cardiac arrest at hospitals, teamwork combines emergency medical work with crisis intervention. Without effective teamwork, emergency medical intervention might fail. Nurses have observed that the emergency code system is so effective that it often brings more staff to the scene than are needed; however, provision is not always made for attending to the emotional needs of anxious family members (Davidhizar & Kirk, 1993). In one hospital, the psychiatric nurses—"surplus" personnel—routinely designate themselves to attend to family members who may otherwise be ignored. Nurses and physicians can be routinely trained to assist in emotional crises as well as medical emergencies (Adamowski, et al., 1993; Bertman, 1991; Hoff, 1995).

CASE EXAMPLE: HOSPITAL EMERGENCY NURSE

What I like about emergency nursing is the chance to follow the patient and develop a relationship. Many people who come to the emergency department don't have a private doctor; they use the hospital emergency service as a family physician.

Any number of people come to the emergency department for social or psychological problems, which are covered over with complaints of abdominal pain, back trouble, or other aches and pains. We even see teenagers for pregnancy testing. Even though there's nothing wrong physically, we never take anyone's problem lightly. We have developed a referral system to a primary care clinic for minor medical complaints so we can concentrate on the emergency function of the emergency department.

In cases of true medical emergency, such as an accident, many people come in extremely upset. For example, if a child has been hurt, the parents need reassurance that everything possible is being done. It's also important to let parents stay with an injured or sick child as much as possible.

In cases of serious injury or accident, it's hard to keep in mind the family's state of emotional upset because we're so busy doing all the necessary procedures to keep the person alive. I think everyone understands and wants us to focus our efforts on necessary life-saving procedures, but at the same time it's important to keep the family posted on the progress being made. I have to keep reminding myself of people's psychological needs in a busy place like this.

One of the hardest problems to deal with in emergency work is the case of battered children. I remember a father who brought in his four-year-old child. He had pushed her down the stairs when she wouldn't eat the steak he had brought home. I have a hard time being helpful to parents like this, but I did make a referral to the social worker.

CASE EXAMPLE: FAMILY PHYSICIAN

I spend only one day a week in the emergency department. When there is a true emergency, there is almost always a crisis as well, because the person's body image is altered in a lot of cases. For example, if someone comes in with the symptoms of a heart attack, I tell the person the facts as gently as I can and try to minimize the negatives: "You may be having a heart attack; you have to be treated in the intensive care unit for a while."

Most of the people who make suicide attempts are not at great risk medically. But I carefully examine what led to the suicide attempt in each case; I assume it must be pressure of some kind. A sympathetic, supportive approach is really important. If the family is involved, I often get caught in between. Sometimes they get angry and ask, "Why are you keeping her here? She'll never do it again!" I make a mental health referral in spite of the family's objections. Besides believing the referral is best for the patient and family, I could get into medical or legal trouble if I didn't follow through.

A fairly typical crisis in the emergency department is the case of an accident victim. The magnitude of the crisis usually depends on the degree of injury. The family always needs help. In our hospital, we take them to as private a place as we can find so we can talk with them freely. Again, it's important to give them straight facts along with sympathy and support.

Another typical situation happened last night. The EMTs attended to a man at home who was in cardiac arrest. They also alerted the hospital emergency department. The man was dead on arrival, and his wife was very upset. Besides her normal grief, she blamed herself for her husband's death because she didn't force

him to follow his doctor's advice and go to the hospital when he first had symptoms. This kind of situation is never easy. . . . Words seem so hollow when one is confronted with the death of a loved one. I sensed disbelief and denial in this woman. One way I've found to approach this sad situation is with the opener: "I have some very bad news to tell you." She cried. I stayed with her and listened to her story. At first, she demanded that I bring her husband back to life. I told her that we couldn't bring him back, and gradually she accepted that. In a case like this, when the woman is blaming herself for her husband's death, I find it helpful to use my medical authority to assure the person that she and the rescue team did everything they could to save her husband. I also try to capitalize on the positive things people did do to help. During the ten minutes I spent with this woman, I learned that her daughter was at home. This was fortunate, because the woman seemed helpless to make arrangements by herself. Another thing I learned was that religion was important to her and her husband. Her involvement in the final anointing helped her accept the reality of her husband's death.

Another thing that's hard for me to deal with is the parents of child abuse victims. I try to control my revulsion and talk with them about what I've found in examining the child and my obligation to report the facts. At first they deny, then they usually cooperate, maybe because I try to be supportive in spite of my feelings about this kind of thing.

There's a lot that can be done in emergency medicine, if we only take the time to do it.

In general, health care practitioners in emergency and acute-care settings need to focus on two key aspects of the crisis management process: (1) the initial contact, and (2) referral and follow-up. These two aspects are interrelated: the likelihood of a person accepting a referral for crisis counseling, physical refuge, AA, or other service following emergency medical treatment (such as after a suicide attempt, rape, battering, or crisis related to drinking) will often be influenced by the health care worker's attitude and recognition of the many facets of the situation. In short, health practitioners in emergency settings are not usually expected to assist people through *all* phases of crisis resolution. Effective crisis management, however, does require assessment of the emotional aspects of events threatening health and life and referral for further assistance (Hoff & Rosenbaum, 1994). Besides clinical skills in crisis management, workers in emergency settings also need an up-to-date resource file with procedures to assure follow-up when referrals are made (Hoff, 1983). Social workers usually coordinate such resources.

In the scenarios cited by this emergency nurse, we see the impact of health care policy on a particular health practice situation. Since the historic election in South Africa, the United States holds the dubious distinction of being the only industrialized nation without comprehensive health insurance for its citizens. The challenge of combining emergency medical treatment and crisis intervention protocols is compounded by the misuse of emergency medical centers for routine prenatal care and common ailments that should be treated in physicians' offices or primary health care settings. On the assumption that health care is a right, not a privilege, and that primary care is less costly than in tertiary settings, some services must be publicly supported (Feingold, 1994; Rachlis & Kushner, 1994).

Summary

Health and assistance to people whose health is threatened constitute a major domain of social life. The loss or threat of losing life, limb, or healthy self-image are occasions of crisis for many. Most often, people who are thus threatened come to the attention of general health providers (e.g., nurses and physicians) and frontline workers such as rescue teams, caseworkers, and others close to people's daily struggles. The potential of workers in these entry points to health and social service systems is enormous, as is the cost-saving in human and financial terms when crisis assessment and intervention are routine parts of practice in these settings.

References

Action for mental health. (1961). New York: Basic Books. (Commissioned by the U.S. Congress.)

Adamowski, K., Dickinson, G., Weitzman, B., Roessler, C., & Carter-Snell, C. (1993). Sudden unexpected death in the emergency department: Caring for the survivors. *Canadian Medical Association Journal, 149*(10), 1445–1451.

Anders, R. L. (1977). When a patient becomes violent. *American Journal of Nursing, 77*, 1144–1148.

Becktell, P. J. (1994). Endemic stress: Environmental determinants of women's health in India. *Health Care for Women International, 15*(2), 111–122.

Benson, H., & Klipper, M. A. (1976). *The relaxation response.* New York: Avon Books.

Bertman, S. L. (1991). *Facing death: Images, insights, and interventions.* Washington: Hemisphere.

Borysenko, J. (1987). *Minding the body: Mending the mind.* Reading, Mass.: Addison-Wesley.

Bredenberg, P. (1991). *Who cares? Social support and women with breast cancer.* Unpublished doctoral dissertation. Syracuse University, Syracuse, NY.

Brody, H. (1988). *Stories of sickness.* New Haven: Yale University Press.

Boston Women's Health Book Collective. (1992). *The new our bodies, ourselves.* New York: Simon & Schuster.

Caplan, G. (1964). *Principles of preventive psychiatry.* New York: Basic Books.

Childs, R. E. (1985). Maternal psychological conflicts associated with the birth of a retarded child. *Maternal Child Health Nursing, 14*(3), 175–182.

Chernin, K. (1985). *The hungry self: Women, eating, and identity.* New York: Harper & Row.

Chopra, D. (1993). *Ageless body, timeless mind.* New York: Harmony.

Conrad, P., & Kern, R. (Eds.). (1990). *The sociology of health and illness: Critical perspectives* (3rd ed.). New York: St. Martin's Press.

Dally, A. (1992). *Women under the knife: A history of surgery.* New York: Routledge.

Davidhizar, R., & Kirk, B. (1993). Emergency room nurses: Helping families cope with sudden death. *Journal of Practical Nursing, 43*(2), 14–19.

Ehrenreich, J. (Ed.). (1978). *The cultural crisis of modern medicine.* New York: Monthly Review Press.

Ehrenreich, B., & English, D. (1979). *For her own good: 150 years of the experts' advice to women.* New York: Anchor Books.

Farberow, N. L. (1981). Suicide prevention in the hospital. *Hospital and Community Psychiatry, 32*, 99–104.

Feingold, E. (1994). Health care reform—more than cost containment and universal access. *American Journal of Public Health, 84*(5), 727–728.

Fiedler, J. L., & Wight, J. B. (1989). *The medical offset effect and public health policy: Mental health industry in transition.* New York: Praeger.

Foster, G., & Anderson, B. G. (1978). *Medical anthropology.* New York: Wiley.

Fuller, B., & Foster, G. M. (1982). The effects of family/friend visits vs. staff interaction on stress/arousal of surgical intensive care patients. *Heart and Lung, 11*(5), 457–463.

Fullerton, C. S., McCarroll, J. E., Ursano, R. J., & Wright, K. M. (1992). Psychological responses of rescue workers: Fire fighters and trauma. *American Journal of Orthopsychiatry, 32*(3), 371–378.

Galanti, G. (1991). *Caring for patients from different cultures: Case studies from American hospitals.* Philadelphia: University of Pennsylvania Press.

Gammon, J. (1993). Which way out of the crisis? Coping strategies for dealing with cancer. *Professional Nurse, 8*(8), 488–493.

Garrison, J. (1974). Network techniques: Case studies in the screening-linking-planning conference method. *Family Process, 13*, 337–353.

Hansell, N. (1976). *The person in distress.* New York: Human Sciences Press.

Hoff, L. A. (1983). Interagency coordination for people in crisis. *Information and referral, 5*(1), 79–89.

Hoff, L. A. (1993). Review essay: Health policy and the plight of the mentally ill. *Psychiatry, 56*(4), 400–419.

Hoff, L. A. (1995). *Violence issues: An interdisciplinary curriculum guide for health professionals.* Ottawa: Health Canada. Health Services Directorate.

Hoff, L. A., & Miller, N. (1987). *Programs for people in crisis: A guide for educators, administrators, and clinical trainers.* Boston: Northeastern University Custom Book Program.

Hoff, L. A., & Rosenbaum, L. (1994). A victimization assessment tool: Instrument development and clinical implications. *Journal of Advanced Nursing, 20*(4), 627–634.

James, C. R., Stall, R., & Gifford, S. M. (Eds.). (1986). *Anthropology and epidemiology.* Dordrecht, Holland & Boston, USA: Reidel.

Jamison, K. R., Wellisch, D. K., & Pasnaw, R. O. (1978). Psychosocial aspects of mastectomy. 1. The women's perspective. *American Journal of Psychiatry, 135*, 432–435.

Johnson, A. B. (1990). *Out of bedlam: The truth about deinstitutionalization.* New York: Basic Books.

Kavanagh, K. J. (1988). The cost of caring: Nursing on a psychiatric intensive care unit. *Human Organization, 47*(3), 242–251.

Kleeman, K. M. (1989). Families in crisis due to multiple trauma. *Critical Care Nursing Clinics of North America, 1*(1), 23–31.

Kruger, S. (1992). Parents in crisis: Helping them cope with a seriously ill child. *Journal of Pediatric Nursing, 7*(2), 133–140.

Kuenzi, S. H., & Fenton, M. V. (1975). Crisis intervention in acute care areas. *American Journal of Nursing, 75*, 830–834.

Landy, D. (Ed.). (1977). *Culture, disease, and healing.* New York: Macmillan.

La Fond, J. Q. (1992). *Back to the asylum.* Oxford and New York: Oxford University Press.

Lindemann, E. (1979). *Beyond grief.* New York: Jason Aronson.

Lugina, H. I. (1994). Factors that influence women's health in Tanzania. *Health Care for Women International, 15*(1), 61–68.

Lynn, J., & Childress, J. F. (1991). Must patients always be given food and water? In C. Levine (Ed.), *Taking sides: Clashing views on controversial bioethical issues,* 4th ed. (pp. 118–126). Guilford, Conn.: Dushkin Publishing Group.

Maxwell, M. B. (1982). The use of social networks to help cancer patients maximize support. *Cancer Nursing, 5*, 275–281.

McCarroll, J. E., Ursano, R. J., Wright, K. M., & Fullerton, C. S. (1993). Handling bodies after violent death: Strategies for coping. *American Journal of Orthopsychiatry, 63*(2), 209–214.

McElroy, A., & Townsend, P. K. (1985). *Medical anthropology in ecological perspective.* Boulder & London: Westview Press.

Millman, M. (1978). Medical mortality review: A cordial affair. In H. D. Schwartz & C. S. Kart (Eds.), *Dominant issues in medical sociology* (pp. 288–244). Reading, Mass.: Addison-Wesley.

Moore, K. W., & Schwartz, K. S. (1993). Psychosocial support of trauma patients in the emergency department by nurses, as indicated by communication. *Journal of Emergency Nursing, 19*(4), 297–302.

Navarro, V. (1994). The future of public health in health care reform. *American Journal of Public Health, 84*(5), 729–730.

Parkes, C. M. (1975). *Bereavement: Studies of grief in adult life.* Middlesex, England: Penguin Books.

Penman, D. T., Bloom, J. R., Fotopoulos, S., Cook, M. R., Holland, J. C., Gates, C., Flamer, D., Murawski, B., Ross, R., Brandt, U., Muenz, L. R., & Pee, D. (1987). The impact of mastectomy on self-concept and social function: A combined cross-sectional and longitudinal study with comparison groups. *Women and Health, 11*(3/4), 101–130.

Polak, P. (1967). The crisis of admission. *Social Psychiatry, 1*, 150–157.

Polak, P. (1976). A model to replace psychiatric hospitalization. *Journal of Nervous and Mental Disease, 162*, 13–22.

Polak, P. (1971). Social systems intervention. *Archives of General Psychiatry, 25*, 10–117.

Pruchno, R. A., & Potashnik, S. L. (1989). Caregiving spouses: Physical and mental health in perspective. *Journal of the American Geriatrics Society, 37,* 697–705.

Ptacek, L. J. (1982). Respite care for families of children with severe handicaps: An evaluation study of parent satisfaction. *Journal of Community Psychology, 10,* 222–227.

Putting people first: The reform of mental health services in Ontario. (1993). Toronto: Ontario Ministry of Health.

Rachlis, M., & Kushner, C. (1994). *Strong medicine: How to save Canada's health care system.* Toronto: HarperCollins.

Richardson, B. K. (1987). Psychiatric inpatients' perception of seclusion room experience. *Nursing Research, 36*(July-August), 234–238.

Schain, W. (1980). Patients' rights in decision making: The case for personalism vs. paternalism in health care. *Cancer, 46,* 1035–1041.

Seeman, M., & Seeman, A. Z. (1992). Life strains, alienation, and drinking behavior. *Alcoholism, 16*(2), 199–205.

Shalev, A. Y., Schreiber, S., Galai, T., & Melmed, R. N. (1993). Post-traumatic stress disorder following medical events. *British Journal of Clinical Psychology, 32* (Part 2), 247–253.

Shipes, E., & Lehr, S. (1982). Sexuality and the male cancer patient. *Cancer Nursing, 5,* 375–381.

Skorupka, P., & Bohnet, N. (1982). Primary caregivers' perceptions of nursing behaviors that best meet their needs in a home care hospice setting. *Cancer Nursing, 5,* 371–374.

Smith, D. R. (1994). Porches, politics, and public health. *American Journal of Public Health, 84*(5), 725–726.

Solomon, M. Z., O'Donnell, L., Jennings, B., Guilfoy, V., Wolf, S. M., Nolan, K., Jackson, B. A., Koch-Weser, D., & Donnelley, S. (1993). Decisions near the end of life: Professional views on life-sustaining treatments. *American Journal of Public Health, 83*(1), 14–23.

Sontag, S. (1978). *Illness as metaphor.* New York: Farrar, Straus & Giroux.

Spector, R. E. (1991). *Cultural diversity in health and illness.* (3rd ed.). Norwalk, Conn.: Appleton & Lange.

Sugg, N., & Inui, N. K. (1992). Primary care physicians' response to domestic violence: Opening Pandora's box. *Journal of American Medical Association, 267* (23), 3157–3160.

Surgeon General's workshop on violence and public health: Report. (1986). Washington, D.C.: Health Resources and Services Administration.

Werner-Beland, J. A. (Ed.). (1980). *Grief responses to long-term illness and disability.* Reston, Va.: Reston.

Zborowski, M. (1952). Cultural components in responses to pain. *Journal of Social Issues, 8,* 16–30.

CHAPTER TWELVE

THREATS TO OCCUPATIONAL AND RESIDENTIAL SECURITY

B asic human needs include success in one's ascribed and achieved social roles, and a secure, stable dwelling place. Meeting these needs implies:

- The ability and opportunity to be creative and productive in a way that is meaningful to us and accepted by others
- Membership in a supportive community that values our presence and contribution
- Enough material supplies to maintain self-sufficiency and protection from the elements

As discussed in the last chapter, a serious change in health status threatens a person's self-image as well as the ability to be self-supportive. Underscoring the interacting relationship between health, occupational, and general social security, many people—especially in the United States where there is no comprehensive health care system—remain in unfulfilling jobs that can literally make them sick (Illich, 1976) to keep from losing insurance coverage. If they lose their jobs, the loss of insurance as well adds to their stress, fear, and insecurity about the future. In turn, these additional stressors affect one's health status and ability to function at precisely the time of greatest need. When occupation-based stress intersects with domestic issues, depression is not uncommon (Phelan, et al., 1991). This includes stress from overwork by people who cannot afford to build regular leisure time into their lives (Schor, 1993). Generally, job security is the fundamental means of maintaining residential security, since housing constitutes most people's major financial liability. The most extreme response to job loss is violence by the dismissed employee against the employer and others, a phenomenon more common in the United States.

These intertwined hazards around health, occupational, and residential security are compounded for those with a prior history of mental illness (Hoff, et al., 1992) and for victims of violence, especially women and children. Most people look forward to the comfort and security of returning to a secure dwelling after a day's work or returning to welcoming co-workers after a vacation or business trip. When occupational and residential status are threatened, however, a person's status may be dramatically changed from:

- Home to streets
- Having a job to the unemployment lines or poverty
- A sense of self-sufficiency to unexpected dependency
- A sense of security to uncertainty about where the next meal is coming from or where the next night will be spent—on someone's couch? in a welfare hotel? a shelter? the mean streets?

In the following pages, the principles and techniques of crisis intervention that frontline workers can apply on behalf of people in crisis around housing and occupational loss are discussed. People need to mourn the losses that characterize these transitions—some of which are life-threatening. And they need the hope that comes from advocacy and social change to alleviate the conditions that deprive people of jobs and home and widen the gap between the rich and poor of the world.

Occupational Changes

Promotion, Success, and Economic Security

Promotion and success do not seem to be hazardous events or occasions for crisis, and for many they are not. But suicide studies reveal that promotion can be the "last straw" that leads some people to decide to commit suicide. The person who is promoted to a prestigious position may feel incapable of performing as expected in the new role. An anticipated promotion can also be a crisis point, as a new position in a company brings increased responsibility as well as higher rank and status; it also requires a change in role relationships among peers. If the move is from ordinary staff worker to a management position, the person may fear loss of acceptance by the peer group he or she leaves (Kanter, 1977).

The combination of loss of familiar supportive relationships at work and the challenge of unfamiliar work becomes too much to handle. A person's vulnerability to crisis in these circumstances is affected by several factors:

1. The general openness of communication within the company or agency
2. The person's ability to openly discuss questions and fears with a trusted confidante, since expressing worries about self-confidence, for example, might jeopardize the promotion
3. The person's perception of self and how one should perform in a given role—especially difficult for perfectionists

The "Success Neurosis" and Sex Roles.   A crisis stemming from promotion has also been called the "success neurosis," which is frequently seen in women who view themselves as occupying second-rate or second-best positions. If they have worked primarily in the role of housewife and mother, they may suddenly become immobilized when other opportunities arise. This can happen even when they have openly expressed a desire for new opportunities.

Crises associated with promotion and success are usually "quiet crises." People in this kind of crisis are not acutely upset but feel generally anxious and depressed and express bewilderment about being depressed. They feel disappointed that they cannot measure up to their own expectations; they know they have every reason to be happy. They cannot relate their feelings of depression to their lack of self-confidence and rigid expectations of themselves. A deep fear of failure may lead to the idea of suicide in the event that the person really does fail.

Anxiety, depression, and suicidal thoughts may move a person in this kind of crisis to seek help. Usually, he or she will go to a local crisis clinic or private therapist. Several crisis counseling sessions are often sufficient for the person to:

• Express underlying fears, insecurity, and disappointment with self
• Gain a realistic perspective on his or her abilities
• Grow in self-confidence and self-acceptance
• Use family and friends to discuss feelings and concerns openly rather than viewing such expressions as another failure

---

CASE EXAMPLE: ANGIE

Angie, age thirty-seven, had been doing volunteer work with the mental health association in her community. One of her special projects was helping handicapped people run a confection stand for local Parks and Recreation Department events. Because of the high quality of her work—which she could only acknowledge self-consciously—her friends urged her to open and manage her own coffee house. She finally did so, and the project was a glowing success. Angie suddenly found herself in the limelight, a situation she had not anticipated. She could not believe it would last. After a few months, she began feeling tense and depressed and thought vaguely about suicide. She talked with her physician about her problem and was referred to a psychiatrist for help.

Short-term crisis counseling may reveal deeper problems of low self-esteem, rigid role expectations, inflexible behavior patterns, and habitual reluctance to communicate feelings of distress to significant people. Psychotherapy should be offered and encouraged, since these people are high risks for suicide if other crisis situations arise (Greenspan, 1983). But in addition to offering individual assistance, as crisis workers and as a society we need to examine the structures and differential expectations and rewards that place women at greater risk of failing in their career aspirations. For example, executive women (unlike executive men) who want to avoid being "derailed" from the career ladder typically must jump through two hoops: traditional masculine behavior and traditional feminine behavior (Morrison, White, & Van Velsor, 1987). This is a new version of the old adage: women must be twice as good to get half as far. One consequence of such stress might be an obsession with work, to the detriment of a healthy balance between work and other activities (Schaef & Fassel, 1988). Although women have made progress in traditionally male-dominated professions like law, medicine, and engineering, many encounter a "glass ceiling" that prevents their promotions in those fields and keeps their pay lower than that of male colleagues. Further, they are vulnerable to the same gender-based harassment and abuse as women in traditionally female-dominated professions such as nursing (Phillips & Schneider, 1993). Finally, despite their high professional status, they shoulder the same dual burden that most women carry: they do the bulk of unpaid domestic work such as child care.

Promotion and success can result in another kind of crisis: one between spouses when a woman earns more than her husband. Traditionally, girls and women have been socialized to play inferior roles, and boys and men are taught to think of themselves as failures if they do not earn more than women. The price for maintaining these stereotypes is very high for both men and women. For some men married to successful women, the risk of early death from heart disease is eleven times greater than in other marriages (Rubenstein, 1982, p. 37). A study of egalitarian marriages (versus those in which a woman holds a stereotypical female job) revealed that the chance of divorce was twice as high, while psychological and physical abuse also was higher (Rubenstein, 1982, p. 38). These findings are supported by other studies of violence (e.g., Dobash & Dobash, 1979).

The origins of such crises can be traced to cultural values and the tradition that men do public work and are paid well for it, while women do private work and are not paid at all (Etheridge 1978; Waring, 1990). When women do work outside the home, they are often expected to do so in traditionally female, nurturant or supportive jobs such as nursing, teaching, and clerical work (Foner, 1994; Kavanagh, 1988; Reverby, 1987). Since the majority of women work outside the home for economic, psychological, and social survival, the points of stress and potential crises are numerous as long as traditional values prevail. For many of these women, the cost of caring is very high (Facione, 1994; Kessler & McLeod, 1984; Sommers & Shields, 1987) and will get higher as the number of elderly and people with AIDS increases, unless men begin to assume equal responsibility for the caring work of society. Crisis counseling or therapy is indicated for individual men and women struggling with these issues. The long-term results, however, will be limited if there is not simultaneous attention directed to the social change strategies relevant to these crises of sociocultural origin (see Chapter Two).

Institutional Barriers to Promotion and Economic Security. Aside from regressive cultural values about men, women, and work, there are institutional barriers to promotion for millions of workers: ethnic minorities and poor women (Sidel, 1986). Disregard for minorities and women is expressed concretely in persistent and alarming job bias, despite civil rights legislation. Thus, values and the profit motive support race, class, age, and sex discrimination, which in turn reinforce traditional values (Seager & Olson, 1986; World Federation of Public Health Associations, 1986). Such social problems can lead to homelessness, child neglect, marital discord, bitterness, withdrawal from the mainstream of social life, drug abuse, suicide, and violence.

Numerous studies (see Chapter Two) underscore the work of Caplan (1964), Hansell (1976), and others documenting the need for intactness of one's social, cultural, and material supplies in order to avoid personal crisis. Pearce and McAdoo (1982), writing for the National Advisory Council on Economic Opportunity regarding the "feminization of poverty," state:

> The typical outcome of a marital breakup in a family with children is that the man becomes single, while the woman becomes a single parent. . . . Men generally do not become poor because of divorce, sex-role socialization, sexism, or, of course, pregnancy. Indeed, some may lift themselves out of poverty by the same means that women plunge into it: the same divorce that frees a man from the financial burdens of a family may result in poverty for his ex-wife and children.

This situation is dramatized by the fact that within a year of divorce, the standard of living for most women decreases significantly and for men it increases. The largest percentage of poor women and children are members of racial minorities, which underscores the combination of race, gender, and class bias. As a group, women in the United States still earn only seventy cents to every dollar earned by men, despite the Equal Pay Act passed in 1965. To offer psychotherapy or crisis counseling alone without job training, day care, and advocacy for adequate housing represents a misunderstanding of the problem, its origins, and solutions. Rather than recycling these old problems, a fresh look upstream to their source holds the most promise for reducing crisis proneness and long-term negative outcomes for victims of discrimination. [See Figure 11.1.]

Paid and Unpaid Work

Worldwide, in labor statistics jargon, *work* is defined as paid work. In Africa, for example, 60 to 80 percent of agricultural work is done by women, though it is not included in official labor force counts. In Canada, according to 1992 data, household work, two-thirds of which is done by women, accounts for 41.4 percent of national output. As Mollison (1993, p. 15A) states:

> The economy would shudder if homemakers stopped doing unpaid work. Families would have to choose between recruiting other unpaid volunteers, hiring replacements, or settling for a life in which unfed, ignorant children and grouchy, unkempt adults struggled for survival under burned-out light bulbs and amid mountains of stinky socks.

In sum, women probably will not achieve equality in the paid work force until men do an equal share of society's unpaid—but nevertheless very necessary—work. Statistics compiled for the 1985 U.N. Decade for Women Conference in Nairobi, Kenya reveal that women do two-thirds of the world's work (not counting unpaid child care), earn one-tenth of the world's income, and own less than one-hundredth of the world's property. As Waring (1990) notes, if women's work "counted," official labor statistics and potentially the entire social landscape could be transformed. In the United States, a national debate is in progress about "reforming welfare as we know it." Few would contest the negative—even damaging—outcomes of intergenerational welfare dependency for some recipients. To yield its intended results, however, this debate should make visible the public denigration of women's work in rearing children alone—often as a result of abuse and because many divorced fathers do not pay child support. Success in welfare reform would also link the worldwide correlation of teenage motherhood and general birth rates with equity in women's economic and educational status. Contrary to popular perception, adolescent pregnancy is not just a racial minority issue; rather, it reflects poverty and the increasing unwillingness of teens to defer sexual activity, factors that cross racial boundaries (Desmond, 1994).

This issue is especially urgent because it is connected to the hopelessness and apathy of chronically poor people—especially in inner cities—who are no longer just the "underclass," but are now referred to as the "outerclass." They do not vote, do not report crimes, and do not always send their children to school; often they do not even have a telephone for sending or receiving calls (Canellos, 1994). In such a climate, despair and violence flourish. Perhaps in no instance is the link between personal crisis and socioeconomic and cultural factors more dramatically illustrated. The tandem approach discussed in Chapter Nine most aptly applies here: assisting individuals through traumatic life events like joblessness and unemployment (often based on race and class status), holding them accountable for violence and child supervision, while *simultaneously* engaging them and others to address the roots of their plight (see Crisis Paradigm, Box 3).

Following the Los Angeles riots, Bondi Gabrel, ethnic minority owner of an apartment complex in that riot-torn community, could have abandoned his damaged building. Instead, he *employed* gang members, provided leadership, options, and a vision of another lifestyle. Gang members now, instead of vandalizing property, are paid to guard it. When chosen as "person of the week" by a national television network, Mr. Gabrel said, "This is what happens when you invest in people. . . . We haven't asked for enough." As this example and Medoff and Sklar's (1994) account of the death and life of an urban neighborhood demonstrate, models for such multifaceted approaches are there and they need to be widely replicated (see also, McKinlay, 1990).

Work Disruption

Just as promotion, success, or disadvantaged status can be a source of crisis or threat to health (Verbrugge, 1982), so can disruption or change in work role, especially for a person accustomed to a lifetime of job security. The depression of inner-city neighborhoods is connected to global economic changes and the widespread loss of manufacturing jobs, which had been the mainstay of security for many who are now desperate. As individuals and families struggle to keep or find new jobs, the median family income in large cities like Boston dropped 15.2 percent between 1989 and 1992, compared with 7.9 percent in other cities and 4.8 percent nationwide (Butterfield, 1993, p. 46). Ethnic minority and immigrant groups are the most affected by the loss of manufacturing jobs, many of which have been transferred to countries with cheaper labor and looser laws protecting both workers and the environment.

Western society's attitude toward work, especially in the United States, is highlighted by a tendency to value people in proportion to how much money they earn and to respect them in proportion to the socioeconomic status they derive from their earnings. In other words, many have absorbed the deeply embedded cultural value: "You're worth what you earn." This value system helps fuel the welfare reform debate and the suspicion on the part of the "haves" that the "have-nots" are ultimately responsible for their own misfortune and could remedy that misfortune if they simply tried harder. Such judgments fail to account for the complex relationship between most unemployment situations and either global economics or discrimination based on race, gender, age, disability, or ill health. Usually, the unemployed or underemployed in a changing economy are deeply regretful of their position and struggle continuously to correct it. These complexities are illustrated in the case of one immigrant family:

> Armando and Eliza have two children and two jobs and rarely see each other because Armando's factory job is during the day and Eliza's hospital job is

nights and weekends. But they're not complaining. "For both of us to have jobs, that's the important thing," Armando says. "Because if the jobs go, everything goes." . . . And more and more, the new immigrants—and poor whites and native blacks, too—have to struggle to find any job at all. That's not the way it was in 1976 when Armando and Jack and their seven brothers and sisters arrived with their mother and a paraplegic father from Cape Verde. Then, factory and mill work was abundant, even if pay was low. "You worked like an animal, but you had food for the table," Jack says. . . . Both families agree that their lives are much more fragile today than ever before—hanging on the instability that pervades work in nearly every field. "That's the very scary thing," Armando adds. "What we have, the way we all live, depends on a job. And today, you cannot depend on a job" (Butterfield, 1993, p. 47).

The dismal job climate is compounded by the fact that the United States is currently in a twenty-one-year low on an index of social health. Sociologist Marc Miringoff of the Fordham Institute for Innovation in Social Policy notes that the United States has seen a widening gap between rich and poor; it has reached the worst recorded levels of child abuse, teen suicide, average weekly earnings, health insurance coverage, and out-of-pocket health costs for those over sixty-five (Dvorchak, 1992). While unemployment figures have dropped, real income adjusted for inflation is down or stagnant, while millions are underemployed or quietly trying to survive. These problems are greatly magnified for ethnic minority groups and aboriginal people in North America. Unemployment, then, whether by firing, layoff, or because of a personal problem like illness, is frequently the occasion of emotional crisis, including violent responses like suicide or murder. While unemployed people must act on their misfortune, they will be much more empowered to do so if they are not inappropriately blamed for their plight.

Regardless of the reasons, the person in crisis because of unemployment is usually in need of a great deal of support. If unemployment originated from personal sources, social support and individual crisis intervention are indicated (Collins, et al., 1992). However, people who are unemployed because of economic recession or discrimination are less likely to feel hopeless and powerless if they are also put into contact with groups devoted to removing the underlying sources of their stress through social change strategies. This includes policy changes that would prevent corporations from simply closing U.S. plants, laying off hundreds of employees, and moving to a country where labor is cheaper without any collaboration with or consideration of the workers who have built their lives around the company. The primary origin of crisis for a worker thus laid off is the profit motive. The appropriate response, therefore, should include linking such a person to groups advocating labor-management policy change (see Crisis Paradigm). In Germany, for example, workers in an automobile manufacturing plant decided on a four-day work week so that *none* lost their jobs.

Standards of personal success for most of us hinge on involvement in work that is personally satisfying and of value to the external community. For example, a fifty-five-year-old man in a middle-management position who is prematurely re-tired may begin to drink or may attempt suicide as a way of dealing with the cri-sis of job disruption. These and other work-related crises are within the common province of personnel directors, occupational physicians and nurses, or anyone the person turns to in distress.

CASE EXAMPLE: RUSSELL AND JENNY OWENS

Russell Owens, age fifty-two, was a civil engi-neer employed for twenty years as a research consultant in a large industrial corporation. When he lost his job because of a surplus of engineers with his qualifications, he tried without success to find other employment, even at lower pay. Family financial needs forced his wife Jenny, age forty-seven, to seek full-time employment as a biology in-structor; she had worked only part-time be-fore. Jenny was grateful for this opportunity to advance herself professionally. She had al-ways regretted the fact that she had never tried to excel at a job, partly because Russell did not want her to work full-time. Gradu-ally, however, Jenny became resentful of hav-ing to support herself, her husband, and their sixteen-year-old daughter, Gwen, in ad-dition to assuming all responsibility for household tasks. She urged Russell to do at

least some of the housework. Since Russell had never helped in this way before, except for occasional errands and emergencies, Jenny's expectations struck a blow to his masculine self-image beyond the sense of failure and inadequacy he already felt from his job loss.

Russell also found it difficult to follow Jenny's advice to seek help with his depres-sion and his increasing dependence on alco-hol. The strain in their marital relationship increased. Jenny eventually divorced Russell, and he committed suicide.

Russell's drinking problem and eventual suicide might have been avoided if immedi-ate help had been available to him at the cri-sis points of job loss and threat of divorce. Such help might also have resulted in a con-structive resolution of Jenny's resentment of Russell concerning the housework.

Rural and Urban Occupational Transitions

Similar dynamics are apparent in the farm crisis. Farmers not only face a threat to their source of livelihood, but also to their way of life. One study revealed that 33.7 percent of family farms were in serious or extreme financial trouble (Olson & Schellenberg, 1986). While it is possible that some farm foreclosures can be traced to individual mismanagement, the problem originates in policies that favor unbridled corporate accumulations of agricultural resources and profits at the expense of individual farm families. For example, federal price supports for farm products are cut back because of a "surplus." Yet in New England, where hundreds of Vermont dairy families have been driven off their farms, there is no milk surplus. Rather, the large amounts of milk at issue are from huge corpo-rate farms in California. It is ironic that, in a country of immigrants who fled Eu-rope and prized the opportunity to earn an honest living on the land, people are now in crisis because public policy favors corporate monopoly over the nation's breadbasket. No doubt the suicides, alcoholism, violence, and family conflicts arising from the farm crisis will continue unless grassroots efforts and public policy (such as that proposed by the Vermont legislature) reverse the conditions causing so much pain and despair among the nation's rural citizens. One such grassroots organization is Farm Aid Rural Management (FARM) in Bismarck, North Dakota. A similar program, The Kitchen Table Alliance, was organized as a countywide community development project in Ontario for farm families in financial, legal, emotional difficulty or crisis to regain their health and productivity. Basically, these groups offer support, advocacy, crisis prevention and referral for these distressed workers and their families.[1]

Although the farm crisis in North America has abated somewhat, similar disruption of a way of life is now occurring in fishing communities worldwide. In poor countries, millions of rural dwellers flock to shanty towns near water, only to continue their grim struggle for survival, often with additional threats of violence in crowded slums. The threat in fishing communities is not only to a way of life taken for granted for generations but to marine life, since over-fishing depletes the fish supply. Support and crisis intervention groups like the Kitchen Table Alliance for farmers are crucial to the health and social welfare of affected fishing community members to prevent suicide, violence, and substance abuse as governments and international agencies address the long-term facets of this issue.

Retirement

Some people look forward to retirement. Others dread it. For many people, retirement signifies loss of status, a reduced standard of living, and a feeling of being discarded by society. The experience is more pronounced when one is forced to retire at an early age due to illness or other disability. It is a time of stress not only for the retired person but for family members, especially wives who do not work outside the home. Suddenly a homemaker has to adjust to having at home all day a husband who often feels worthless and who may have developed few outside interests or hobbies apart from work.

The attitude people hold toward retirement depends on the situation they retire *to*; whether retirement is pleasant or not is also influenced by life style. Key areas of concern in evaluating a person's retirement situation include:

1. Does the person have any satisfying interests or hobbies outside of work? For many, work has been their main focus all of their adult lives, and most of their pleasures are work-related.

[1]Information about the Ontario group, including training program development, is available at 240 George Street, P.O. Box 579, Arthur, Ontario N0G 1A0; telephone (519) 848–2667; FAX (519) 848–3901.

2. Does the person have a specifically planned retirement project? For example, some people plan to study literature, carpentry, or cooking when they retire. For people of means, Elder Hostel offers many such programs.
3. Does the person have a comfortable place to live?
4. Does he or she have enough retirement income to manage without excessive dependence?
5. Is the person in reasonably good health and free to manage without hardship?
6. Has the person been well-adjusted socially and emotionally before retirement?

Even if the retired person's circumstances are favorable in all or most of these areas, retirement can still be stressful. We live in a youth-oriented society, and retirement signals that one is nearing or has already reached old age; after that, death approaches.

For some people, retirement is not an issue or occasion for crisis. They may be self-employed and simply keep working at a pace compatible with their needs and inclinations. Such people usually prepare for a reduced pace and have a healthy attitude toward life in each development phase, including old age. A new view of the life cycle suggests three phases: learning, earning, and returning. Thus, instead of retiring, people have an opportunity to return wisdom and other values to society and to have something returned to them after their years of learning, earning, and caring for others (Schoonover, 1987).

Those who are in crisis as a result of retirement should have the assistance accorded anyone experiencing a loss. They need the opportunity to grieve the loss of their former status, explore new ways of feeling useful, and eventually accept their changed roles.

Residential Changes

Moves across country or to a different continent require leaving familiar surroundings and friends for a place with many unknowns. Even though the person moving may have many problems at home, at least he or she knows what the problems are. Pulling up stakes and starting over can be an exciting venture, an occasion for joy and for gaining a new lease on life—or a source of deep distress and an occasion for crisis.

Consider the young woman who grew up in the country and moves to the city for the first time. She asks herself, Will I find a job? Will I be able to make friends? Will I be unbearably lonely? Will I be safe? Or, the career person looking for opportunities wonders, Will things be any better there? How will I manage not seeing my family and friends very often? And last, consider the immigrant who worries, How will those foreigners accept me? Will I be able to learn the language so I can get along? Who will help me if things go wrong? What if I want to come back and don't have the money?

Anticipated Moves

These are a few of the many questions and potential problems faced by people who plan a move in hopes of improving their situation. Even in these instances, moving is a source of considerable stress. It takes courage to leave familiar territory, even when the move would free one from many negative situations. No matter what the motive for the move, and despite the anticipation of better things to come, people in this transition state often experience a sense of loss.

To prevent a crisis at this time, the person planning and looking forward to a move should avoid denying feelings of loss. Even when a person is moving to much better circumstances, there is usually the loss of close associations with friends or relatives. As in the case of promotion or success, the would-be mover often does not understand her or his depression, which is probably related to the denial of feelings and guilt about leaving friends and relatives. Understanding and expressing these feelings helps the person keep an open relationship with friends left behind and frees the person to use and enjoy new opportunities more fully, unburdened of misplaced guilt or depression.

People who plan and look forward to a move are vulnerable to other crises. Once they reach their destination, the situation may not work out as anticipated: the new job may be less enjoyable than the old one; the escape from a violent city to a farm may seem less secure than expected; new friends may be hard to find; envisioned job opportunities may not exist.

Social isolation and the inability to establish and maintain satisfying social attachments make a person vulnerable to crises and even suicide. People who have satisfying supports can help prevent crises among those who have recently moved and who have not established a reliable social support system. Elderly people, for example, who are moved to a group residential setting have a much improved chance of adjusting well to the change and perceiving it as a challenge if (1) they had a choice in relocation, (2) relocation was predictable and understandable within their meaning system, and (3) they received necessary social support (Armer, 1993). In the Cohousing movement discussed in Chapter Five, diversity by age is one of the goals, with some groups reserving a certain number of units (e.g., five households out of twenty-five) for persons fifty-five and older. A planned move of this sort for people who dread living in housing complexes only for old people could do much to avoid a crisis during this major life transition.

Unanticipated Moves

The potential for crisis is even greater for those who do not want to move but are forced to. Consider the family uprooted to an unknown place because of a job transfer; inner-city dwellers—especially older people—dislocated because of urban renewal; victims of disaster moving from a destroyed community; people evicted because of unpaid rent; mental patients who have been discharged to the community without adequate shelter and social support; battered women and their children who are forced to leave their homes to avoid beating or death; political or war refugees who must leave their homelands; or migrant farm workers who must move each year in the hope of earning a marginal subsistence. Afghan refugee women, for example, not only have lost family members and property, but also face dramatic cultural differences, tripled social burdens, and lack of appropriate mates where they have now settled, in Northern California (Lipson & Miller, 1994).

Thousands of teenagers and young people either run away from home, or they are simply "on the move." Many young people who run away do so because they are physically or sexually abused, or because they have "come out" as gay or lesbian and are wholly rejected by their families. Usually they lack housing, food, and money; many are further exploited sexually or feel forced into prostitution for survival; in extreme cases they are killed by police for petty stealing and vagrancy. Or, there are groups of people who have been relocated by governments. Some of the most dramatic examples of such forced relocation and the long-term damaging effects are the destruction of Boston's West End in the 1950s to build Government Center (Gans, 1962); the 1953 dispatching of eighty-five Inuit people from northern Quebec to the High Arctic where their families were wrenched apart and they endured extreme hardship and deprivation (Aubry, 1994); and the creation of racially segregated communities in South Africa (Sparks, 1990). As a result of these government actions, Boston's former West Enders are still mourning the loss of their homes, while the Inuit and South African majority are still seeking justice. Finally, there is the ordinary traveler who is en route from one place to another and loses money or belongings or is attacked.

In spite of the crisis potential of moves for many, moving can also be an occasion for growth (Singular, 1983). While highly mobile families may have fewer deep friendships, the family unit many feel closer and have a stronger self-concept as a result of successful coping in diverse circumstances. Psychologists counseling people with emotional problems related to relocation identify four phases in coping with a move: (1) decision making—the less a person contributes to the decision, the more potential there is for trouble; (2) preparation—mastering the many details preceding a move; (3) separation from the old community—including acceptance of the sadness and loss involved; and (4) reinvestment—through involvement in one's new community (Singular, 1983, p. 46). These phases are akin to grief work and the rites of passage discussed in Chapters Four and Thirteen.

Helping the Migrant

Where is help available for the people in crisis related to migration? Crisis centers and mental health agencies are appropriate for people who are under great stress before a move as well as those who are anxious and upset afterward. Special programs for stranded youth are on the rise. Social service agencies and services for aging persons should also provide anticipatory guidance and crisis counseling to all groups forced to move because of a planned project such as urban renewal. Unfortunately, such support and counseling is either not available or is not offered regularly.

CASE EXAMPLE: NOREEN ANDERSON

Noreen Anderson, age sixty-one, was confined to her apartment with a serious muscle disease. She was forced to retire at age fifty-eight and had felt lonely and isolated since then. She did not have family in the area but did have many friends. However, they gradually stopped visiting her after she had been confined for a year. Now her apartment building was being converted to condominiums that she could not afford. The heat had been turned off in March (in a cold, northern U.S. city). Everyone in the building had moved out except Noreen, who was unable to move without help. Fortunately, Noreen's telephone was not disconnected. She called various social service agencies for help and was finally referred to a local crisis center.

An outreach crisis counselor went to Noreen's apartment. She expedited an appli-

cation through a federal housing agency for a place for Noreen in a senior citizens' housing project. The counselor also engaged an interfaith volunteer agency to help Noreen pack her belongings and processed a request for supplies through Catholic Charities. Noreen was grateful for the help received after her several desperate telephone calls, but by this time she was depressed and suicidal. The crisis counselor saw her in her new apartment in the senior citizen's housing project for several counseling sessions. She helped Noreen get in touch with old friends again and encouraged the friends to visit on a regular basis. Retired Senior Citizen Volunteers (RSVP) also visited Noreen, which helped relieve her isolation and loneliness. Noreen was no longer suicidal at termination of the counseling sessions.

Traveler's Aid Society. The Traveler's Aid Society has been doing crisis intervention work with people in transit for years. Caseworkers of this agency see travelers at the peak of their distress. The traveler who calls the Society is often without money or resources and is fearful in a strange city. In extreme cases, the person may have been beaten, robbed, or raped. The Traveler's Aid Society caseworker gets in touch with relatives; assures emergency medical services, food, and emergency housing; provides travel money; and assures the traveler a safe trip home. Unfortunately, the Traveler's Aid Society is poorly linked to other crisis services in most communities. It has low visibility as a social service agency, is often poorly funded, and does not operate on a twenty-four-hour basis in most places. A close working relationship with a twenty-four-hour crisis service could remedy this situation. The relative isolation of this agency often results in the Traveler's Aid staff handling suicidal or emotionally upset travelers by themselves, without the support of crisis specialists who should be available.

International Institute and Other Support.   The International Institute and special refugee groups also help people in crisis related to immigration. The Institute's unique contribution is crisis work with refugees and immigrants who do not know the local language. Inability to speak a country's language can be the source of acute crises related to housing, employment, health, welfare, and legal matters. Institute workers, all of whom speak several languages, assist refugees and immigrants in these essential life areas.

There is an International Institute in nearly all major metropolitan areas, where most refugees and immigrants first settle. Health and social service personnel can refer immigrants who are unaware of this service on arrival. The language crisis is so acute for some immigrants that they may be mistakenly judged psychotic and taken to a mental hospital, or they may have to rely inappropriately on their own children for translation. Intervention by a multilingual person is a critical part of care in such cases.

As is the case with the Traveler's Aid Society, this important social service agency has low visibility in the community and is not linked adequately with twenty-four-hour crisis services. Needed linkages may become routine as health and crisis services become more comprehensive and cosmopolitan (Hoff & Miller, 1987; Rachlis & Kushner, 1994).

The actual and potential crises of immigrants and refugees have become more visible as international tensions have grown. People persecuted or sought out for protest seek refuge and political asylum in friendly countries with greater frequency. Cooperation between private and public agencies on behalf of these people is paramount to avoid unnecessary distress and crisis. In addition to legal, housing, language, and immediate survival issues, refugees experience the psychological pain of losing their homeland. No matter how we may have been treated, most of us have a strong attachment to our country of birth. Whether this bond is broken voluntarily or by threat to life, we need an opportunity to mourn the loss and find substitutes for what was left behind.

One way that refugees and immigrants cope with their loss is to preserve their customs, art, language, ritual celebrations, and food habits. These practices provide immigrants with the security that comes from association with their familiar cultural heritage. Sensitivity of neighbors and agency personnel to immigrants' cultural values, along with control of their own ethnocentrism, can go a long way in helping refugees feel "at home." On the other hand, members of host countries need particular sensitivity regarding a practice like female genital mutilation (FGM), which some immigrants wish to continue. This ritual cannot be excused on grounds that it is a cultural norm, since the World Health Organization has declared it a human rights violation; Canada has declared it illegal (see Gullen, 1992 and Chapter Thirteen).

Homelessness and Vulnerability to Violence

Some people live in cardboard boxes, ride the subway all night long, or stay in doorways of public buildings until they are asked by the police to move. Some sleep on steel grates to catch steam heat from below. Some battered women and their children move from shelter to shelter, staying the limit at each because battering does not fit the city's criteria of eligibility for emergency housing; one mother of three finally bought a tent and camped in a city park.

There are an estimated three million homeless people in the United States, while three or four times that many stay with family and friends. Unless drastic action is taken, this figure will increase to nineteen million by the end of the century. The majority of these people are women and children. Besides having no secure place to stay, homeless people are frequent victims of rape or robbery of their few possessions; homeless youth are often victims of child prostitution; among elderly homeless, some are disabled, some are deaf or blind, and some have symptoms of Alzheimer's disease. Contrary to popular perception, a good percentage of the homeless hold low-paying jobs that do not provide enough income to pay inflated rental prices. Many are victims of eviction when apartments are converted to condominiums for upwardly mobile, mostly white professionals. At no time since the Great Depression have homeless people represented such a cross-section of a wealthy Western society.

In industrialized nations, the most visible and highest numbers of homeless people are in the United States. In fact, as the problem continues, many worry that homelessness will become institutionalized as a permanent feature of social life. Several factors that help explain the apparent intractability of this problem are: (1) the growing disparity between rich and poor; (2) the lack of a national health program that includes sufficient coverage for crisis and mental health services; (3) the continuing bias against the mentally ill and the resulting inadequate transitional housing and support services to prevent homelessness (Hoff, et al., 1992; Jencks, 1994; Weitzman, et al., 1992). But the problem is by no means limited to the United States. Worldwide recession and similar bias against the mentally ill occur cross-culturally, and in any society where community values are sacrificed in favor of the individualistic paradigm that dominates in the United States (Bellah, 1986; Hoff, 1993). Perhaps most alarming of all is the fact that children in the United States now constitute the largest segment of homeless people (Davidhizar & Frank, 1992).

Homelessness strips people of their self-respect, denies them their elementary rights as citizens, and blights the future of a nation's greatest resource—children. The crisis of homelessness is dramatized by current happenings in San Francisco under the rubric of the Matrix program. San Francisco law allows a team of city workers from the police, sanitation, and mental health departments to search out the homeless on the streets. When a homeless person is encountered, he or she is questioned and, if possible, arrested or committed involuntarily to a psychiatric facility. If the person is sleeping, the police officer gently taps the individual, who typically reacts in a startled or frightened manner. The mental health professional steps in with a "rapid diagnosis of paranoia, or somehow makes the determination that the person may be a danger to him/herself or others and commits said person to a determined observation period in the hospital. As the hapless individual is taken away, all his belongings are trashed by the . . . Sanitation Engineers" (Dean, 1994, p. 3). Under the Matrix program, a person can be charged with "sleeping in a park at night for lodging." Thus far, 62,000 citations have been issued, with a fine of $79 for each citation. Dean (p. 3) compares the Matrix program to scenarios from World War II:

> Right now, the government of San Francisco is doing things that you think only fascist countries are doing.
>
> Right now, someone who is homeless in San Francisco is being stripped of his/her meager belongings.
>
> Right now, a human being in San Francisco is being caged like a criminal because she/he is homeless.
>
> Right now, Keith McHenry is awaiting trial, which begins on Halloween day, because he chooses to feed the homeless in San Francisco. [McHenry was cited for serving food to the homeless at the United Nations Plaza under auspices of the Food Not Bombs program.]
>
> Right now, there is someone locked in a psych ward in San Francisco because he/she has been "diagnosed as homeless."
>
> Right now, a child in San Francisco is selling his/her body for a meal or shelter.
>
> Right now, in San Francisco, the Matrix program is in effect.
>
> Right now, San Francisco is getting cold.

The victim-blaming practice of attributing homelessness to personal deficits is not supported by research that corrects the methodological flaws of earlier prevalence studies (Link, et al., 1994). This study also suggests that the problem is of greater magnitude than has commonly been assumed. The crisis of homelessness is due primarily to the severe cuts in federal funds to build or rehabilitate low-income housing and to the over-priced real estate market that is generally free of obligation to include low- and moderate-income housing in their speculative ventures. Haphazard policies and bureaucratic ineptness are also responsible. As Jonathan Kozol (1988) relates from his months with the homeless in one of New York's welfare hotels, the city spends $1,900 per month for a family of four, thus supporting enormous profits for a modernized poorhouse. But as Holly, one of Kozol's informants said:

> All this time I had been looking for apartments I was lots of places that I didn't have the money for. . . . $270 a month was my budget limit for rent. . . . I used

to tell the New York City officials, "All the money you will pay for me to stay in a hotel? You can't give me half that money once to pay the rent and rent deposit? I could get me an apartment. You won't ever see me any more."

These problems are all exacerbated in the case of the homeless mentally ill, who are victims of a failed deinstitutionalization program and inadequate community planning (Hoff, 1993; Hoff, et al., 1992; Johnson, 1990).

What do we do for people who have no place to sleep or who are at risk of dying from exposure to the elements in spite of affluence all around them in the richest country in the world? People often react to the homeless who appear on a doorstep or beg for a quarter with embarrassment and discomfort. But regardless of how charitably people respond to individual appeals for help, the crisis of homelessness in a humane, democratic society entails more than goodwill or charity. Although there is still a tendency to blame the victim (Ryan, 1971), people do not choose to be poor or homeless. As Kip Tiernan (1987) of the Elderly Homeless Coalition in Boston says, "I'm tired of conservatives saying piously, 'Ah yes, the poor—they're always with us.' I'm tired of liberals who wave a cot or a sandwich at me when I shout for justice, not charity." As emphasized throughout this book, a crisis of social origin demands a social response. Thus, the interrelated social, cultural, and economic factors—along with discrimination based on race, sex, and age—that precipitate crises of homelessness must be addressed in a comprehensive proactive manner (Rapp & Chamberlain, 1985). We should support individual and communal efforts like those of Moshe Dean and others who write for and sell *SPARE Change*, New England's journal of the streets. Such efforts, however, will never be sufficient to avoid further crises of homelessness without a change in public policies affecting housing (see Figure 11.1, Box 3).

Summary

To be happy, we need some meaningful work to support ourselves and a secure place to live. Many people are threatened with the loss of these basic necessities. Opportunities to assist people in crisis because of occupational or housing loss crosses the social service and health care landscape. Helping people at these initial crisis points can make an enormous difference in the final outcomes of these transition states. Removing the socioeconomic roots of crises like unemployment and homelessness is urgent public business.

References

Armer, J. M. (1993). Elderly relocation to a congregate setting: Factors influencing adjustment. *Issues in Mental Health Nursing, 14*(2), 157–172.

Aubry, J. (1994, March 5). Exiled to a forsaken place. *The Ottawa Citizen*, pp. 1, B1–6.

Bellah, R. (1986). *Habits of the heart: Individualism and commitment in American life*. New York: HarperCollins.

Butterfield, B. D. (1993, December 26). Seeking more in cities with less. *Boston Sunday Globe*, pp. 1, 46–47.

Canellos, P. A. (1994, February 6). The outer class: Angry and alone, America's poorest drift further away. *Boston Sunday Globe*, pp. 1, 24–25.

Caplan, G. (1964). *Principles of preventive psychiatry*. New York: Basic Books.

Collins, C., Tiedje, L. B., & Stommel, M. (1992). Promoting positive well-being in employed mothers: A pilot study. *Health Care for Women International, 13*(1), 77–85.

Davidhizar, R., & Frank, B. (1992). Understanding the physical and psychosocial stressors of the child who is homeless. *Pediatric Nursing, 18*(6), 559–562.

Dean, M. (1994). The beginnings of genocide, or San Francisco's homeless living under the yoke of the Matrix Program. *Spare Change, 3*(7), 3.

Desmond, A. M. (1994). Adolescent pregnancy in the United States: Not a minority issue. *Health Care for Women International, 15*(4), 325–332.

Dobash, R. P., & Dobash, R. E. (1979). *Violence against wives: A case against the patriarchy*. New York: Free Press.

Dvorchak, R. (1992), October 5. Social health 'index' puts U.S. at 21-year low. *Boston Globe*, p. 3.

Etheridge, C. F. (1978). Equality in the family: Comparative analysis and theoretical models. *International Journal of Women's Studies, 1* 50–62.

Facione, N. C. (1994). Role overload and health: The married mother in the waged labor force. *Health Care for Women International, 15*(2), 157–167.

Foner, N. (1994). *The caregiving dilemma: Work in an American nursing home*. Berkeley: University of California Press.

Gans, H. J. (1962). *The urban villagers*. New York: Free Press.

Greenspan, M. (1983). *A new approach to women and therapy*. New York: McGraw-Hill.

Gullen, J. (1992). Report on the first international study conference on genital mutilation of girls in Europe. Ottawa: Family Service Centre.

Hansell, N. (1976). *The person in distress*. New York: Human Sciences Press.

Hoff, L. A. (1990). *Battered women as survivors*. London: Routledge.

Hoff, L. A. (1993). Review essay: Health policy and the plight of the mentally ill. *Psychiatry, 56*(4), 400–419.

Hoff, L. A., & Miller, N. (1987). *Programs for people in crisis: A guide for educators, administrators, and clinical trainers*. Boston: Northeastern University Custom Book Program.

Hoff, M. D., Briar, K. H., Knighton, K., & Van Ry, A. (1992). To survive and to thrive: Integrating services for the homeless mentally ill. *Journal of Sociology and Social Welfare, 29*(4), 235–252.

Illich, I. (1976). *Limits to medicine*. Middlesex, England: Penguin.

Jencks, C. (1994). *The homeless*. Cambridge, Mass.: Harvard University Press.

Johnson, A. B. (1990). *Out of bedlam: The truth about deinstitutionalization*. New York: Basic Books.

Kanter, R. M. (1977). *Men and women of the corporation*. New York: Basic Books.

Kavanagh, K. H. (1988). The cost of caring: Nursing on a psychiatric intensive care unit. *Human Organization, 47*(3), 242–251.

Kessler, R. C., & McLeod, J. D. (1984). Sex differences in vulnerability to life events. *American Sociological Review, 49*, 620–631.

Kozol, J. (1988), *Rachel and her children: Homeless families in America*. New York: Crown.

Link, B. G., Susser, E., Stueve, A., Phelan, J., Moore, R. E., & Struening, E. (1994). Lifetime and five-year prevalence of homelessness in the United States. *American Journal of Public Health, 84*(12), 1907–1912.

Lipson, J. G. (1994). Changing role of Afghan refugee women in the United States. *Health Care for Women International,* 15(3), 171–180.

Lipson, J., & Miller, S. (1994). Changing roles of Afghan refugee women in the United States. *Health Care for Women International, 15*(3), 171–180.

McKinlay, J. B. (1990). The case for refocusing upstream: The political economy of illness. In P. Conrad & R. Kern (Eds.), *The sociology of health and illness* (3rd ed., pp. 502–516). New York: St. Martin's Press.

Medoff, P., & Sklar, H. (1994). *Streets of hope: The fall and rise of an urban neighborhood.* Boston: South End Press.

Mollison, A. (1993, June 27). Unpaid work by homemakers under scrutiny. *St. Paul Pioneer Press,* p. 15A.

Morrison, A. M., White, R. P., & Van Velsor, E. (1987). Executive women: Substance plus style. *Psychology Today, 21*(8), 18–27.

Olson, K. R., & Schellenberg, R. P. (1986). Farm stressors. *American Journal of Community Psychology, 14*(5), 555–569.

Pearce, D., & McAdoo, H. (1982). *Women and children: Alone and in poverty.* Washington, D.C.: National Advisory Council on Economic Opportunity.

Phelan, J., Schwartz, J. E., Bromet, E. J., Dew, M. A., Parkinson, D. K., Schulberg, H. C., Duran, L. O., Blane, H., & Curtis, E. C. (1991). Work stress, family stress, and depression in professional and managerial employees. *Psychological Medicine, 21*(4), 999–1012.

Phillips, S. P., & Schneider, M. S. (1993). Sexual harassment of female doctors by patients. *New England Journal of Medicine, 329*(26), 1936–1939.

Rachlis, M., & Kushner, C. (1994). *Strong medicine: How to save Canada's health care system.* Toronto: HarperCollins.

Rapp, C. A., & Chamberlain, R. (1985). Case management for chronically mentally ill. *Social Work, 30*(5), 417–422.

Reverby, S. (1987). *Order to care.* Cambridge: Cambridge University Press.

Rubenstein, C. (1982). Real men don't earn less than their wives. *Psychology Today, 16,* 36–41.

Ryan, W. (1971). *Blaming the victim.* New York: Vintage Books.

Schaef, A., & Fassel, D. (1988). Hooked on work. *New Age Journal,* January-February, 42–48, 57–63.

Scheper-Hughes, N., & Lovell, A. M. (1986). Breaking the circuit of social control: Lessons in public psychiatry from Italy and Franco Basaglia. *Social Science and Medicine, 23*(2), 159–178.

Schoonover, P. (1987). Personal communication.

Schor, J. B. (1993). *The overworked American: The unexpected decline of leisure.* New York: Basic Books.

Seager, J., & Olson, A. (1986). *Women in the world: An international atlas.* New York: Simon & Schuster.

Sidel, R. (1986). *Women and children last: The plight of poor women in affluent America.* New York: Penguin.

Singular, S. (1983). Moving on. *Psychology Today, 17,* 40–47.

Sommers, T., & Shields, L. (1987). *Women take care.* Gainesville, Fla.: Triad.

Sparks, A. (1990). *The mind of south Africa: The story of the rise and fall of apartheid.* London: Mandarin.

Tiernan, K. (1987, November 1). They're elderly and homeless and falling through the cracks. *Boston Sunday Globe,* p. A29.

Verbrugge, L. M. (1982). Work satisfaction and physical health. *Journal of Community Health, 7*(4), 262–283.

The Violence Against Women Survey. (1993, November 19). *The Daily.* Ottawa: Statistics Canada.

Waring, M. (1990). *If women counted: A new feminist economics.* New York: HarperSanFrancisco.

Weitzman, B. C., Knickman, J. R., & Shinn, M. (1992). Predictors of shelter use among low-income families: Psychiatric history, substance abuse, and victimization. *American Journal of Public Health, 82*(11), 1547–1550.

World Federation of Public Health Associations. (1986). *Women and health: Information for action issue paper.* Washington, D.C.: American Public Health Association.

CHAPTER THIRTEEN

STRESS AND CHANGE DURING LIFE PASSAGES

How are the terms *transition or passage* and *status* and *role change* related? What do they mean for people in crisis? *Transition* refers to passage or change from one place or stage of development to another. *Status* designates the place of individuals and groups with respect to their prestige, rights, obligations, power and authority within a society. People are evaluated socially by their contribution to the common good and by other criteria such as birth, marital alliance, sex, race, age, sexual identity, wealth, and power. One's status is related to but different from one's *role*: status refers to *who* a person is, while role refers to *what* a person is expected to *do* within a given sociocultural milieu (Zelditch, 1968, p. 251).

What do these social concepts have to do with people in crisis in the clinical sense? It is, after all, a normal part of human life to grow and develop through childhood, adolescence, middle age, old age, to death. It is also common to marry, give birth, and lose one's spouse. Anthropologists and psychoanalysts for years have referred to these transition states as "life crises" (Erikson, 1963; Freud, 1950; Giovannini, 1983; Kimball, 1960). There is a difference, however, in the anthropological concept of life crisis and its common usage by crisis intervention clinicians, even though, as Golan (1981, p. 7) states, there is something in common between the two conceptions of high-stress situations. In anthropology, "life crisis" refers to a highly significant, expectable event or phase in the life cycle that marks one's passage to a new social status, with accompanying changes in rights and duties. Traditionally, such status changes are accompanied by rituals (such as puberty and marriage rites) designed to assist the individual in fulfilling new role expectations and to buffer the stress associated with these critical—though normal—life events. In traditional societies, families and the entire community, led by "ritual experts," are intensely involved in the life passages of individual community members. This *anthropological* concept of life crisis corresponds roughly to the "anticipated" crises discussed in the clinical literature on crisis (see "The Origins of Crisis" in Chapter Two). "Crisis" in its *clinical* meaning flows from the tradition of Caplan (1964) and others, who emphasize the sudden onset and brief duration of acute emotional upsets in response to identifiable traumatic events. In this sense, adolescence, marriage, giving birth, and entering middle age are not crises except in extraordinary circumstances, such as when the bridegroom fails to show up, or the expected infant is stillborn—unanticipated traumatic events that accompany the transition. Transition states are "critical" life phases, not necessarily traumatic, but with the *potential* for activating an "acute emotional upset" in the clinical sense. They are turning points, social and psychological processes involving the challenge of successfully completing social, developmental, and instrumental tasks, for example:

• Changing social role, such as single to married
• Changing image of self, such as young to middle aged, healthy to sick
• Gathering material resources to support a new family member

As "turning points" in the developmental process, these "life crises" fit the classic definition of crisis as a period of both danger and opportunity. They also highlight the importance of social, cultural, and material supplies (Caplan, 1964) necessary for individuals to avoid acute emotional upset. Another connection between the anthropological and clinical definitions of crisis is the fact that individuals in acute emotional upset do not exist in a social vacuum; they are members of cultural communities. People in crisis are therefore influenced by social expectations of how to behave and by values guiding their interpretation of expected and unexpected life events—factors that figure strongly in the way one resolves a particular emotional crisis.

Thus, if it is unclear *who* a person is, *what* he or she is expected to do, or *how* the person fits into familiar social arrangements based on cultural values, status or role ambiguity is activated. Status and role ambiguity can create so much stress that a person with conflicting or changed roles may withdraw from social interaction or may try to change the social structure to redefine the anxiety-provoking statuses (Douglas, 1966; Weiss, 1976; Zelditch, 1968). For example:

• If pregnant teenage girls sense that they are expected to drop out of high school, they are more likely to be poorly educated, unemployed, dependent on welfare, and to marry early, which enhances their potential for future crises.
• If widowed people sense that they are a threat to social groups of married people, they may feel cut off from social support and thereby increase their risk of emotional crisis around traumatic events.
• If children of parents feuding around divorce are not allowed to see their

grandparents, they may ask, Who is my family? The deprived grandparent may ask, What have I done wrong?

Rites of Passage: Traditional and Contemporary

An important means of reducing the stress and minimizing the chaos associated with such role ambiguity is the constructive use of ritual. One of the most dramatic differences between traditional and urban or industrialized societies is the relative importance of ritual and the separation between the sacred and profane. With an increase in industrialization comes a corresponding increase in secularization and decrease in sacred ceremonialism. In his classic work, *Rites of Passage,* van Gennep (1960, p. 11) distinguished three phases in the ceremonies associated with an individual's "life crises": rites of separation (prominent in funeral ceremonies), transition rites (important in initiation and pregnancy); and rites of incorporation (prominent in marriage). A complete schema of rites of passage theoretically includes all three phases. For example, a widow is *separated* from her husband by death; she occupies a *liminal* (transitional) status for a time, and finally is *reincorporated* into a new marriage relationship (Goody, 1962).

These rites protect the individual during the hazardous process of life passages, times considered potentially dangerous to the person if not supported by the community. Ritual thus makes public what is private and makes social what is personal, and gives the individual new knowledge and strength (LaFontaine, 1977; Turner, 1967, p. 50). For example:

- A person who loses a loved one needs a public occasion to mourn.
- A couple who are intimate and cohabiting desire social approval (often through marriage).
- A dying person who is anointed has new knowledge of the imminence of death and greater strength to accept death.
- A divorced person needs community support following a failed marriage—in short, a ritual for public recognition and acceptance of a new role.

Rites of passage are not developed to the same extent by all societies (Fried & Fried, 1980). Until recently, it was generally assumed that rites of passage are relatively unimportant in modern societies: public and private spheres of activity and various social roles (such as worker, parent, or political leader) are more clearly separated than in traditional societies and hence in less need of ritual specification. However, there is no evidence that people in a secular urban world have less need for ritualized expression during transition states (Kimball, 1960, pp. xvi–xvii). The modern discarding of ritual can be understood in part as a move toward greater freedom of the individual. Ritual can be a powerful mechanism for maintaining the status quo in traditional and contemporary societies (Durkheim, 1915);

less ritual implies more personal freedom. Thus, while some rituals protect the individual during stressful transitions, they have a social purpose as well. For example, the traditional Samburu of Kenya, a polygynous gerontocracy [society rule by elders] kept young men in a marginal position relative to the total society and forbade them to marry until around age thirty, an institution known as "moranhood." This ritual preserved the concentration of power and wives among the older men (Hoff, 1978; Spencer, 1965, 1973). The following example illustrates a contemporary negative ritual.

CASE EXAMPLE: AMERICAN COLLEGE CAMPUS

Thirty miles from Reno, under a star-filled desert sky, a lone pick-up truck grinds to a halt alongside the Pyramid Lake Highway. Three men slide out of the cab and stagger to the back of the truck. All wear black felt hats adorned with a yellow patch that depicts the setting sun. The three grin at the sight that greets them: five youths, their clothing flecked with vomit, are sprawled across the truck bed like bags of cement.

The five are ordered to get up, and four struggle to comply by easing their way down from the tailgate to the road. One remains on the truck bed, a dark-haired giant wearing a thick Fu Manchu mustache. The three youths with hats are amused and clamber aboard to wake him. They laugh drunkenly as they shake him. Suddenly, one youth tears open the limp young man's coat and

puts an ear to his chest. All laughter ceases. The only sound is the whistling wind that bends back the sagebrush as it passes.

The dead youth was a twenty-three-year-old University of Nevada football player. His death concluded a three-day drinking spree required for admission into a suspended, but still active, campus club called the Sundowners. . . . A second Sundowner pledge was hospitalized the same night. His blood alcohol count registered .456 (a person is legally drunk with a .10 reading).

A grand jury investigating the case determined that the five pledges had been pummeled, ridiculed, cursed, and intimidated by approximately ten of the thirty Sundowner members . . . with the apparent encouragement of the membership (Nuwer, 1978).

The practice of hazing has come under increasing scrutiny over the past decade. Several states have passed antihazing legislation. In Massachusetts, for example, the law forbids any dangerous initiation activities, requires pledges to be informed of the law, and specifies punishment of violators or those who fail to report hazing. These laws were written on the premise similar to child abuse dynamics: if one is abused, one learns to abuse others. It appears that this negative rite of passage has moved from fraternity houses to the football field in some communities, where demonstrating teamwork requires urinating on a teammate (Pierce, 1992, p. 86). And increasingly on U.S. college campuses, binge drinking is indulged in by thousands of young people. In a contemporary twist on traditional rites of passage, these young people (not unlike their Samburu brothers or Somali sisters) feel pressured to drink in order to "belong" in a new environment without the usual supports of family and neighborhood. Wherever hazing occurs, students have poorer grades, reduced career motivation, and increased drop-out rates—all challenges for school and parents' groups to create positive rituals for students under stress who have a powerful need to belong.

Another ritual under scrutiny is female genital mutilation. Sometimes referred to as female circumcision, unlike male circumcision, the operation damages or destroys a woman's normal sexual response and causes life-threatening physical complications. The World Health Organization has condemned the practice as a human rights violation (Hosken, 1981) affecting an estimated 90 to 100 million women and girls in African, Far Eastern and Middle Eastern countries. Novelist Alice Walker's (1992) fictionalized account, *Possessing the Secret of Joy,* has made the practice and its context of gender-based oppression widely visible in the Western world. Canada has declared the practice illegal, while Somali immigrant physicians and others in North America advocate for elimination of the practice and the education of health professionals in how to deal sensitively with women presenting their daughters for the ritual in Western medical settings (Gullen, 1992). However, as with teen pregnancy and similar issues, this practice is intricately tied to socioeconomic and educational equity for women worldwide (Ngugi, 1965).

CASE EXAMPLE: MARRIAGE AMONG THE SAMBURU

The social value imbuing everything in Samburu society is *nkanyit*. This keystone of Samburu morality includes notions of respect, honor, shame, duty, politeness, avoidance, and decency, with the overriding emphasis on respect. A woman is taught to respect, fear, and avoid the elders from an early age. Her training induces her to accept the difficulties of marriage to an elder two to three times older than herself, a situation that makes the marital strains more understandable. As in most societies, girls and women are valued less than boys and men; all girls are brought up with the idea of being good wives, an investment for their kin and husbands.

After marriage, a woman rarely goes home again, as this would endanger the tenuous stability of the marriage even more. Samburu women learn very early their inevitable lot of subordination and that the reputation of the clan hinges on their good behavior, not unlike the sexual double standard elsewhere. These notions are reinforced through the marriage ritual. Spencer characterizes the marriage ritual as a form of brainwashing and marriage for the average woman as the single crisis of her life (Hoff, 1978; Spencer, 1976, 1973).

CASE EXAMPLE: MARRIAGE FOR CONTEMPORARY NORTH AMERICAN WOMEN

Unlike their Samburu sisters, marriage and especially the ritual of the wedding day itself are high points in the lives of many contemporary women. Like their Samburu sisters,

however, many girls and women today still view themselves as failures if they cannot marry and retain a husband. Caught up in the emotional high of the wedding ritual

Case Example, cont.

with dreams of living happily ever after, the average bride is unconscious of the social significance of the ritual of being "given away" by her father and relinquishing her own name to assume that of her husband (Chapman & Gates, 1977). Many women willingly interrupt or delay careers to support their families through unpaid and devalued household work. Many are happy and secure in their role and testify that their dreams have come true. Millions, however, are battered, as the marriage license seems to have been transformed for some into a "hitting license" (Straus, Gelles, & Steinmetz, 1980); they feel trapped and become convenient

objects of violence (Browne, 1987; Dobash & Dobash, 1979; Hoff, 1990). Or they become "displaced homemakers" (Jacobs, 1979; Lopata, 1973). Many women are left behind for younger women, especially during middle age, when women often are considered "over the hill," while men become more "distinguished." Often this occurs after women have sacrificed education and career opportunities in order to fulfill the social expectation of building a stable home. Among women heading households alone, 55 percent are poor (Newberger, Melnicoe, & Newberger, 1986, p. 708).

These examples suggest that ritual serves to maintain society or various subgroups in a state of traditional equilibrium with each person behaving according to accepted roles. As discussed in earlier chapters, however, maintaining traditional social roles, often reinforced through the negative use of ritual, can exact a considerable price from certain individuals, for example, more heart disease and suicides for men, social isolation or death for adolescents by suicide or manslaughter, and battering or poverty for women. The case examples also illustrate a continuum between traditional and contemporary rites of passage and suggest that people in all times and places need ritual. But what kinds of rituals are needed, and under what circumstances should they take place? How can ritual be helpful for the individual in transition as well as for society?

Ritual holds a paradoxical place in a secularized society. On the one hand, it is viewed as a sign of an earlier stage of social evolution (Moore, 1992). On the other hand, certain rituals are retained without critical examination of their expression in contemporary life. In modern life, three approaches to ritual are observed: (1) ritual is often denied any relevance; (2) some of its most oppressive and destructive aspects for individuals remain from ancient tradition or are recycled to include the abuse of alcohol, guns, or cars, and medical technology to prolong life; (3) when ritual is observed, it is highly individualized, as in the rite of psychotherapy, in which the fifty-minute session and other practices are observed. Such rituals are complemented by medicalization and its focus on individuals rather than groups in modern urban societies.

These interpretations of ritual, however, are in the process of change. Meaningless and destructive rituals are being dropped entirely or are being questioned. For example, many women today retain their last names after marriage, and *both* parents of the bride *and* groom (rather than only the father of the bride) participate in the marriage ceremony. Similarly, cultural awareness is replacing the condemnation of "savage" customs of "primitive" peoples (Fanon, 1978; Paul, 1978). Barbaric rituals, oppression, and violence are no longer seen as the province of any one society, traditional or modern.

Our task as crisis workers is to consider the place of ritual during critical turning points of life, particularly as it relates to crisis prevention. Whether or not critical life passages also become occasions of emotional crisis will depend on

1. What the individual does to prepare for anticipated transitions
2. The nature and extent of social support available to the individual during turning points
3. The occurrence of unanticipated hazardous events (such as fire, accident, illness, or loss of job) during critical phases of life
4. Our creativity as crisis workers in helping individuals and families develop positive contemporary rites of passage where there are few or none

Traditional and contemporary rites of passage are compared and the continuity between them illustrated in Table 13.1. The successful passage of individuals through critical stages in the developmental process depends on a combination of personal and social factors (Panchuck, 1994). Transition states highlight the dynamic relationship between the individual, family, and society (see "Privacy, Intimacy, Community" in Chapter Five). For example, adolescents who choose marriage or parenthood even though they are not ready for those responsibilities, may become liabilities to society and may face more complex problems during later stages of development. On the other hand, the reason they are personally unfit might be traced to inadequate support from adults and to the complex social, economic, and cultural factors that affect adolescents and their families (Leach, 1994; Newberger, Melnicoe, & Newberger, 1986).

The role of individuals and families during transition states demands the successful completion of several tasks. For instance, among the traditional LoDagaa in Ghana (Goody, 1962), widows are metaphorically buried by being dressed in premarital "fibres" to signify that they are again adolescents without husbands. They are also fed, as a symbolic last supper of husband and wife, and as a test of the widow's possible complicity in her husband's death. The widow's acceptance of food is equivalent to an oath to the ancestors of her innocence. The widow cooks porridge and flicks some on her husband's shrine to show that she has not committed adultery. These rituals are dramatic in that they involve not only the individual and the family but the entire community.

In contrast, in contemporary society there is the stereotype of the widow who sets the table every night for her dead husband. A possible reason for this behavior may be that the widow had no social, public occasion to cook her "last supper." She lacks the necessary community support to separate from her previous

TABLE 13.1. RITES OF PASSAGE IN COMPARATIVE PERSPECTIVE.

Life Passage	Traditional Rites*	Contemporary North American Rites	
		Unexamined or Questionable	Newly Emerging or Suggested
Birth	Attended by family and/or midwife; birth occurs in natural squatting position Death risk is high if there are complications	Medicalized birth: pubic shaving, ultrasound, drugs, episiotomy or forceps, horizontal position Absence of family and friends unless specially arranged Death risk in the U.S. is the highest among 15 developed countries	Natural childbirth aided by husband's or friends' coaching in home or birthing center, attended by midwife with back-up medical care for complications Death risk is low when attended by properly trained midwife and medical backup is available for special cases
Adolescence	Puberty rites	Hazing and binge drinking on college campuses Religious rites of confirmation and Bar and Bat Mitzvah† Obtaining driver's licenses†	Supervised college initiation Support and education groups in high schools, churches, and colleges, such as those concerning menstruation, sexuality, driving responsibly without drinking, and parenthood Relating traditional religious rites to modern life
Intimate relationships: beginnings and endings	Betrothal and marriage rites; required remarriage of widow; or remarriage may be forbidden	Bridal showers; stag parties† Traditional marriage rites	Egalitarian marriage ceremony and contract Consciousness-raising groups for men and women regarding traditional versus egalitarian male and female roles Divorce ceremonies Support groups for the divorced or for parents without partners

*These rites vary widely among societies. No attempt is made to summarize them here; they are cited to illustrate continuity with modern practice. For an introduction to traditional transition rituals and further references, see Fried and Fried (1980).
†These rites are not always used to their greatest positive potential.

role, abandon her private illusion that her husband is still alive, and proceed to a new role without her husband. This example illustrates the tremendous importance of moving beyond the individual and the family to such social creations as widow-to-widow clubs—a contemporary substitute for the elaborate death rituals of traditional societies.

Life Passage	Traditional Rites*	Contemporary North American Rites	
		Unexamined or Questionable	Newly Emerging or Suggested
Middle Age	Not generally ritualized; general increase in social value and respect by community; post-menopausal women may be regarded as asexual	Labeling of menopause as "illness"; individual psychotherapy and drugs for depression; estrogen replacement therapy for women Men past youth become more "distinguished"; women are often devalued further	Education and peer support groups for menopausal women Support groups for couples to redefine marriage relationship to avoid "empty nest" and other midlife crises
Old Age	Not generally ritualized; general increase in social value and respect by family and community Infirm elderly are cared for by family	Forced retirement Institutional placement for care	Economic and social policies to support care of elderly at home; respite services for caretakers Senior citizen programs such as part-time or shared jobs
Death	Usually elaborate, extended rituals involving family and entire community	80 percent die in institutions with restricted family involvement Mortician has become the main "ritual expert" Children often barred from death and burial rituals Prescription of tranquilizers to survivors after death of a loved one	Social support to aid in grief work Hospice care for the dying; support for family to care for dying member at home Support groups for cancer patients Inclusion of children in death and burial rituals Enhancement of funeral director's role to assist with grief work Widow-to-widow and other self-help groups for survivors

Golan (1981, pp. 21–22) outlines the specific tasks to be accomplished by individuals and families during transition states. Her division of "material-arrangemental" tasks (such as exploring resources and choices in the new role) and psychosocial or affective tasks (such as dealing with feelings of loss and longing for the past) corresponds to the emotional, cognitive, and behavioral steps in effective crisis coping discussed in Chapter Four. However, the effectiveness of these individual and family coping strategies greatly depends on the social and cultural setting. If a society is poor in constructive ritual, if familiar, secure routines and supports in an old role are not replaced, and if there is little awareness of the need for social support, even the strongest individuals may be unnecessarily scarred during passage through life's developmental stages. The challenge of moving on to a new stage of development or role becomes a threat: "Will I succeed or fail?" "What will people think if I fail?" "No . . . I don't think I can face having this baby—not without the help of its father." "Life just isn't worth living if I can't keep on working. . . . I'm worth more dead than alive."

Keeping in mind the traditional and contemporary rites of passage and their relationship to stress and crisis in modern society, we can discuss the hazards and opportunities of these normal passages from birth to death. During these passages, crisis counselors and health and mental health professionals can be thought of as contemporary "ritual experts" (see Crisis Paradigm, Box 3, lower circle).

Birth and Parenthood

Parenthood places continuous demands on a person from the time of conception until at least the child's eighteenth birthday. Parents must adjust to include an additional member in their family group. Such adjustment is especially difficult for first-time parents, even when they assume the role of parenthood willingly and regard their children as a welcome burden. The unique pleasure and challenge of bearing and nurturing a child through childhood into adult life usually outweighs the ordinary problems of parenthood.

Some parents fall into their role unwillingly or use it to escape less tolerable roles. Consider, for example, the adolescent who seeks relief from a disturbed family home and uses pregnancy as an avenue of escape, or the woman who may have more children than she can properly care for emotionally and physically. Some women have been socialized to view themselves as having no other significant role than that of mother and wife. Others do not limit their pregnancies because of religious beliefs forbidding artificial contraception. Still others lack the knowledge and means to limit their pregnancies. Unwanted children and their parents are more crisis prone than others. Emotional, social, and material poverty are important contributors to their crisis vulnerability.

All parents, whether or not their children were wanted, are under stress and strain in their parental role. Parenthood requires a constant giving of self. Except for the joy of self-fulfillment and watching a child grow and develop, the parent-child relationship is essentially nonreciprocal. Infants, toddlers, and young children need continuous care and supervision. In their natural state of dependency, they give only the needy love of a child who says, in effect, I am helpless without you, take care of me, protect me.

Some children, in fact, are not only dependent and needy but for various reasons are a source of grief to their parents. Their difficult behaviors, for example, trouble at school or drug abuse, often signal trouble in the parents' marriage or in the entire family system. Sometimes parents try to deal with these troubles by themselves, struggling for a long time with whatever resources they have. Often they are ashamed to acknowledge that there is a problem with the child. They view any problem as a reflection of their own failure. Still other parents may not have access to child and family resources for help, either because the resources do not exist or because they cannot afford them.

Chronic problems of parenthood often persist until a crisis occurs and finally forces parents to seek outside help. Common examples of ongoing problems are a child's getting into trouble with the law, running away from home, becoming pregnant during adolescence, truancy, being expelled from school, or making a suicide attempt.

Parents usually seem surprised when these problems occur, but evaluation of the whole family often reveals signs of trouble that were formerly unobserved or ignored. Teachers, recreation directors, pastors, truant officers, and guidance counselors who are sensitive to the needs of children and adolescents can help prevent some of these crises. They should urge parents to participate in a family counseling program *early*, at the first sign of a problem. It is important for counselors and parents to keep in mind that even if preventive programs are lacking, it is never too late to act. An acute crisis situation provides, once again, the opportunity for parents and child to move in the direction of growth and development and for the parents to fulfill their needs for generativity.

Common Crisis Points for Parents

Common points of crisis for parents include the following:

Death of a Child. Crisis often occurs after the death of a child not only because of the parents' acute loss but because the death requires parents to reorder their expectations about the normal progression of life to death—that parents usually precede their children in death. Thus, the loss of a child is like no other death experience. Some claim it is felt more acutely than loss of a spouse. It is also keenly painful to accept the fact that death has cut off the child's passage through life. Besides being a profound loss, death of a child threatens the parents' perception of parenthood and the normal life cycle (Covington & Theut, 1993; Knapp, 1987; Walsh & McGoldrick, 1991).

The sudden death of infants is known as crib death. The exact cause of these deaths is still unknown, hence the medical designation: sudden infant death syndrome (SIDS). With no warning signs, parents or a baby-sitter will find the infant dead in its crib. They bring the infant to the hospital emergency department in a desperate, futile hope of reviving it. The parents or caregiver have fears and guilt that they may somehow have caused the death. The fact that emergency service staff may seem suspicious or appear to blame the parents complicates this crisis.

Indeed, the emergency staff must rule out the possibility of child battering, which they cannot do without examination.

Whether or not the child was battered, emergency personnel should withhold judgment. Parents in either case are in crisis and need understanding and support. Those in crisis over sudden infant deaths should be offered the opportunity to express their grief in private and with the support of a nurse. Hospital chaplains can often assist during this time and should be called in accordance with the parents' wishes. Parents should also be given information about self-help groups of other parents whose infants died suddenly in their cribs.

The most widely known and used group for parents whose infants have died is the Sudden Infant Death Syndrome Foundation. This is a national organization with chapters in all states and major cities. The program includes support from other parents, counseling from maternal-child nurse specialists, education through films, and a speakers bureau with medical and lay experts on the topic.[1]

The following case example illustrates the crisis of SIDS for parents and shows how negative outcomes of this crisis might have been avoided through crisis intervention by the pediatrician and others.

CASE EXAMPLE: LORRAINE

I can't begin to tell you what my life was like before Doris at our counseling center helped me. Six months ago, my second child died from crib death. She was two months old. When Deborah stopped breathing at home, I called the rescue squad. They resuscitated her and took her to the hospital. Deborah was kept in the intensive care unit for two months. Finally, the hospital and doctor insisted that we take her home. When we did, she died the very same day. I was completely grief stricken, especially since I am forty-one years old and had waited so long to have a second child. Our other child, David, is seven. I just couldn't accept the fact that Deborah was dead. My husband and the doctors kept telling me to face reality, but I kept insisting on an answer from the pediatrician as to why Deborah had died. I began having chest pains and problems breathing.

Several times my husband called the ambulance and had me taken to the hospital for elaborate heart tests. My doctor told me there was nothing physically wrong with me.

I went home and things got worse. My husband became impatient and annoyed. I worried day and night about doing something wrong with David and eventually causing his death. The school principal finally called me to say that David was having problems at school. I realized I was being overly protective, but I couldn't help myself. The school recommended that we go to a child guidance clinic with David. I resisted and went back instead to my pediatrician and insisted once again on knowing the cause of Deborah's death. The pediatrician was apparently tired of my demands and recommended that I see a psychiatrist. I felt he was probably right but also felt we couldn't af-

[1]Further information about SIDS is available from the National SIDS Foundation, Inc., 10500 Little Patuxent Parkway, Suite 420, Columbia, MD 21044; telephone (800) 221-SIDS.

Case Example, cont.

ford a psychiatrist; we had spent so much money on medical and hospital bills during the past year. I became so depressed that suicide began to seem like my only way out. One night after an attack of chest pain and a crying spell, I was so desperate that I called the suicide prevention center. The counselor referred me to the local counseling center where I saw Doris.

With Doris' help, I discovered that I was suffering from a delayed grief reaction. Through several counseling sessions, I was

able to truly mourn the loss of my child, which I had not really done through all those months of trying to be brave as my doctor and husband wanted me to be. Doris and I included my husband in some of the sessions. On her recommendation, I finally joined a group of other parents whose infants had died of crib death. I began to understand my fear of causing David's probable death and could finally let go of my overprotectiveness of him.

While crib death has special features, the death of other children is also traumatic and requires similar support and opportunities for grief work. In their study of mothers' and fathers' grief resolution, Kachoyeanos and Selder (1993) identified three processes: "presencing" the child through memory, reactivating the trauma of loss, and identifying missed options.

The Compassionate Friends is a self-help group offering friendship and understanding to bereaved parents after the death of a child whether by illness, murder, accident, or suicide. This international organization was founded by a pastor in England and now has over 200 chapters around the United States.

Birth of a Stillborn Child.   The response of a mother at this crisis point is similar to that of mothers giving birth to a handicapped child: anger, loss, guilt, and questioning (see Chapter Eleven). Mothers ask, Why did this have to happen to me? What did I do wrong? What did I do to deserve this? Parents' need for grief work and the critical role of medical and hospital personnel is highlighted in the case of Gerry.

CASE EXAMPLE: GERRY HENDERSON

Gerry Henderson, age twenty-nine, gave birth to a stillborn child. Immediately after delivery, the child was taken out of the delivery room. Gerry never saw the baby; she was asleep from the anesthetic given her. Together with hospital authorities, Gerry's husband Tom, who was numb and frightened, made arrangements to cremate the baby without consulting Gerry. The baby was not given a name. No one from the family at-

tended the burial service. Tom was convinced that this was the best way to spare his wife and family any unnecessary grief.

When Gerry woke up and these facts were announced to her, she was beside herself with shock and grief, but Tom thought it best not to talk about the matter. Gerry was essentially alone with her grief. The nurses had a hard time handling their own grief and so were unable to offer Gerry support.

Case Example, cont.

When Gerry returned home, her cousin invited her for a visit. The cousin had just had a new baby herself. Gerry felt she could not possibly face seeing another woman's live and healthy baby without breaking down. She was urged, however, to make the visit by her mother-in-law and husband who said, "After all, you have to face reality sometime." Gerry refused to go to her cousin's house, though this caused further strain between her and her husband. Gerry's grief and tension reached a point that she began hearing the sound of a baby crying at various times during the day and during her sleepless nights. Since she knew there was no baby, Gerry was afraid she was going crazy. She was barely able to complete simple household chores.

After a week of lonely agony, Gerry walked into a nearby crisis clinic, where she cried inconsolably and poured out her story to a counselor. Tom was asked to come in as well. Through several crisis counseling sessions, it became apparent that Tom was as shocked and grief stricken as his wife, but believed that the only way to handle the infant's death was to "act like a man," not talk about his grief, and try to keep going. The cremation and not naming the baby were Tom's symbolic way of trying to wash away the problem. Gerry's mother-in-law and cousin joined in one of the counseling sessions. They were helped to understand the importance of not forcing Gerry to relate to another child while she was actively grieving the loss of her own.

After Gerry and Tom did their grief work with the counselor's help, Gerry was able to resume a normal life without the child she had anticipated. Eventually, she also could relate to her cousin and her cousin's child without hostility.

The lack of contemporary rites of passage for mourning and dealing with death in hospitals is highlighted by another recent example:

CASE EXAMPLE: INFANT DEATH

A woman gave birth to twins who both died about ten minutes after birth. The parents were not religious and struggled alone with their decision about how to mark the short life and early death of their children. Their grief work was not helped by the fact that people kept referring to the infants as "stillborn." To the mother especially, it was very important for people to realize and acknowledge that she had given birth to live, not dead, infants.

Miscarriage is another common source of misunderstanding. Because many women miscarry without knowing it, some regard all miscarriages as the simple passing of body fluids. An insensitive remark such as, "You can always try again," fails to take into account the mother's bonding with the unborn life or that she may not want to try again. A mother needs to mourn this loss within the framework of the meaning the pregnancy had for her and her family, in spite of others' possible dismissals of the event as relatively unimportant (see Borg & Lasker, 1981).

Similarly, women who have an abortion need to grieve the loss regardless of the moral and religious conflicts that may accompany the event (Teichman, Shenhar, & Segal, 1993). Despite continued public controversy over abortion, for most women faced with an unwanted pregnancy, abortion is rarely a matter of good versus evil, but rather the lesser of two evils in the face of daunting odds.

The Medicalization of Birth. The potential crises surrounding birth and parenthood are colored further by controversy about caesarean births. Traditionally, caesarean birth was selected when there was risk of life for the child or mother (less than 10 percent of births). Rates of caesarean births in some U.S. hospitals are now well over 25 percent. There is perhaps no event arising from birth and parenthood that shows more sharply the difference between traditional societies and Western societies. Birth in North America has come to be identified as an elaborate medical event in which mothers turn over the unique birthing process to physicians, drugs, and surgery. The hazards of medicalizing the natural event of birth are increasingly challenged (Jordan, 1993; Mitford, 1993). The development of birthing centers and the increasing use of midwives is an outgrowth of public debate over birth as a natural event (Boston Women's Health Book Collective, 1992; Inch, 1984). Ideally, the management of birth should be in natural settings with trained midwives with obstetrical consultation available for medical complications during birth to avoid the possible crisis of unnecessary death. Such medical intervention is required in only a small percentage of total births. For most births, medicalization is itself a hazard to be avoided (Jordan, 1993).

Illness of a Child. Similar intervention is indicated for parents whose children are seriously ill, have had a serious accident, or are dying. The modern, relaxed visiting regulations in most hospital wards for children have reduced the crisis possibility at this time for both parents and child. Parents are encouraged to participate in their child's care so that the child feels less isolated and anxious about separation from parents, and the parents feel less threatened about their child's welfare.

Divorce and Single Parenthood

The high rate of divorce in North America has stabilized. The parent who gains custody of the children has the responsibility of rearing them alone, at least until remarriage; the other parent experiences a loss of his or her children. The loss is more acute if the divorced parents live in different cities or different parts of the country. If the loss is accompanied by a sense of relief, guilt usually follows. To assuage guilt, the relieved parent may shower the children inappropriately with material gifts or accuse the other parent of being too strict, inattentive, or uncaring. This crisis point of parenthood can be anticipated whenever the divorce itself is a crisis for either parent. Divorce counseling can help avoid future crisis.

The increase of no-fault divorce laws and attention to the needs of children in divorce settlements will also help prevent crises for parents, children, and grandparents. While divorce affects children of all ages, preschoolers are at greatest risk following divorce. However, as already discussed, it is not so much the divorce itself as it is the manner in which parents conduct themselves, and the poverty (especially for women), that cause the greatest stress on children of divorced parents (Newberger, Melnicoe & Newberger, 1986, p. 689–691; Sidel, 1986). Existing laws do not adequately address the crisis of divorce, as attested by the incidence of child-snatching by the parent denied custody. Another problem faced by many mothers is the awarding of custody to fathers on the basis of their greater financial security, even when these fathers have not been the primary caretakers of the children (Chesler, 1986). While the increasing interest of fathers in parenting their children is applauded, to award them custody primarily on a class basis is a cruel punishment of mothers, who have assumed the major burden of child care throughout history.

This growing practice highlights the need for social change to address women's economic inequality. As Newberger, Melnicoe, and Newberger (1986, p. 709) write, "If working wives and female heads of household were paid the wages of similarly qualified men, about half the families living in poverty would not be poor." This economic disparity is exacerbated by the fact that many fathers abandon parenting altogether after divorce (Sidel, 1986, p. 104) and the majority of divorced women receive no alimony or child support (Newberger, Melnicoe, & Newberger, 1986, p. 693).

Teenage Parenthood. The problems and hazards of single parenthood are increased for a teenager with no job and an unfinished education. The infants of teen mothers are also at increased risk of death, battering, and other problems exacerbated by the poverty of most adolescent parents (Newberger, Melnicoe, & Newberger, 1986, pp. 681–685). Increasingly, teenage mothers do not automatically drop out of high school because of pregnancy, do not marry only because they are pregnant, and do not give up their babies. Hospitals and social service agencies are now establishing collaborative programs with high schools that include an emphasis on health, sex education, parenthood, and career planning. There is also growing recognition that the prevalence, problems, and hazards of teenage pregnancy will not subside until values and opportunities for women in society change. Counselors and others working with young mothers—many of whom are from low-income or troubled homes—repeatedly note that these girls see mothering as their only chance for fulfillment. Life seems to offer them no prospect of happiness through career or an education. Indeed, there is still widespread social, cultural, and economic reinforcement of the notion that a woman's major value to society is her capacity for motherhood, a view bolstered by Freudian psychoanalytic theory (see Chodorow, 1978). A young woman may sense that she has little chance to contribute anything else to society, and says in effect, "But I can produce a baby." Thus, a girl may not plan to conceive, but once pregnant she finally finds meaning in her life; she now will be important and necessary—at least to a helpless infant. Current efforts to reform welfare will probably fail if they do not consider these issues and emphasize the joint responsibility of mothers and fathers for the children they produce (Eyre & Eyre, 1993).

Stepfamilies and Adoption

While divorce and teen pregnancy rates are high in North America, so are rates of remarriage and the increasing presence of blended families. As with any major transition, families in these situations face many challenges and need support through crises in order to reap the potential riches of new family structures while avoiding the pitfalls, especially for children. There is now a growing body of literature on this topic, including the need for communitywide approaches to helping such families (e.g., O'Callaghan, 1993).

Adoption is another parenting issue ripe with opportunity and danger for the child, parents, and entire groups. One married woman who could not bear a child and wanted to adopt sacrificed her marriage because her husband wanted no children. A single person desiring parenthood usually faces many more challenges during the approval process than a heterosexual couple with the same desire. Anyone, married or single, who attempts interracial adoption in the United States must navigate not only the usual hurdles but also the national debate on the topic. The National Association of Black Social Workers, for example, disapproves of such adoptions, comparing it to cultural genocide. The other side of this argument, while acknowledging the importance of racial identity, emphasizes the common humanity and needs of all children for nurturance and love in a stable family—needs that are rarely met in institutional settings or with frequent shifts between foster families (Bartholet, 1993; Bates, 1993).

Lesbian and Gay Parenthood

The contemporary stresses of parenthood include those of gay, lesbian, and bisexual parents. There is probably no group of parents more misunderstood than gay parents. The myth and fear is that gay parents will bring up their children to be gay. Another myth is that gay men are much more likely than straight men to abuse children. As a result, lesbian and gay parents may lose custody of their children for no other reason than their sexual identity. Gay people of both sexes may be denied adoption if their sexual identity is known. For example, community protest in Massachusetts resulted in the removal of a foster child from the home of two gay foster parents, only to have the child abused six months later in a "normal" foster home. Crises around gay parenthood might decline with reflection on the following facts: The vast majority of parents are heterosexual; yet these straight parents have reared millions of gay people. The necessary role models of either sex and sexual identity exist for *all* children in many social contexts besides the home. Also, the majority of child sexual abusers are heterosexual male relatives (Raymond, 1992; Williams, 1992).

Surrogate Parenthood

In a landmark decision, the New Jersey supreme court declared that paying a woman to have a baby constitutes illegal baby selling and perhaps is criminal and

potentially degrading to women. Nevertheless, legal, ethical, and emotional controversy over this technological response to the desire of childless couples for children will probably continue, with proponents citing the Bible in support of their
position and opponents noting that the last time human beings were bred for transfer of ownership was during slavery (Arditti, Klein, & Minden, 1984; Corea, 1985).
The parenting issues of infertility and the right of procreation are cited as rationales justifying surrogacy. However, infertility rates are highest among low-income
racial minority groups, due in part to greater exposure to various hazards, while
lower rates among affluent women are traced largely to later age at attempting
pregnancy. Surrogate babies, therefore, are usually born to poor women and paid
for by affluent white couples. In the United States, the price of a surrogate arrangement is usually $10,000 for the mother, with another $15,000 going to the spon-
soring agency (late 1980s figures); women in Third World countries are paid much
less or nothing at all. Also, while procreation is a right, this right cannot be exercised at the expense of the primordial right of a woman to the child she has nur-
tured and birthed. The *preventive* approach to the infertility that has spawned
surrogacy includes removal of environmental and workplace hazards (see Chavkin,
1984 and Chapters Ten and Twelve), and child care provisions that would allow
career women to have children at earlier ages without compromising their jobs
(Gerson, 1986). The continuing controversy in wealthy countries surrounding this
issue is illustrated in the 1993 report of a Royal Commission on New Reproductive Technology in Canada. While the Commission was mired in controversy for
years, it did reach consensus on some issues such as tighter licensing standards and
the banning of surrogate motherhood and sex-selection techniques (Mickleburgh,
1993; Krishnan, 1994).

The complexity of this issue is compounded by a resurgence of nineteenth-
century natalism that emphasizes the biological reproduction role of women. Natalism's seductive power is dramatized in the stories of two Montreal couples who
began in vitro technology; one couple followed through for years at enormous financial and personal cost, while the other dropped out in favor of adoption and
a more global (versus individualistic) approach to their desire to care for children (see *The Technological Stork*, Canadian Film Board). But among those parents
who in good faith choose adoption, after weathering the crisis of infertility, some
are confronted with the loss of their adopted child to biological parents whose
rights are almost always favored by courts, sometimes apparently irrespective of the
child's best interests. One couple who faced this crisis made meaning out of their
loss by advocating for a change in laws that more fairly protect the rights of all concerned in such cases—and succeeding in their efforts.

Fatherhood in Transition

A discussion of parenthood is incomplete without considering the changing notion of fatherhood, especially in regard to prevention of parent-child crises. The
changing role of fathers is related to several factors: (1) the necessity for most moth-

ers to work outside the home; (2) financial and other risks of single parenting to all concerned; (3) increasing realization of the benefits to children of being reared by two parents rather than one; (4) growing awareness by fathers of what they miss emotionally through marginal involvement in parenting. However, there are strains in this transitional process (Shapiro, 1987). Several factors work against contemporary fathers assuming a more active role in child rearing: (1) continued sex-role socialization at home and in school (Sadker & Sadker, 1994); (2) continued gender-based inequality in the paid labor force; (3) the tenacious notion that it is more appropriate for a mother than a father to take time from a job on behalf of family needs (Thurer, 1994); (4) lack of role models for male participation in child care; (5) gender-based stereotypes in such professions as nursing and child development; (6) some women's continued ambivalence about men's active participation.

Since child care is the only arena in which women routinely have exercised control, it is unlikely that they will readily give it up so long as their limited access to other areas of power continues. Language is a barometer of our success here; that is, we still hear that mothers "take care of their children," while fathers "baby-sit" or "watch" them. In North America and worldwide, the poverty of children usually mirrors the poverty of their mothers. A 1993 U.N. Human Development Report on thirty-three countries that keep gender-based statistics reveals that no country (including rich nations like Canada, Germany, Switzerland, and the United States) treats women as well as it treats men. And a social health index measuring, among other items, child poverty and teen suicide puts the United States at a twenty-one-year low (Dvorchak, 1992), reinforcing earlier studies citing the U.S. lag behind Western European countries in policies and practice that address the needs of working parents. Poverty and inadequate child-care services are not just issues for welfare mothers; they adversely affect increasing numbers of intact families and struggling parents. Some corporations are also realizing greater business returns, more employee satisfaction, and reduced absenteeism as a result of providing child-care benefits. As Ruddick (1989) suggests, children, women, men, and the whole social order would benefit by balancing domestic and public work between women and men.

Adolescence and Young Adulthood

Opinion regarding the age span of adolescence varies in different cultures and according to different theorists. The Joint Commission on Mental Health of Children in the United States considered youth up to age twenty-five in the program it recommended for youth in the 1970s. The extent of adolescence is influenced by such factors as: (1) length of time spent in school, (2) age at first marriage, (3) parenthood or the lack of it, (4) age at first self-supporting job, and (5) residence (with or apart from parents). In general, adolescence can be considered in two stages—early and late. Late adolescence overlaps with young adulthood, particularly for those who prolong vocational and educational preparation into their early and middle twenties.

Developmental Challenges and Stress

During early adolescence, the major developmental task is achievement of "ego identity" (Erikson, 1963). Adolescents and young adults must give up the security of dependence on parents and accept new roles in society, including responsibility in the work world and achieving a capacity for intimacy. The adolescent struggles with the issue of independence and freedom from family. On the one hand, the young person is very much in need of the family's material and emotional support. On the other hand, he or she may resent the continued necessity of dependence on parents. Interdependence—a balance between excessive dependence and independence—is a mark of growth during this stage.

Developmental tasks during late adolescence include finding and adjusting to a place in the world apart from immediate family and developing a capacity for intimacy in one's chosen sex role. These tasks may involve finding and holding a satisfying job; succeeding in college, technical training, or graduate school; and choosing and adjusting to a life style such as marriage or communal living.

Success with the developmental tasks of adolescence depends on what happened during one's infancy and childhood, including transitions such as toilet training, weaning, and starting school. An unhappy childhood is the usual precursor to unhappiness for an adolescent or young adult. Successful completion of the tasks of adolescence or young adulthood can be accomplished only if parents know when to let go and do not prevent the young person from making decisions she or he is capable of making independently. Young people today simultaneously face new opportunities and terrifying threats, often with insufficient support in either instance.

U.S. society has been described as youth oriented. This does not mean that Americans particularly value younger people; instead, it shows a devaluation of older people. In fact, the necessary services for both normal and troubled young people are grossly lacking in many communities. For example, many schools do not have guidance counselors or school social workers. The youthful population in every community should have access to emergency hostels where young people abused by their parents or seeking refuge from conflict can go. There should be housing for youthful offenders in special facilities with a strong community focus—not with hardened criminals. And all schools should provide suicide prevention programs (see Chapters Six and Seven).

Sexual Identity Crisis

As already noted in the chapters on suicide and violence, many adolescents today are at increased risk of destructive behaviors toward self and others, while gay, lesbian, and bisexual youth are at even greater risk, especially of suicide. Though complex factors intersect during all adolescent crises, homophobia in mainstream North America is commonly assumed to underpin the crises and chronic problems faced by gay youth. Williams (1992, 1986), an anthropologist who has studied among Native people of North American, Pacific, and Southeast Asian cultures, points out how these people revere androgynous members of the community as "higher" because the spirit from which all life (human, animal, plant) emanates has blessed the person with *two* spirits; hence the person is respected as a "double person" with particular roles and contributions to make in religion, the family, the workplace, and the community at large. Thus, "difference is transformed—from *deviant* to *exceptional*—becoming a basis for respect rather than stigma" (Williams, 1992, p. 267). From his field work with the Lakota, for example, Williams notes that the *berdache* (androgynous men) are the first choice to become adoptive parents when there is a homeless child—a marked contrast to nearly universal policy in most North American jurisdictions forbidding such adoption allegedly to prevent sexual molestation.

Blumenfeld (1992) shows the enormous costs of homophobia to *all*—those who are stigmatized, victimized, and deprived of an opportunity to live peaceful and fruitful lives, as well as those who have accepted the notion that these "different" people are also evil. But the highest price is paid by adolescents during the vulnerable developmental stage of discovering their sexual identity in a homophobic mainstream society and coming to terms with who they are without engaging in self-destructive behaviors. Figure 13.1 illustrates the sexual identity crisis that many lesbian, gay, and bisexual youth experience. It depicts the Crisis Paradigm applied to this at-risk group of adolescents, highlighting both the danger and opportunity to move beyond homophobia toward a more egalitarian value system as espoused by many pre-Columbian native communities. (See also Blumenfeld & Lindop, 1994.)

Helping Young People

Parents, teachers, pastors, youth directors, guidance and residence counselors, and school nurses are in powerful positions to help or hinder young people in their quest for identity and a meaningful place in society (Novello, 1993; Van Ornum & Mordock, 1987). Help may mean simply being available and attentive when a young person is upset and wants to talk; offering information the young person needs in order to make decisions about career, education, or marriage; guiding young people in the use of counseling and other resources when they find themselves in a crisis; or acting as a youth advocate in instances of neglect, abuse, or other injustice.

The crisis intervention principle of doing things *with*, rather than *to* and *for*, troubled people is particularly important when trying to help the young (see Chapter Four). Since a major developmental task of adolescence is finding a unique

FIGURE 13.1. SEXUAL IDENTITY CRISIS.

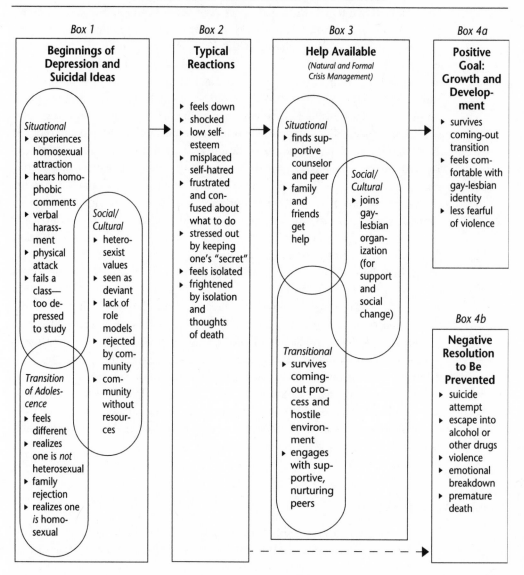

Box 1

Beginnings of Depression and Suicidal Ideas

Situational
▸ experiences homosexual attraction
▸ hears homophobic comments
▸ verbal harassment
▸ physical attack
▸ fails a class—too depressed to study

Social/Cultural
▸ heterosexist values
▸ seen as deviant
▸ lack of role models
▸ rejected by community
▸ community without resources

Transition of Adolescence
▸ feels different
▸ realizes one is *not* heterosexual
▸ family rejection
▸ realizes one *is* homosexual

Box 2

Typical Reactions

▸ feels down
▸ shocked
▸ low self-esteem
▸ misplaced self-hatred
▸ frustrated and confused about what to do
▸ stressed out by keeping one's "secret"
▸ feels isolated
▸ frightened by isolation and thoughts of death

Box 3

Help Available
(Natural and Formal Crisis Management)

Situational
▸ finds supportive counselor and peer
▸ family and friends get help

Social/Cultural
▸ joins gay-lesbian organization (for support and social change)

Transitional
▸ survives coming-out process and hostile environment
▸ engages with supportive, nurturing peers

Box 4a

Positive Goal: Growth and Development

▸ survives coming-out transition
▸ feels comfortable with gay-lesbian identity
▸ less fearful of violence

Box 4b

Negative Resolution to Be Prevented

▸ suicide attempt
▸ escape into alcohol or other drugs
▸ violence
▸ emotional breakdown
▸ premature death

place and achieving healthy interdependence, a counselor's inattention to this principle can defeat the purpose of the helping relationship. Certainly, a young person in trouble may need a caring adult to help make certain decisions. But the same principle applies here as in work with troubled adults: the troubled person should participate in any decision affecting him or her unless that is clearly impossible under certain circumstances. Then the counselor should be ready and available to act on the person's behalf. Some adults assume that young people are incapable of making any decisions or of accepting any responsibility. In contrast, others force adolescents to make decisions and assume responsibilities they may not be ready for. Either attitude causes trouble. Crises and ongoing problems such as drug abuse, delinquency, and violence can often be avoided when young people have the support they need to meet the demands of this phase of development.

CASE EXAMPLE: NORA STAPLES

Nora Staples, age seventeen, and her sister Jennifer, age sixteen, moved to a large city 300 miles from their home in order to get away from their abusive father. Their elderly grandparents invited Nora and Jennifer to stay with them, despite their cramped living quarters and dire financial straits. Nora and Jennifer's parents had divorced when the children were eleven and ten respectively. Their mother left the area after the divorce, and the girls had not seen her since. For four years, Nora and Jennifer stayed with an aunt and uncle who lived near their father's home.

When Nora was fifteen and Jennifer fourteen, their father insisted that they live with him. He expected them to cook and keep house, which they did without complaint; they were afraid of what he would do if they rebelled. On weekends, their father went on drinking binges. Every month or two after such a binge, he would put both girls out of the house and lock the door; they would then go back to their aunt and uncle's house for a few days until their father insisted they come home again. The aunt and uncle were finally threatened by the father if they ever took the girls in again. When they heard this, Nora and Jennifer hitchhiked to their grandparents' home.

Two weeks after arriving at her grandparents' home, Nora began talking about shooting herself. The grandmother called a local crisis clinic and persuaded Nora to talk with the counselor. Indeed, Nora had obtained a gun and was seriously considering suicide. She felt angry with her father, though she had never let him know that. She also felt guilty about leaving him, although she couldn't bear to be with him any longer. Now she felt she was a burden to her grandparents and saw no point in going on. Nora agreed, however, to come to the crisis clinic for counseling to deal with her problem. She also agreed to a plan to dispose of the gun with the help of her grandparents and the police. Nora's grandparents were helped to deal with their anger and disgust with their son for the way he had treated Nora and Jennifer.

In spite of her problems, Nora managed to graduate from high school with honors at age seventeen and was offered a scholarship by a nearby private college. She was undecided about whether to start college immediately or get a job to help support herself while living with her grandparents.

The service plan for Nora and her grandparents included the following:

1. Individual counseling sessions for Nora to deal with her anger and misplaced guilt regarding her father, to help her make a decision about college or work, and to explore alternatives other than suicide as a way out of her despair.

2. Family counseling sessions for Nora, her grandparents, and her sister Jennifer to help them deal together with their feelings about the situation, to find ways of supporting one another, and to find a solution to the problem of crowded living quarters.
3. Collateral conferences with the Child Welfare Department to obtain financial support for Nora and Jennifer and to enable the grandparents to find a larger residence.

Nora, Jennifer, and their grandparents were also advised of their rights and of the resources available to them to press charges of neglect against the father if he came to take the young women away with him, as they suspected he would do within weeks.

By the end of eight individual counseling sessions and six family sessions, Nora was no longer suicidal. She had learned that the scholarship would be available to her the following year if she chose to delay going to college. She therefore decided to stay with her grandparents for a year and get a job to help support herself. One factor in this decision was Nora's realization, through counseling, that she was very resentful of having had to assume so much responsibility for her father and his needs. She said she wanted the chance to live in peace and quiet with a family for a while. Also, she felt deprived, as a result of her disturbed home situation, of the opportunity to live the way most teenagers do.

She also gained the strength and courage to file charges against her father when he came to demand that she and Jennifer return to his home. A restraining order was obtained, and he was directed by a family court to make regular support payments to Nora and Jennifer while they continued to live in their grandparents' home. Custody of Nora and Jennifer was vested with their grandparents.

A six-month follow-up contact revealed that Nora was much happier and had decided to go ahead with college plans. She was advised of college counseling services available to her should she become upset and suicidal again.

Young women like Nora and Jennifer need special support to avoid crisis during their passage through adolescence. If adolescents come from troubled families, we should pay particular attention to the social and family approaches discussed in Chapter Five. The role of grandparents in such situations is becoming more common as drug abuse, joblessness, and poverty among parents leave many children—even infants—without the family support they need. Grandparents are not only essential in these cases but also need extra support themselves as they "weather the storm" of resumed parenting roles during a major transition state of their own (Newby, 1993). On the other hand, grandparents who feel useless and discarded may gain a new lease on life by tending to the needs of children within familial and community circles. A loosening of the dominant nuclear family structure, enhancement of extended family roles, and community developments such as Cohousing (see Chapter Five) can serve not only distressed children but the community at large.

But even if family disturbance, rejection, and deprivation are not apparent, many young people complain that they do not feel *listened* to. Parent effectiveness training should begin in high school and include a focus on listening, loving, and giving, as well as discipline and nonviolent positive control approaches. Adult guidance from schools, churches, and recreation directors should supplement family support with creative approaches (Brendtro, Brokenleg, & Van Bockern, 1990; Canter & Canter, 1988). Hazing tragedies, teenage gangs, binge drinking, and similar negative group associations attest to the tremendous need of young people for peer belonging and acceptance along with adult guidance. Dangerous hazing activities are remarkable for their destructiveness and for their lack of any mature adult influence. While rites of passage for adolescents are necessary, the challenge is to develop contemporary alternatives that reflect sensitivity to adolescents' simultaneous needs for support, guidance, independence, and group belonging. For example, when considering the current threat of AIDS and of adolescents' continuing abuse of alcohol, groups such as Students Against Drunk Driving or discussion sessions on AIDS and responsible sexual behavior can function as contemporary "rites of passage" during this critical developmental phase (see Crisis Paradigm, Box 3, lower circle).

Helping a Family in Crisis

More consistent efforts are also needed within social service and mental health agencies for family approaches to the problems of adolescents. The interrelated stresses and crises of parents and their children, along with several intervention strategies, are illustrated in the following example of a family in crisis.

CASE EXAMPLE: THE PAGE FAMILY

Donald Page, age forty-four and Ann Page, age thirty-nine, had been married for twenty years and had four children: Alice, age twenty; Michael, eighteen; Betsy, fourteen; and Gary, nine. Donald worked in a local automobile factory. After two years in military service, he returned home as a disabled veteran. Ann had worked as a secretary prior to their marriage and returned to work when her husband joined the service. When Donald returned, the Pages moved to a small farm on the outskirts of a large city. They leased the farmland and Donald stayed at home most of every day doing odd jobs around the farm. He did few routine household chores, even though Ann worked full-time outside the home. The Pages had a bleak social life and, in general, their marriage and family life was strained.

The Page children felt isolated because it was difficult to see their friends except during school hours. Alice had a baby at age seventeen and dropped out of her junior year in high school. She and her mother quarreled constantly over responsibility for the baby, who lived in the family home. After two years of this fighting, Alice's parents asked her to find a place of her own, which she did. Meanwhile, Ann threatened to report Alice to child welfare authorities if she didn't start assuming more responsibility for her child. Ann really wanted to keep

Case Example, cont.

Alice's baby herself, for she had wanted another child. Alice also talked about giving her baby away to her mother.

Meanwhile, Betsy was reported to be having problems in school, and teachers suspected her of taking drugs. Betsy had been belligerent at home, refusing to do chores and staying out late. Finally, Betsy ran away from home and was returned by police after three days. Donald and Ann were advised by police and school authorities to seek help for Betsy. They did not follow through and continued alone in their struggle to control her behavior. Michael tried to help both Betsy and his parents, but he felt pulled between the two parties. Gary was the "spoiled" child, and occasionally asked why everyone was fighting all the time.

When Betsy's school problems heightened, she was threatened with expulsion and a week later ran away again. This time when police found her, she threatened suicide if she was taken home. Police took her to a community mental health emergency service where she saw a crisis counselor; she begged to be placed in a detention center rather than go back home.

After several hours with Betsy, the counselor was able to persuade her that she could help her and her family make things more tolerable at home and that a detention center was no place for a girl her age—at least not until other alternatives had been tried. Meanwhile, Betsy's parents were called and asked to come to the crisis clinic. Betsy felt hopeless about anything changing at home, although she expressed the wish that somehow things could get better. Two situations she particularly hated were: (a) her father and mother fighting about what she could and couldn't do and whom she could and couldn't see, and (b) her mother's and Alice's constant fighting about Alice's baby. If these situations at home didn't change, she said she just wanted to die.

The Pages agreed to a contract for eight crisis counseling sessions that were to involve the entire family, including Alice. One of the sessions was with the parents, Alice, and Betsy only. Another session was with the parents, Betsy, the school guidance counselor, principal, and homeroom teacher. Goals of the counseling sessions included:

1. Improving communication among all members of the family and cutting out the contradictory messages Betsy was receiving
2. Helping family members detect signs of distress among themselves and learning to listen and support one another when troubled
3. Working out a mutually agreeable program of social outlets for Betsy
4. Working out a plan to divide the chores in a reasonable and consistent way among all family members
5. Arriving at an agreeable system of discipline that included rewards and punishments appropriate to various behaviors
6. Helping Alice make satisfying decisions regarding herself and her baby
7. Developing a plan to work cooperatively with Betsy's teachers and the guidance counselor to resolve Betsy's problems in school

Family members agreed on various tasks to achieve the above goals. For example, Donald and Ann would set aside some private time each day to discuss their problems and disagreements about discipline—out of the children's range of hearing. Betsy agreed to follow through on certain chores around the house. If she failed to do so, Ann agreed not to pick up after her and to discuss disciplinary measures with Donald. Alice would seek individual counseling to assist her in making a decision about herself and her child.

Two of the counseling sessions were held in the home, which the counselor observed was quite crowded. One result of this meeting was that the family found ways of ensuring individual privacy in spite of cramped quarters.

The threats of Betsy's suicide attempt and school expulsion were crisis points that moved Donald and Ann to work on underlying problems in their marriage. These problems made parenthood more difficult than it might otherwise have been. After eight crisis counseling sessions, the Page family existence was much less disturbed but by no means tranquil. However, Betsy was no longer in danger of being expelled from school, and she at least preferred her home to a detention house. Donald and Ann Page agreed to marriage counseling for themselves after termination of the crisis counseling contract in an effort to make their future years as parents less burdensome. The attention directed to dealing with marriage and family problems may decrease the chance that Betsy will follow in her sister's footsteps and become pregnant out of wedlock.

Intimate Relationships: Beginnings and Endings

Intimate relationships are important; a break in intimate attachments can lead to crisis. In this section, the beginnings and endings of intimate relationships are discussed briefly as one of the major transition states.

Intimacy as a Basic Need

An intimate relationship refers to any close bond between two people in which there is affection, reciprocity, mutual trust, and a willingness to stand by each other in distress without expectation of reward. The emphasis in this definition is on psychological and social intimacy, although a sexual relationship may also exist. Whether one is married, single, or living with someone of the same or opposite sex, intimate relationships are essential to a happy, productive life. Sexual relationships alone do not necessarily imply intimacy as here defined (see "Assessment Forms" in Chapter Three).

Intimate relationships—the social and emotional bonds between people—constitute a significant portion of the fabric of society. Some of the more common of these relationships and intimacies are courtship, marriage, and deeply committed friendships outside marriage. Entering into such a relationship is a major event with important social and psychological ramifications. Common endings include divorce or widowhood. While these endings of intimate relationships are highly visible, other, less official disruptions of close bonds can be equally traumatic and often produce crisis.

At the beginning and ending of an intimate relationship the people involved undergo a change in role and status: from single state to married, from spouse to divorcee, from associate to friend, or from friend to forgotten one. When beginning a new intimate relationship, an old, secure role must be abandoned and replaced by a new and unfamiliar one. If the person changing roles is lacking in personal and social resources, taking on a new role may be the source of crisis. Often a role change results in feelings of loss and of mourning what one has given up. When the familiar role of lover, spouse, or trusted friend ends, a person may lose a sense of security. He or she may experience crisis because a basic needed attachment is severed and may again face the challenge of role and status change. Thus, transitions into and out of supportive intimate relationships are among the more common occasions of crisis for many people.

Besides couples who begin and end intimate relationships, couples who choose to remain childless also experience strain. Reasons for remaining childless include support for zero population growth, inability to cope with the responsibility of parenthood, and difficulty in finding adequate day-care facilities for children. Childless couples often meet with social disapproval from others who assume that the basic purpose of marriage is procreation. In effect, the message is: you can have intimacy if you assume the social responsibility of producing and rearing children. The National Alliance for Optional Parenthood is working on gradually changing the public's attitude toward childless marriage.

Gay and lesbian couples face similar disapproval, despite the movement to ensure equal rights for gay people. Various municipal and other jurisdictions, for example, have recently guaranteed gay couples the same employment insurance benefits as other couples. Gay men in particular often face additional threats to intimate attachments related to AIDS.

Excessive Dependence on Intimate Attachments

Since intimacy with others is an integral part of our lives, deep emotion and importance are attached to intimate relationships. Our feelings about these attachments affect our thoughts and behavior. For example, some people have unrealistic expectations of those they love and may behave in unusual ways when the bond between loved ones is threatened or severed (Vaugh, 1987). In contrast, some people have such deep fear of possible rejection that they repeatedly resist offers of friendship, love, and, intimacy. Crisis can occur at the beginning of attachments or when the intimate relationship is disrupted, as in divorce, death of a spouse, or betrayal by a friend.

Halpern (1982) discusses "addictions" to people—the excessive need to be attached to someone special—as well as the dynamics of ending such an addiction: breaking away, and appreciating the beauty and positive aspects of solitude. Remembering Halpern's maxims and those described in other self-help books can help buffer the crisis potential when breaking out of addictive or destructive relationships. For example:

1. You can live—and possibly live better—without the person to whom you are attached.
2. A mutual love relationship should help one to feel *better*, not worse, about oneself.
3. Guilt is not reason enough to stay in a relationship.
4. Some people die of destructive relationships. Do you want to be one of them?
5. If someone says, "I'm not ready for a relationship," or, "I'm not going to leave my spouse," or "I don't want to be tied down," believe it.
6. The pain of ending a relationship, like other crises, will not last forever. In fact, it will not last as long as the pain of sustaining it.
7. We are whole and valuable as individuals apart from particular relationships.
8. When we end a destructive relationship, we open our lives to new possibilities.

Singles, Isolation, and Divorce

Considered within the privacy, intimacy, and community dynamic (see Chapter Five), an excessive dependency on intimacy usually results in a neglect of basic needs for privacy and community. On the other hand, attachments to people who are not good for us can be fostered by the threat of social isolation.

Social opportunities, especially for the single person who has moved recently to a new community, are often lacking. In many communities, social events are organized around couple relationships. Consequently, a single person may find it extremely difficult or impossible to feel comfortable in a tightly knit society that demands that people participate as couples. Many communities now have singles organizations where single people of any age can make friends and enjoy a wide range of social activities. However, despite the existence of these clubs, it is still difficult for a single person to establish satisfying social relationships after changing location. Fortunately, the single state is now being accepted by many as a fulfilling lifestyle, which makes it easier for the single person to establish social contacts in a new community.

If a person is not single by choice and is unable to make friends easily, he or she is likely to be crisis prone. Psychotherapy may be indicated if the person is chronically unhappy or depressed about being single; if living alone, that person is also a greater risk for suicide. In general, the risks of isolation and crisis responses like suicide are greater when the person is single because of divorce, separation, or widowhood.

Divorce is particularly hazardous when the burden of care and support of young children falls entirely on one parent and when older people divorce and their value system has no place for divorce. Until very recently, divorce in the latter category was rare. It is now increasing rapidly and is overwhelmingly initiated by men. The crisis potential of these nonmutual divorce actions is high because of:

- Lack of expectation
- Contradiction of deeply held values
- Widespread absence of social support structures for these special groups

Consider the following example of what divorce can mean to an older person.

CASE EXAMPLE: HELEN

Helen, age sixty-four, was not allowed to continue working in the same government agency as her husband Tom when they married thirty-five years ago. It was understood and accepted then that a husband should have the advantage of career development and the wife should tend the home and children. Giving up her fledgling career as a civil servant was not a problem for Helen, as it was also understood and expected that marriage was for a lifetime and that her future economic support was secure. When Helen was sixty, Tom, then age sixty-four, left her for a woman twenty-five years his junior. Helen felt devastated and suicidal, going over and over with her friends and two adult children that somehow it must have been her fault. She said repeatedly that Tom's death would have been preferable to a divorce.

Helen had a hard time acknowledging to anyone but her family and closest friends that she was divorced. She felt ashamed and frequently referred to herself as a widow. Helen could not understand how her daughter Caroline, also divorced, could be so apparently unruffled by the event (Caroline

had no children, worked as a writer, and preferred her single life). At age sixty, Helen's only marketable job skill was baby-sitting. She was also a good gardener and cook but had no paid work experience in these fields. Besides being mateless at age sixty, Helen barely escaped homelessness. By a stroke of luck, she obtained the marital home and was able to rent one room so she could pay taxes and utilities. There was no legal provision, however, for her to receive benefits from her husband's pension.

In spite of these hardships, Helen scraped by, came out of her depression after two years, and now takes advantage of senior citizen travel packages and attends adult education classes. She is attractive, charming, and dearly loved by her friends and family; she acknowledges at times that she may be better off without Tom in spite of occasional loneliness. Two years ago, Helen turned down the marriage proposal of a courtly but sickly man, age eighty. While she was fond of this man, she resisted tying herself down to what she anticipated would eventually turn into a nursing role, especially after adjusting to her new freedom.

The harsh realities of the single life are contradicted by stereotypes of swinging singles with a carefree existence. The single state without children does provide greater freedom to pursue one's career or engage in other activities, but the hazards of single parenthood speak for themselves. Every lifestyle has its advantages and trade-offs; for example, greater freedom and less responsibility may be balanced against greater insecurity in old age. Pollner (1982), through an analysis of film, exposes the popular belief that men are much better off single than married. Social research in the last century, beginning with Durkheim (1915), consistently reveals that marriage in fact is more advantageous and ego-protective for men than it is for women (Oakley, 1981). On the other hand, women and men who have never married are better adjusted and are less at risk for suicide than those who have lost a spouse by any means. The hazards to individuals in these transition states would be modified by contemporary rites of passage such as divorce ceremonies and acceptance into widows' clubs. Lacking such social supports can leave single people in a permanent liminal (transitional) state (van Gennep, 1960), as they are never quite reincorporated into the community in their new role.

Middle Age

The term "middlescence" has been applied to those past adolescence but not yet senescent. Stevenson (1977, p. 1) identifies two stages in this period of adult life: middlescence I, the core of the middle years between thirty and fifty, and middlescence II, the new middle years extending from fifty to seventy or seventy-five. This division contrasts with the U.S. Census Bureau and popular opinion, which define middle age as the time between the ages of forty-five and sixty-four. Until very recently, little attention has been paid to the middle years except in the negative sense of stereotypes about being "over the hill," sexually unattractive, unhappy, and depressed (Anderson & Stewart, 1994; Golan, 1981; Levinson, et al., 1978; Panchuck, 1994.) People in midlife are literally caught in the middle: they have major responsibilities for the young and the old. They are the primary figures in society's major institutions: family, business, education, health and social service, religion, and politics. Besides doing most of the regular work of society, they are also its major researchers, with the understandable result that they have focused their research primarily on groups other than themselves.

Because of the relative lack of attention given to the midlife period, it is not surprising that many popular notions about midlife are the result of myth and folklore. Considering also the influence of medicalization, this major life passage is often recast as a "disease" to be "treated." The reality is that most people in midlife:

- Are happier than they were when younger
- Lead highly productive and satisfying lives
- Have stable jobs and have met the major challenges of education and parenthood
- Are securely settled in a community in purchased rather than rented housing
- Enjoy a network of satisfying social relationships

- Have more disposable income and financial security than either the young or old
- Enjoy good health and feel physically and mentally vigorous

In general, middle-agers today have more options than in earlier times because they are healthier. Census data reveal that North American and Western European women age forty-five can expect to live thirty-five more years, and men twenty-nine more years. Popular beliefs about middle age lag behind these statistical predictions.

Many, however, experience midlife as a threat. If a person at midlife is married and has children, familiar parenting roles may no longer fill one's day; spousal roles may need redefining (Maltas, 1992). If not single by choice, a middle-ager may see the chances for marriage as decreasing. Men may be threatened by a diminished sex drive and leveling off of career advancement opportunities. Women in careers face the same threat; women without careers must meet the challenge of returning to school or resuming an interrupted career. The onset of menopause may threaten a woman's sense of feminine identity and attractiveness. Both men and women may perceive their lives at middle age as quickly slipping away before they achieve what they want for themselves and others.

The success of men and women in dealing with these midlife changes depends on:

- Their psychological health and general outlook on life
- Lifelong preparation for this stage of human development
- Social support and economic security

Some people are trapped into the false security of living as though life were an unending fountain of youth. Such people may avoid healthy preparation for the developmental tasks of midlife. Or, if they are socially isolated and lack the financial assets necessary to pursue education and leisure activities, midlife can increase their crisis proneness. In spite of the advantages middle-aged people have, this developmental passage is as hazardous as other transitions, though it is not as hazardous as popular stereotypes would have us believe.

Among all the myths associated with middle age, none is more widespread than that of female menopause as a disease. Significant efforts to undo this stereotype include publications such as *Our Bodies, Ourselves* by the Boston Women's Health Book Collective (1992), which has been translated into many foreign languages. It is now widely accepted that menopause is a natural transition state, not a disease, in spite of bodily and mental changes such as hot flashes and a changing view of self past child-bearing age. Not only does menopause not require medical intervention for distress in the majority of cases, but estrogen replacement therapy, so popular in the past, is linked with various complications and remains controversial (MacPherson, 1987). Menopause support groups now sometimes take the place of estrogen replacement therapy during this important transition state. In such groups, women receive factual information (which is often rare and imprecise from the mainstream gynecology profession) and support in coping with the physical, social, and psychological changes accompanying the cessation of menstruation (MacPherson, 1985, 1992).

Men undergoing the climacteric could benefit from similar support groups. Coming to terms with middle age could influence the behavior of men who cope with changes in themselves by establishing liaisons with younger women.

Old Age

It has been said that we are as old as we feel. Many of the issues discussed regarding middle age apply to old age: psychological outlook, social support, and economic security are critical factors affecting the crisis proneness of old people. The issues concerning retirement, noted in Chapter Twelve, also apply to many elderly people, and many are at special risk for crisis. For example, minority elders have lower incomes than white elders; three-fourths of the elderly below poverty level are female; older women earn one-third the wages or salaries of older men; low-income elderly are much more likely to have limiting chronic conditions than high-income elderly (Estes, 1986). Also, with the federal cutbacks in domestic programs since 1981, greater burdens of caring for increasing numbers of elders fall on women (Doress & Siegal, 1987; Sommers & Shields, 1987).

The needs of elders are being addressed through the work of advocates for the elderly such as senior legislators, the Gray Panthers, the Older Women's League, the American Association of Retired Persons, and increasing numbers of individuals. A recent emphasis on gerontologic research and graduate training programs in universities also can contribute to the long-range welfare of the elderly. Many of the myths about old age are an extension of those about middle age: old age is a disease, and old people are uniformly needy, dependent, and asexual.

Attitudes Toward the Elderly

Despite increased political advocacy and advances in gerontological research, ageism and stereotypes about old people persist. Cultural values and the policies and practices flowing from them do not change rapidly. Old people are not as highly valued in mainstream North American society as they are, for example, in some Native communities and most non-Western societies. Recent social emphasis on the small nuclear family has virtually displaced the extended family arrangement in most Western societies. Grandparents, aunts, and uncles are no longer integrated into a family home. Children, therefore, routinely have only two adults (their parents) as role models and supporters. In cases of death, desertion, or divorce, children are even more deprived of adult models. Fortunately, this is changing with attempts to get children and old people together, for example, through nursing home visits by groups of children.

Older people experience even greater hardship than children do by their exclusion from the nuclear family. They feel—and often are—unwanted. Often they are treated as guests and have no significant role in matters of consequence in their children's families. When older people, because of health or other problems, do live with their grown children, additional tensions arise. The older person may become impatient and irritable with the normal behavior of the grandchildren. Space is sometimes insufficient to give everyone some privacy, or the old person may seem demanding and unreasonable (Killeen, 1990).

Services for the Elderly

Stress can be relieved and crisis situations prevented when special public health and social services are available to families caring for an older person. In some areas of North America, outreach workers from the public office for aging make regular contacts with older people in their homes. Names of needy people are obtained from pastors, welfare, and mental health workers.

Outreach service such as this is very helpful in preventing crises and avoiding institutionalization. Contrary to public perception, only 5 percent of old people in the United States live in nursing homes, and even people 100 years and older are often highly engaged in living (Clayton, et al., 1993). Where public services are lacking, the lives of many older people can take on a truly desperate character (see "Abuse of Elders" in Chapter Eight). The situation is particularly acute for the older person living alone who (for physical or psychological reasons) is unable to get out. Senior citizen centers now exist in nearly every community. Every effort should be made to encourage older people to use the services of these centers. This may be the only real source for keeping active physically and for establishing and maintaining social contacts. Such physical and social involvement is essential to prevent emotional, mental, and physical deterioration. Some people will need help in order to use these services: money and transportation to get there or counseling to convince them to use the service.

Other services for the elderly in the United States and Canada include, for example:

- Retired Senior Citizen Volunteers (R.S.V.P.), a group available for various kinds of volunteer tasks
- Phone Line, which maintains a roster of names of shut-in people (elderly or disabled) and calls to assure the person's safety and contact with a helping agency
- Meals on Wheels, an organization that makes and delivers hot meals to the incapacitated

- Help Your Neighbor—and similar public and private organizations available to the isolated and distressed

    Visiting nurses are another key resource. Often a nurse can detect stress or suicidal tendencies. A fast-growing service in the United States, Program for All-Inclusive Care for the Elderly (PACE), aims to keep frail elderly people in their homes while providing medical and housekeeping support. In addition to the above services for older people, all agencies for the aging should maintain active contact with the local crisis center for consultation and direct assistance in acute crisis situations.

CASE EXAMPLE: ANTONE CARLTON

Antone Carlton, age seventy-seven, lived with his wife Martha in a run-down section of a city. Antone was nearly blind, and both legs had been amputated due to complications of diabetes. Antone and Martha survived on a poverty-level income. Martha, age sixty-eight, was able to take care of Antone. Then she was hospitalized and died of complications following abdominal surgery. Antone was grief stricken. After Martha's death, a visiting nurse came regularly to give Antone his insulin injection and arrange for help with meals.

    One day, Antone's house was broken into, and he was beaten and robbed of the few dollars he had. The nurse found Antone with minor physical injuries, but he was also depressed and suicidal. The local crisis center was called and an outreach visit made. The crisis outreach team assessed Antone as a very high risk for suicide. Antone, however, insisted on remaining in his own home. The services of Help Your Neighbor were enlisted for Antone, especially to provide for an occasional visitor. Homemaker services were also arranged. A week later, Antone was beaten and robbed again, but he still refused to move out of his home. The nurse inquired about a senior citizen housing project for Antone. They refused to accept anyone as handicapped as Antone, although he did consider leaving if he could move to such a place. After a third robbery and beating a few weeks later, Antone agreed to move to a nursing home.

Institutional Placement of the Elderly

    In Antone's case, a nursing home placement was a means of resolving a crisis with housing, health care, and physical safety. However, admission to a nursing home is itself an occasion for crisis for nearly every resident. Also, while some people do well in a nursing home, for many, institutionalization marks the beginning of a rapid decline in physical and emotional health. A new nursing home resident will invariably mourn the loss of his or her own home or apartment and whatever privacy it afforded, no matter how difficult the prior circumstances were. New residents resent their dependence on others, regardless of how serious their physical condition may be. These problems are less acute for those who need intermediate-level care; their health status does not require such complete dependence. In domiciliary-level care, residents remain independent and are much less subject to crisis.

If a person has been placed in a nursing home by family members, he or she may feel unloved and abandoned. Some families do abandon an old parent, often not by choice, but because they cannot handle their own guilt feelings about placing the parent in a nursing home, no matter how necessary that placement might be.

The most stressful time for a nursing home resident is the first few weeks after admission. The new resident's problems are similar to those of people admitted to other institutions: hospitals, detention facilities, or group homes for adolescents. Crisis intervention at this time will prevent many later, more serious problems such as depression, suicidal tendencies, withdrawal, refusal to participate in activities, and an increase in physical complaints. Studies reveal that a significant number of elderly people simply give up after retirement or admission to a nursing home and die very soon thereafter (Seligman, 1974). Hopelessness in these cases is the forerunner to death. Elderly people admitted to nursing homes should be routinely assessed for suicide risk.

Besides having to deal with feelings of loss, resentment, and rejection, some people placed in nursing homes do not get a clear, honest statement from their family about the need for and nature of the placement. This contributes further to the person's denial of his or her need to be in the nursing home.

Nursing staff who are sensitive to this crisis of admission to a nursing care facility are in a key position to prevent some negative outcomes. The newly admitted resident—along with his or her family—should be provided ample opportunity to express feelings associated with the event. Family members should be persuaded to be honest with the resident about the situation. Family members will feel less guilty and more able to maintain the social contact needed by the resident if they do not deny reality. Staff should actively reach out to family members, inviting them to participate in planning for their parent's or relative's needs in the nursing care facility. This will greatly relieve the stress experienced by an older person during the crisis of admission and adjustment. It will also reduce staff crises. When families are not included in the planning and have no opportunity to express their own feelings about the placement, they often handle their stress by blaming the nursing staff for poor care. This is a desperate means of managing their own guilt as well as the older person's complaints about the placement.

Besides the crisis of admission, other crises can be prevented when nursing care facilities have (1) activity programs in keeping with the age and sociocultural values of the residents, (2) programs involving the residents in outside community events, and (3) special family programs. Unfortunately, the quality of nursing care facilities frequently reflects a society's devaluation of older people. Funding is often inadequate, which prevents employment of sufficient professional staff.

Retirement and the realization of old age are times of stress but need not lead to crisis. Societal attitudes toward old age can change so that this stage of life can be anticipated by more and more people as another opportunity for human growth. In some societies, retired people are called on regularly to work several weeks a year when full-time workers go on vacation. There are many other opportunities in progressive societies for older people to remain active and involved. Many crises in the lives of elderly citizens can be avoided if they are accorded more honor and some post-retirement responsibilities.

How we treat our elderly citizens can account for the marked difference in death rituals in traditional and modern urban societies: in modern societies many people are dead *socially* (by forced retirement or familial rejection) long before physical death occurs. Therefore, society need only dispose of the body—no rituals are needed to transfer social functions (Bloch, 1971; Goody, 1962). This cross-cultural observation invites further consideration of death, the final passage.

Death

Death is the final stage of growth (Kübler-Ross, 1975). It marks the end of life and is the most powerful reminder we have that we have only one life to live and that to waste it would be folly.

Death has been a favorite topic of writers, poets, psychologists, physicians, and anthropologists for centuries. Volumes have been written by authors such as Aries (1974), Bertman (1991), Feifel (1977), Fulton, et al. (1978), Glaser and Strauss (1965), Mitford (1963), Kastenbaum and Aisenberg (1972), Kübler-Ross (1969, 1975), and others. There is even a science of thanatology (study of death and dying). Yet death is still a taboo topic for most people, which is unfortunate because it means the loss of death as a "friendly companion" to remind us that our lives are finite. Such denial is the root of the crisis situation that death becomes for many. Vast and important as the subject of death is, consideration of it here is limited to its crisis aspect for health and human service workers.

Attitudes Toward Death

Death is not a crisis in itself, but becomes one for the dying person and survivors because of the widespread denial of death as the final stage of growth. As Tolstoy wrote so eloquently in *The Death of Ivan Ilych*, the real agony of death is the final realization that we have not really lived our life, the regret that we did not do what we wanted to do, that we did not realize in and for ourselves what we most dearly desired. This fact was borne out in research by Goodman (1981), who compared top performing artists' and scientists' attitudes toward death with a group who were not performing artists or scientists but were similar in other respects. She found significant evidence that the performing artists and scientists were less fearful of death, more accepting of death, and much less inclined to want to return to earth after their death if they had a chance. Having led full and satisfying lives, they were able to anticipate their deaths with peace and acceptance. They had "won the race with death."

The denial of death, so common in U.S. society, is a far greater enemy than death itself. It allows us to live our lives less fully than we might with an awareness and acceptance of death's inevitability. Through the works of Elisabeth Kübler-Ross (1969, 1975) and many others, we have made progress in dealing with death openly. However, many health professionals and families still are reluctant to discuss the subject openly with a dying person.

This is changing through the promotion of living wills, advance directives regarding the use of extraordinary treatment, and the public debate about physician-assisted suicide. For many, the assisted suicide issue is primarily one of maintaining control over one's last days and not suffering unnecessary pain. More and more physicians and nurses are concerned about the influence of technology on the care of the dying and the undertreatment of pain (Solomon, et al., 1993), and they avail themselves of courses on death and dying (see Bertman, 1991). Increased public awareness, a more realistic approach to death, and a loosening of denial's grip is now evident as people consider (especially through media attention) the prospect of dying in an institution attached to tubes and with no control over or conscious awareness of the process. As Dubler (1993) notes, the culture of medical institutions must change to accommodate the notion of negotiated death. The Patient Self-Determination Act passed by Congress in 1990 facilitates such change by requiring health care institutions to inform patients of their rights to make advance medical directives. The Act encourages people to think about what treatment they wish if terminally ill. It also assures compliance with their wishes for the kind of death they envision. The AIDS crisis makes the need to come to terms with death more urgent than ever (see Chapter Fourteen).

Many problems and crises associated with death, dying people, their families, and those who attend them in their last days might be avoided if death were faced more directly. As noted by Kübler-Ross (1969, 1975), Fagerhaugh and Strauss (1977), and others, nurses, physicians, ministers, and family need to become open, communicative companions to those who are dying. However, nurses and physicians often avoid talking openly with dying people about their condition. Dying patients pay a high emotional price when this happens. The numerous examples of avoidance cited in Kübler-Ross's classic book, *On Death and Dying* (1969), still apply in many situations unless the staff has had extensive sensitization to the practices she recommends.

The inability or refusal to come to terms with death is a critical issue for crisis workers in general, not just on behalf of the dying. Why? Because death, as suggested in earlier chapters, is a kind of prototype for *all* crisis experiences. That is, many crises arise directly from the death of a loved one. But all crises and life passages are like a "minideath" in the *loss* experience common to them all. The successful resolution of crisis, then, is crucially connected to the process of coming to terms with loss. Helping others through their losses and helping them find new roles, new relationships, and emotional healing depends heavily on whether we are comfortable with the topic of death and our own mortality. A healthy attitude toward our own death is our most powerful asset in assisting the dying through this final life passage and comforting their survivors.

In a culture without strong ritual and social support around dying, the major burden of positively dealing with death falls on individuals. Crisis workers and health professionals associated with death in their professions can make their work easier by attending courses on death and dying, which are widely offered on college campuses. Sensitization to death and its denial in modern society is also aided by reading literary and other works on the topic (Cutter, 1974; Fried & Fried, 1980; Goodman, 1981; Goody, 1962; Rosenthal, 1973; Tolstoy, 1960. Intensive workshops focusing on our own denial of death through sensitizing exercises are another means of forming death awareness. Such workshops have provided the stimulus for some to become aware of the preciousness of every moment (Bertman, 1991). Coming to terms with our own death not only can change our life and eventual death but lays the foundation for assisting others through death.

Helping a Dying Person

In U.S. society, most people whose deaths are anticipated die in institutions such as hospitals or nursing homes, not in their own homes. Proportionately more people with AIDS, however, die at home. Rosenthal (1973), a young poet dying of leukemia, struck out against the coldness and technology that awaited him along with death in a hospital. He tells his remarkable story of facing death and living fully until that time in *How Could I Not Be Among You?* (1973). On learning of his imminent death from leukemia, Rosenthal checked out of the hospital, moved to the country, and did the things he wanted to do before dying.

Many others are not able to die in self-chosen circumstances; most will spend the last phase of their lives in hospitals or nursing homes. These dying people deserve to have the shock of their terminal illness tempered by those who attend them. Crisis intervention for a person who has learned of a diagnosis of fatal illness begins with awareness of one's own feelings about death. Next in the helping process is understanding what the dying person is going through. Wright (1985) refers to the acute, chronic-living, and terminal phases of a person's response to a life-threatening illness. Family members and everyone working with the dying will recognize the phases of dying as described by Kübler-Ross (1969) from her interviews with over 200 dying patients.

Kübler-Ross identifies five stages of dying: denial, anger, bargaining, depression, and acceptance. All people do not necessarily experience all the stages, nor do these stages occur in a fixed, orderly sequence. Kübler-Ross's work is most useful for sensitizing health and hospice workers to some of the major issues and problems faced by the dying.

1. *Denial:* Typically, denial is expressed with, "No, not me," on becoming aware of a terminal illness. People deny even when they are told the facts explicitly. Denial is expressed by disbelief in X-ray or other reports, insistence on repeat

examinations, or getting additional opinions from other doctors. Denial is the basis for the persistence of quack remedies. But denial may be necessary as a delaying mechanism so the person can absorb the reality of his or her terminal illness. During this phase, the person is withdrawn and often refuses to talk. Nurses, physicians, ministers, and social workers must wait through this phase and let the person know that they will still be available when he or she is finally ready to talk. Pressing a person to acknowledge and accept a bitter reality before he or she is psychologically ready may reinforce the need for defensive denial. Self-help groups (such as those sponsored by Omega and the AIDS Action Committee in the Boston area) are a contemporary substitute for traditional rites of passage through this important transition state.

2. *Anger:* When denial finally gives way, it is often replaced by anger: "Why me?" This is more difficult for hospital staff and family to deal with than denial, as the person often expresses the anger by accusations against the people who are trying to help. The person becomes very demanding. No one can do anything right. He or she is angry at those who can go on living. Nurses are frequently the targets of anger. It is important for them to understand that the anger is really at the person's unchosen fate, not at themselves. They must support the patient—not retaliate or withdraw—recognizing that the anger must be expressed and will eventually pass.

3. *Bargaining:* Faced with evidence that the illness is still there in spite of angry protests, the person in effect, says, "Maybe if I ask nicely, I'll be heard." This is the stage of bargaining, which goes on mostly with God, even among those who do not believe in God. Bargaining usually consists of private promises: "I'll live a good life," or "I'll donate my life and my money to a great cause." During this phase, it is important to note any underlying feelings of guilt the person may have or any regrets that life has not been lived as idealized. The dying person needs someone who can listen to those expressions of regret.

4. *Depression:* During this stage of dying, people mourn the losses they have borne: losses of body image, income, people they loved, joy, or the role of wife, husband, lover, or parent. Finally, they begin the grief of separation from life itself. This is the time when another person's presence or touch of the hand means much more than words. Again, acceptance of one's own eventual death and the ability to be with a person in silence is the chief source of helpfulness at this time.

5. *Acceptance:* This follows when anger and depression have been worked through. The dying person becomes weaker and may want to be left alone more. It is the final acceptance of the end, awaited quietly with a certain expectation. Again, quiet presence and communication of caring by a touch or a look are important at this time. The person needs to have the assurance that he or she will not be alone when dying and that any wishes made, such as in advance directives, will be respected. Messages of caring will give such assurance.

Awareness and understanding of our own and of the dying person's feelings are the foundation of care during the crisis of terminal illness and death. Crisis intervention with families of dying people will also be aided by such awareness and understanding. Since dying alone is a dying person's greatest fear, communication with families is essential. Families should not be excluded from this final phase of life by machines and procedures that unnecessarily prolong physical life beyond conscious life. Family members who help by their presence will very likely become more accepting of their own future deaths. Denial of death and death in isolation do nothing to foster growth.

The Hospice Movement

One of the most significant recent developments aiding the dying person is the hospice movement founded by a physician, Cecily Saunders (1978), in London in 1967. Sylvia Lack (1978), also a physician, extended the hospice concept to the United States (McCabe, 1982). The hospice movement grew out of awareness of the needs of the dying, and concern that these needs could not be met adequately in hospitals engaged primarily with curing and acute-care procedures. A main focus of the hospice concept is the control of pain and provision of surroundings that will enhance the possibility of dying as naturally as possible. The growing emphasis on palliative care research and service extends this concept.

Lack has identified ten components of hospice care (McCabe, 1982, p.104):

1. Coordinated home care with inpatient beds under a central, autonomous hospice administration
2. Control of symptoms (physical, social, psychological, and spiritual)
3. Physician-directed services (due to the medical nature of symptoms)
4. Provision of care by an interdisciplinary team
5. Services available twenty-four hours a day, seven days a week, with emphasis on availability of medical and nursing skills
6. Patient and family regarded as the unit of care
7. Provision for bereavement follow-up
8. Use of volunteers as an integral part of the interdisciplinary team
9. Structured personnel support and communication systems
10. Patients accepted into the program on the basis of health care needs rather than ability to pay

The hospice movement is a promising example of a new awareness of death in modern society and the importance of supporting the rights of the dying. The pivotal place of this service for the dying is underscored by the AIDS crisis and by increasing numbers of other people who may prefer to die at home. As more people select hospice care, however, the need for respite for families and more hospital-based hospices will also increase (Wegman, 1987). Assistance for the dying person is supported by the "Dying Person's Bill of Rights," adopted by the General Assembly of the United Nations (1975, p. 99).

I have the right to be treated as a living human being until I die.

I have the right to maintain a sense of hopefulness however changing its focus may be.

I have the right to be cared for by those who can maintain a sense of hopefulness, however changing this might be.

I have the right to express my feelings and emotions about my approaching death in my own way.

I have the right to participate in decisions concerning my care.

I have the right to expect continuing medical and nursing attention even though "cure" goals must be changed to "comfort" goals.

I have the right not to die alone.

I have the right to be free from pain. I have the right to have my questions answered honestly.

I have the right not to be deceived.

I have the right to have help from and for my family in accepting my death.

I have the right to die in peace and dignity.

I have the right to retain my individuality and not be judged for my decision, which may be contrary to beliefs of others.

I have the right to discuss and enlarge my religious and/or spiritual experiences, whatever these may mean to others.

I have the right to expect that the sanctity of the human body will be respected after death.

I have the right to be cared for by caring, sensitive, knowledgeable people who will attempt to understand my needs and will be able to gain some satisfaction in helping me face my death.

Throughout our lives, hazardous events and transitions can be occasions of crisis, growth, or deterioration. So in death, our last passage, we may experience our most acute agony or the final stage of growth. Whether or not we "win the race with death" depends on:

- How we have lived
- What we believe about life and death
- The support of those close to us during our final life crisis

Summary

Life passages are minideaths. In each of these transition states, we leave something cherished and familiar for something unknown and threatening. We must mourn what is lost in order to move without terror to whatever awaits us. Preparation for transitions—whether from one role to another, one stage of life to another, or from life to death—is helpful in averting acute emotional crisis during passage. To assist us in this all-important life task, we need contemporary ritual experts, that is, mature, caring people who are willing to support and protect us from tumultuous waves that might block our successful passage. These modern-day ritual experts are crisis counselors, members of self-help groups, pastors, health professionals, family, neighbors, and friends—people who care about people in crisis.

References

Anderson, C. M., & Stewart, S. (1994). *Flying solo: Single women at midlife*. New York: W.W. Norton.

Arditti, R., Klein, R. D., & Minden, S. (Eds.). (1984). *Test-tube women*. London: Pandora Press.

Aries, P. (1974). *Western attitudes toward death from the middle ages to the present*. Baltimore: Johns Hopkins University Press.

Bartholet, E. (1993). *Family bonds: Adoption and the politics of parenting*. Boston: Houghton Mifflin.

Bates, J. D. (1993). *Gift children: A story of race, family, and adoption*. New York: Tichnor & Fields.

Borg, S., & Lasker, J. (1981). *When pregnancy fails*. Boston: Beacon Press.

Bertman, S. L. (1991). *Facing death: Images, insights, and interventions*. Washington: Hemisphere.

Bloch, M. (1971). *Placing the dead*. London: Seminar Press.

Blumenfeld, W. J. (Ed.). (1992). *Homophobia: How we all pay the price*. Boston: Beacon Press.

Blumenfeld, W. J., & Lindop, L. (1994). *Family, schools, and students' resource guide*. Boston: Massachusetts Department of Education, Safe Schools Program for Gay and Lesbian Students.

Blumenfeld, W. J., & Raymond, D. (1993). *Looking at gay and lesbian life* (2nd ed.). Boston: Beacon Press.

Boston Women's Health Book Collective. (1992). *The new our bodies, ourselves*. New York: Simon & Schuster.

Brendtro, L. K., Brokenleg, M., & Van Bockern, S. (1990). *Reclaiming youth at risk*. Bloomington, Ind.: National Education Service.

Browne, A. (1987). *When battered women kill*. New York: Free Press.

Buehlman, K. T., Gottman, J. M., & Katz, L. F. (1992). How a couple views their past predicts their future: Predicting divorce from an oral history interview. *Journal of Family Psychology 5*(3/4), 295–318.

Canter, L., & Canter, M. (1988). *A proven step-by-step approach to solving everyday behavior problems* (Rev. ed.). Santa Monica, Calif.: Lee Canter & Associates.

Caplan, G. (1964). *Principles of preventive psychiatry*. New York: Basic Books.

Chapman, J. R., & Gates, M. (1977). *Women into wives: The legal and economic impact of marriage*. Beverly Hills: Sage.

Chavkin, W. (Ed.). (1984). *Double exposure: Women's health hazards on the job and at home*. New York: Monthly Review Press.

Chesler, P. (1986). *Mothers on trial: The battle for children and custody*. Seattle: Seal Press.

Chodorow, N. (1978). *The reproduction of mothering*. Berkeley: University of California Press.

Clayton, G. M., Martin, P., Poon, L. W., Lawhorn, L. A., & Avery, K. L. (1993). Survivors of the century. *Nursing and Health Care, 14*(5), 256–260.

Corea, G. (1985). *The mother machine*. New York: Harper & Row.

Covington, S. N., & Theut, S. K. (1993). Reactions to perinatal loss: A qualitative analysis of the National Maternal and Infant Health Survey. *American Journal of Orthopsychiatry, 63*(2), 215–222.

Cutter, F. (1974). *Coming to terms with death.* Chicago: Nelson-Hall.

Dobash, R. P., & Dobash, R. E. (1979). *Violence against wives: A case against the patriarchy.* New York: Free Press.

Doress, P. B., & Siegal, D. L. (1987). *Ourselves, growing older.* New York: Simon & Schuster.

Douglas, M. (1966). *Purity and danger.* London: Routledge & Kegan Paul.

Dubler, N. N. (1993). Commentary: Balancing life and death—proceed with caution. *American Journal of Public Health, 83*(1), 23–25.

Durkheim, E. (1915). *Elementary forms of the religious life.* London: Hollen St. Press.

Dvorchak, R. (1992, October 5). Social health 'index' puts U.S. at 21-year low. *Boston Globe,* p. 3.

Erikson, E. (1963). *Childhood and society* (2nd ed.). New York: W.W. Norton.

Estes, C. L. (1986, June 30). Older women and health policy. Paper presented at Women, Health, and Healing Summer Institute, University of California, Berkeley.

Eyre, J., & Eyre, R. (1993). *Teaching your children values.* New York: Simon & Schuster.

Fagerhaugh, S. Y., & Strauss, A. (1977). *Politics of pain management.* Menlo Park, Calif.: Addison-Wesley.

Fanon, F. (1978). Medicine and colonialism. In J. Ehrenreich (Ed.), *The cultural crisis of modern medicine* (pp. 229–251). New York: Monthly Review Press.

Feifel, H. (Ed.). (1977). *New meanings of death.* New York: McGraw-Hill.

Freud, S. (1950). *Totem and taboo.* London: Routledge & Kegan Paul.

Fried, N. N., & Fried, M. H. (1980). *Transitions: Four rituals in eight cultures.* New York: W.W. Norton.

Fulton, R., Markusen, R., Owen, G., & Scheiber, J. J. (Eds.). (1978). *Death and dying.* Reading, Mass.: Addison-Wesley.

General Assembly of the United Nations. (1975). Quoted in *American Journal of Nursing, 75,* 99.

Gerson, K. (1986). Briefcase, baby, or both? *Psychology Today, 20*(11), 30–36.

Giovannini, M. (1983). Personal communication.

Glaser, B. G., & Strauss, A. (1965). *Awareness of dying.* Chicago: Aldine.

Golan, N. (1981). *Passing through transitions.* New York: Free Press.

Goodman, L. M. (1981). *Death and the creative life.* New York: Springer.

Goody, J. (1962). *Death, property, and the ancestors.* London: Tavistock.

Gullen, J. (1992). Report on the first international study conference on genital mutilation of girls in Europe. Ottawa: Family Service Centre.

Halpern, H. (1982). *How to break your addiction to a person.* New York: McGraw-Hill.

Hoff, L. A. (1978). *The status of widows: Analysis of selected examples from Africa and India.* Master's dissertation, London: London School of Economics.

Hoff, L. A. (1990). *Battered women as survivors.* London: Routledge.

Hosken, F. (1981). Female genital mutilation and human rights. *Feminist Issues, 1*(3), 3–23.

Inch, S. (1984). *Birth rights.* New York: Pantheon.

Jacobs, R. H. (1979). *Life after youth.* Boston: Beacon Press.

Jordan, B. (1993). *Birth in four cultures* (4th ed.). Prospect Heights, Ill.: Waveland Press.

Kachoyeanos, M. K., & Selder, F. E. (1993). Life transitions of parents at the unexpected death of a school-age and older child. *Journal of Pediatric Nursing, 8*(1), 41–49.

Kastenbaum, R., & Aisenberg, R. (1972). *The psychology of death.* New York: Springer.

Killeen, M. (1990). The influence of stress and coping on family caregivers' perceptions of health. *International Journal of Aging and Human Development, 30*(3), 197–211.

Kimball, S. T. (1960). Introduction: *Rites of passage.* A. van Gennep. Chicago: University of Chicago Press. (French edition 1909).

Knapp, R. J. (1987). When a child dies. *Psychology Today, 21*(7), 60–67.

Krishnan, V. (1994). Attitudes toward surrogate motherhood in Canada. *Health Care for Women International, 15*(4), 333–358.

Kübler-Ross, E. (1975). *Death, the final stage of growth.* Englewood Cliffs, N.J.: Prentice-Hall.

Kübler-Ross, E. (1969). *On death and dying.* New York: Macmillan.

Lack, S., & Buckingham, R. W. (1978). *First American hospice.* New Haven, Conn.: Hospice.

LaFontaine, J. (1977). The power of rights. *Man, 12,* 421–437.

Leach, P. (1994). *What our society must do—and is not doing—for our children today.* New York: Knopf.

Levinson, D. J., Darrow, C. N., Klein, E. N., Levinson, M. H., McKee, B. (1978). *The seasons of a man's life.* New York: Knopf.

Lopata, H. (1973). *Widowhood in an American city.* Cambridge, Mass.: Schenkman.

Maltas, C. (1992). Trouble in paradise: Marital crises of midlife. *Psychiatry, 55*(2), 122–131.

MacPherson, K. (1992). Cardiovascular disease prevention in women and noncontraceptive use of hormones: A feminist analysis. *Advances in Nursing Science, 14*(4), 34–49.

MacPherson, K. (1985). Osteoporosis and menopause: A feminist analysis of the social construction of a syndrome. *Advances in Nursing Science, 7*(4), 11–22.

MacPherson, K. (1987). Osteoporosis: The new flaw in woman or in science? *Health Values, 11*(4), 57–62.

McCabe, S. V. (1982). An overview of hospice care. *Cancer Nursing, 5,* 103–108.

Mickleburgh, R. (1993, November 30). Prohibit surrogate mothers, report says—Controls urged for technology. *Globe and Mail,* pp. 1, A6–7.

Mitford, J. (1993). *The American way of birth.* New York: Dutton.

Mitford, J. (1963). *The American way of death.* New York: Simon & Schuster.

Moore, T. (1992). *Care of the soul: A guide for cultivating depth and sacredness in everyday life.* New York: Walker.

Newberger, C. M., Melnicoe, L. H., & Newberger, E. (1986). *The American family in crisis: Implications for children.* Special Issue: *Current Problems in Pediatrics, 16*(12), 670–739.

Newby, D. (1993). Intergenerational caregiving: Transition from grandparent to parent. Unpublished doctoral dissertation, Boston College, Boston.

Ngugi, W. (1965). *The river between.* London: Heinemann.

Notarius, C., & Markman, H. (1988). *We can work it out: Making sense of marital conflict.* New York: Putnam.

Novello, J. (1993). *What to do until the grown-up arrives.* Kirkland, Wash.: Hogrefe & Huber.

Nuwer, H. (1978). Dead souls of hell week. *Human Behavior,* October, 53–56.

Oakley, A. (1981). *Subject women.* New York: Pantheon.

O'Callaghan, J. B. (1993). *School-based collaboration with families.* San Francisco: Jossey-Bass.

Panchuck, P. (1994). *The midlife experience of contemporary women: Views along the midway.* Unpublished doctoral dissertation, Leslie College, Boston.

Papernow, P. L. (1993). *Becoming a stepfamily: Patterns of development in remarried families.* San Francisco: Jossey-Bass.

Paul, J. A. (1978). Medicine and imperialism. In J. Ehrenreich (Ed.), *The cultural crisis of modern medicine* (pp. 271–286). New York: Monthly Review Press.

Pierce, C. P. (1992, November 1). Hazing: A foul becomes personal. *Boston Sunday Globe,* p. 86.

Pollner, M. (1982). Better dead than wed. *Social Policy, 13*(1), 28–31.

Raymond, D. (1992). "In the best interests of the child": Thoughts on homophobia and parenting. In W. J. Blumenfeld (Ed.), *Homophobia: How we all pay the price* (pp. 114–130). Boston: Beacon Press.

Rosenthal, T. (1973). *How could I not be among you?* New York: G. Braziller.

Rubenstein, C. (1982). Real men don't earn less than their wives. *Psychology Today, 16,* 36–41.

Ruddick, S. (1989). *Maternal thinking.* Boston: Beacon Press.

Sadker, M., & Sadker, D. (1994). *Failing at fairness: How America's schools cheat girls.* New York: Charles Scribner's Sons.

Saunders, C. (1978). Hospice care. *American Journal of Medicine, 65,* 726–728.

Seligman, M.E.P. (1974). Giving up on life. *Psychology Today, 7,* 80–85.

Shapiro, J. L. (1987). The expectant father. *Psychology Today, 21*(1), 36–42.

Sidel, R. (1986). *Women and children last: The plight of poor women in affluent America.* New York: Penguin.

Solomon, M. Z., O'Donnell, L., Jennings, B., Guilfoy, V., Wolf, S. M., Nolan, K., Jackson, R., Koch-Weser, D., Donnelley, S. (1993). Decisions near the end of life: Professional views on life-sustaining treatments. *American Journal of Public Health, 83*(1), 14–23.

Sommers, T., & Shields, L. (1987). *Women take care.* Gainesville, Fla.: Triad.

Spencer, P. (1965). *The Samburu.* London: Routledge & Kegan Paul.

Spencer, P. (1973). *Nomads in alliance.* Oxford, U.K.: Oxford University Press.

Stevenson, J. S. (1977). *Issues and crises during middlescence.* New York: Appleton-Century-Crofts.

Straus, M. A., Gelles, R. J., & Steinmetz, S. (1980). *Behind closed doors: Violence in the American family.* New York: Anchor Books.

Teichman, Y., Shenhar, S., & Segal, S. (1993). Emotional distress in Israeli women before and after abortion. *American Journal of Orthopsychiatry, 63*(2), 277–288.

Thurer, S. L. (1994). *The myths of motherhood: How culture reinvents the good mother.* Boston: Houghton Mifflin.

Tolstoy, L. (1960). *The death of Ivan Ilyich.* New York: New American Library.

Turner, V. (1967). *The forest of souls.* Ithaca, N.Y.: Cornell University Press.

van Gennep, A. (1960). *Rites of passage.* Chicago: University of Chicago Press (French edition 1909).

Van Ornum, W., & Mordock, J. B. (1987). *Crisis counseling with children and adolescents.* New York: Continuum.

Vaugh, D. (1987). The long goodbye. *Psychology Today, 21*(7), 37–42.

Walker, A. (1992). *Possessing the secret of joy.* New York: Harcourt Brace Jovanovich.

Walsh, F., & McGoldrick, M. (Eds.). (1991). *Living beyond loss: Death in the family.* New York: W.W. Norton.

Wegman, J. A. (1987). Hospice home death, hospital death, and coping abilities of widows. *Cancer Nursing, 10*(3), 148–155.

Weingarten, K. (1994). *The mother's voice: Strengthening intimacies in families.* New York: Harcourt Brace Jovanovich.

Weiss, R. S. (1976). Transition states and other stressful situations: Their nature and programs for their management. In G. Caplan & M. Killilea (Eds.), *Support systems and mutual help: A multi-disciplinary exploration* (pp. 213–232). New York: Grune & Stratton.

Williams, W. L. (1992). Benefits for nonhomophobic societies: An anthropological perspective. In W. J. Blumenfeld (Ed.), *Homophobia: How we all pay the price* (pp. 258–274). Boston: Beacon Press.

Williams, W. L. (1986). *The spirit and the flesh: Sexual diversity in American Indian culture.* Boston: Beacon Press.

Wright, L. K. (1985). Life-threatening illness. *Journal of Psychosocial Nursing, 23*(9), 7–11.

Zelditch, M. (1968). Status, social. In D. L. Sills (Ed.), *International encyclopedia of the social sciences.* New York: Macmillan & Free Press.

CHAPTER FOURTEEN

PEOPLE WITH AIDS: PERSONAL, COMMUNITY, AND GLOBAL PERSPECTIVES

"Working with Ted changed my life. . . . I'll never be the same."

hospice volunteer

"Having AIDS is a blessing in a way. . . . It opened my spiritual being."

42-year-old man with AIDS

"It's so humiliating to be so dependent on people. . . . I think I'll kill myself."

23-year-old man with Kaposi's sarcoma, dying of AIDS

"The nurses really want to be here. . . . Lance forced himself to eat one of the chocolate chip cookies I made because, he said, 'You made it just for me.'. . . I almost cried, there was such a bond there."

psychiatric liaison nurse

"Through this experience, I have found me."

volunteer with AIDS Action Committee

"I can't move my legs at night, but if I touch even one person, then maybe it will help them be good to my boy who lost his mother to this horrible disease."

woman dying of AIDS

These statements from people with AIDS and those who help them dramatize the *opportunity* and the *danger* of a crisis, which, more than any other, may symbolize a much larger crisis of the modern world: persistent and growing inequalities that leave the poor, people of color, and women disproportionately at risk for AIDS.

This final chapter elaborates on the meaning of these vignettes and related experiences in socioeconomic and cultural perspective. This chapter also reveals that when judgment and avoidance replace understanding and assistance, the resulting fear, prejudice, and ignorance can add insult to injury for individuals and families in crisis because of AIDS. Finally, the AIDS crisis and its demand for a humane and effective response dramatize the need to address related societal crises that precede and follow affliction with AIDS: unequal access to health care, homelessness, malnutrition, and inadequate health care, social services, and family support.

AIDS: Illustration of the Crisis Paradigm

The Crisis Paradigm (see Figure 14.1) informing this book describes the experience of people in crisis and the process of using the opportunities a crisis provides and avoiding its dangers. Earlier chapters have shown that success in crisis work requires understanding the origins of a particular crisis experience and tailoring intervention strategies to these distinct yet interrelated sources. AIDS is not only a crisis of global proportions; it also typifies life crises as a whole and cuts across the ramifications of crises already discussed: loss, grief, and mourning; suicide by despairing people with AIDS; antigay violence; social network support; family and community crises; status changes in health, residence, and occupation; and finally, life-cycle transitions and death.

The traumatic event of being diagnosed with a fatal disease reverses the natural progression of life-span development, forcing the person with AIDS to face death at a life phase when energy, independence, sexuality, and community involvement are at their peak rather than in decline. A person who tests positive for the virus (HIV) that causes AIDS may feel similarly overwhelmed. Add to this the prevalence of AIDS among groups already despised or disadvantaged (gay and bisexual men, blacks and Hispanics, intravenous drug users) because of sex-role prejudice and the effects of racism and poverty, and AIDS can be viewed as not only the most tragic epidemic of this century but as the paradigmatic or typical life crisis—for those suffering from AIDS, for those caring for them, and for the global community. Not only for the individuals confronting AIDS, but for all of us, perhaps no other crisis will present greater danger or opportunity for the human community.

As AIDS progresses into its second decade, with no vaccine on the horizon and a shrinking commitment to disadvantaged groups in which rates are highest, public health officials and activists are taking another look, even though they described the Ninth International Conference on AIDS as "lacking a guiding sense of meaning and spirit" (Mann, 1993, p. 1378). The fastest-growing rates of AIDS are among women between fifteen and forty-four—especially women of color; an increasing number of cases are appearing in Africa and Asia, where poverty abounds. Rates among persons fifty and older are also increasing. However, even

FIGURE 14.1. CRISIS PARADIGM.

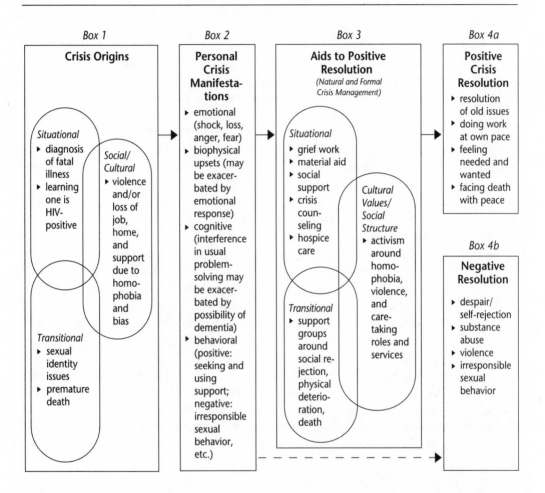

Crisis origins, manifestations, and outcomes, and the respective functions of crisis management in interactional relationship applied to a person with AIDS or testing HIV-positive. The arrows pointing from 'origins" to positive resolution illustrate the *opportunity* for positive outcomes of the AIDS crisis; the broken line at bottom depicts the potential *danger* of the AIDS crisis in the absence of appropriate aids to individuals and responses by society.

as dire statistics are cited, the lack of meaning and spirit Mann cites may signal a gradual paradigm shift to the view that AIDS is not primarily a medical-scientific issue, but rather, it is an issue of *justice:* factors placing people at risk of chronic immunodeficiency are primarily *social* and *political* (Murphy, 1994). Citing the work of immunologist Root-Berstein (1993), Murphy, a Canadian activist and policy analyst, declares that AIDS itself is not a disease, but a medical construct including a growing list of almost thirty associated diseases. As such, Murphy asserts it is not an epidemic but a by-product of poverty, malnutrition, and chronic exposure to such diseases as malaria and tuberculosis. In essence, AIDS is endemic, a view supported in mainstream analysis at international AIDS conferences. For example, Jonathan Mann of the International AIDS Center at the Harvard School of Public Health (1993, p. 1379) states:

> The central insight gained from over a decade of global work against AIDS is that societal *discrimination* [emphasis added] is fundamentally linked with vulnerability to HIV. The spread of HIV in populations is strongly influenced by an identifiable societal risk factor: the scope, intensity, and nature of discrimination practiced within the particular society. The HIV pandemic flourishes where the individual's capacity to learn and to respond is constrained. Belonging to a discriminated-against, marginalized, or stigmatized group reduces personal capacity to learn and to respond.

At the Tenth International Conference on AIDS in Tokyo, Professor Mann reiterated this theme: "Those at highest risk are those whose rights are least realized and whose dignity is least protected" (Radin, 1944, p. 10). Mann stressed that curtailment of AIDS is also in a nation's economic interest (given the cost of caretaking and loss of productive workers), though some listeners still question the wisdom of mixing health and human rights issues.

These perspectives provide support for the overall message of this chapter: AIDS as a crisis for individuals is intertwined with the sociocultural origins depicted in the Crisis Paradigm informing this book. Let us examine this crisis from the perspective of people with AIDS and those who help them, keeping in mind the link between their personal pain and the underlying social and cultural factors that leave them disempowered and vulnerable. (See standard texts for historical overview and medical/nursing facets: Shilts, 1987; Durham & Cohen, 1987; Barth, Pietrzak, & Ramler, 1993; Hughes, Martin, & Franks, 1987.)

CASE EXAMPLE: DANIEL

Daniel is a thirty-eight-year-old bisexual man who has been diagnosed with AIDS for eighteen months and is now living in a hospice managed by the local AIDS Action Committee (AAC). Pneumocystis pneumonia was the occasion for Daniel's several hospitalizations in the past eighteen months. He is down from his usual 185 pounds to 130, has periodic bouts of nausea and diarrhea, and some neurological involvement that affects his gait. Once a successful health care worker and artist, Daniel lost his job because of federal cuts in domestic programs and could not find another. Getting AIDS further reduced his employability. He is now without

employment, receives Social Security disability payments, and is eligible for food stamps.

Daniel says that he was "cancelled by Medicaid three times for no reason. . . . When I left the hospital I had no money, no job, no apartment. . . . I'm still struggling with the VA for the benefits coming to me. If it weren't for AAC, I would have been out on the street. With the trouble I've had getting care, especially an awful social worker, I got a dose of what the elderly and the homeless go through. You know, I say 'forget your cure.' What would I ever want to come back [from death] for? Homelessness? Poverty? I have no regrets. . . . I used to be seen as a

Case Example, cont.

pillar of strength, then people saw me as sick and no longer there for them, but slowly they're coming back. So, I don't have a regular job anymore, but now I'm a teacher and counselor [helping other people with AIDS], and I work three hours volunteering at a local men's shelter. I also do liaison work at the hospital where I was a patient. Yes, I get weak, but now I do what I can when I can and as much as I can. There's not the same pressure as before. . . . As long as I don't set expectations, there's no disappointment.

CASE EXAMPLE: SOPHIA

Sophia, age thirty, has a four-year-old son whom she placed with relatives as an infant because she could not care for him properly as long as she was addicted to drugs. Although she has had symptoms for about four years, Sophia was diagnosed with AIDS only two years ago. She suffers from night sweats, thrush, shingles, chronic fatigue, abscesses, a platelet disorder, and central nervous system involvement, including seizures and memory loss. Through her twelve years of addiction, Sophia worked as a waitress and a prostitute to support her drug habit. "It's hard to realize that all the things I dreamed about if I was drug free can't be now because of AIDS. . . . I thought having a baby would help me get my act together. I was wrong, but I would never hurt my son. . . . I don't take pride in too many things I've done, but I spared Michael by putting him in a stable environment. I'm not sorry I had Michael because he's what keeps me going now. . . . If it weren't for him, I probably would have killed myself already. I'm not through doing what has to be done—helping other drug users, and letting my son know me better. And I do a lot of talks for doctors and nurses about AIDS.

Michael and I spend every weekend together. . . . I'm making some videos for him so he will remember who I was and how much I love him. He knows to say no to drugs. . . . Behind every addict, you know, there is a child, a lover. It's people's responsibility to set aside their biases, to take care. . . . I have my problems, but at least I can care for someone else's pain, maybe because I've been close to pain. Some say they should lock up prostitutes, but don't tell me it's my fault that a man rides around in his Mercedes-Benz looking for sex instead of being faithful to his wife. I have wonderful friends. . . . When the memory problems get worse I'll give one of them power of attorney because my family judges me very harshly—for my addiction, prostitution, and now AIDS. . . . plus, I'm a lesbian—and if I left it to them, they would put out all the people who care about me when I'm dying. None of my family come to see me when I'm in the hospital. It's sad. I've spent half my life finding myself and now I'm going to die, but I have an opportunity to plan my time and get closure, and that's good.

Daniel and Sophia are at peace;[1] indeed, talking and being with them is an inspiration. Both are doing meaningful work. At his young age, Daniel feels he has

---

[1]Daniel and Sophia are now dead, but they live on because in spirit they are everyman and everywoman.

accomplished much of his life's work, though he still wants to write his memoirs. Dan does not seem to be afraid of death. When asked if he would commit suicide if his symptoms included a new crisis point, dementia, he said "No . . . it could be tough, though, because I've always been very independent and self-sufficient. . . . I had to fight like hell to get what I have now, but if it came to the point where I needed more care and they don't respond, well, I'm going anyway."

As Daniel's neurological symptoms progressed, his struggle to remain at peace intensified. He also was stressed by the fact that some of his friends could not face the reality of his approaching death, but instead of expressing their pain and impending loss, they either avoided him or made fleeting visits saying they "didn't have time to talk." Daniel's occasional angry outbursts toward his friends may be displacements of the anger he feels about dying but which is difficult to express because it implies a contradiction to his "caretaker" and "nice guy" image of himself. Sophia readily expresses her sadness and pain but says her work is not done yet, so she keeps going and no longer feels like killing herself.

How did Daniel and Sophia arrive at the peace and acceptance they experience in spite of constant physical pain and knowledge that they are dying? By what process did Daniel win his fight to get where he is? How did Sophia come to manage her ultimate life crisis in a constructive manner and finally give up her addiction to drugs? The Crisis Paradigm (see Figure 14.1.) illustrates the process of dealing with the crisis of AIDS and how people with AIDS can capitalize on the opportunity this tragic event offers and avoid the danger inherent in crisis. The following discussion elaborates on the paradigm using the AIDS crisis experience and illustrations from the lives of Sophia and Daniel. It shows what people with AIDS have in common with others such as victims of violence or man-made disaster whose crises originate primarily from the sociocultural milieu.

Crisis Origins

Although AIDS was initially viewed as a "gay" disease, people now generally recognize that HIV makes no distinction based on race, class, sex, age, religion, or sexual identity. For those it strikes, a diagnosis of AIDS is an unanticipated, traumatic event of overwhelming proportions. With the growing belief that more than half of HIV carriers will eventually develop AIDS unless new treatments are found, we may only have seen the tip of the iceberg, particularly if endemic conditions of poverty, malnutrition, and widening disparities between rich and poor nations are not alleviated. Individuals, of course, can modify behaviors such as drug use or unprotected sex that place them at greater risk, especially if a person's cultural heritage is considered in prevention programs (Bayer, 1994). However, as in the case of other epidemics, history reveals that *public health* measures— not medicines—have had the greatest impact in saving and lengthening lives. Thus, even among groups in the wealthy United States, in the so-called outerclass, education in risk-reduction behaviors must be combined with economic and other change—in other words, the intertwined *origins* of the problem must be addressed simultaneously.

The current state of medical knowledge and the lack of a cure or vaccine also amounts to an almost certain prediction of death for most AIDS patients within months or a few years. However, as Haney (1988, p. 251), a person with AIDS, notes, prediction about how long the person has to live "is simply a game of statistics and fortune telling. Doesn't it make more sense to help the person with AIDS to focus on the possibilities of living with AIDS rather than on a negative self-fulfilling prophecy?" As with any statistical predictors, then, we must remember that there are always individual exceptions to the pattern. A few people have lived well beyond the predicted time of death. And we also know that *how* one lives with AIDS depends heavily on one's socioeconomic status, particularly access to health care and social services. As noted in Chapter Two, the timing of a life event influences its effect. In the case of AIDS, facing the final transition—one's own or that of friends—during youth or early middle age reverses the natural order of things and demands extraordinary support. And families of persons dying with AIDS must come to terms with the reversal of their natural expectation to precede rather than follow their children in death.

Despite some progress in establishing gay rights, another developmental challenge concerns the issue of coming out. If a gay man is comfortable with his own identity but has not come out to his family and then contracts AIDS, old issues may resurface as he informs his family of his illness. His homosexual orientation will be implied even if he does not reveal it. This revelation constitutes either a new developmental challenge for him and his family centering on sexual identity, or instigates further loss through rejection by family members who cannot accept having a homosexual son (see Figure 14.1, Box 1, lower circle; also, Figure 13.1). In the cases of both Daniel and Sophia, their families have not come to terms with the lifestyles and sexual orientation of their children. The support of a group like PFLAG (Parents and Friends of Lesbians and Gays) might have helped change their views. As sad as it is, though, that Daniel and Sophia must do without family help during their terrible illness, they do not allow family rejection to exacerbate their problems; rather, they avail themselves of alternative sources of support—loyal and trusted friends.

Once a person is diagnosed as having AIDS, other events often follow: loss of job, home, friends, and sometimes family. But these losses are closely tied to the social-structural and cultural factors noted above, unlike temporary homelessness due to a fire or the unexpected death of a loved one from an illness that is not stigmatized (Sontag, 1978) (see Figure 14.1, Box 1, right circle). Complicating this facet of the AIDS crisis is the lack of a comprehensive plan for health and housing for the poor, sick, and disadvantaged, either in the United States or in most poor countries. This general social problem is exacerbated for people with AIDS because of continuing homophobia and the predominance of individualistic versus broader public health approaches to the issue. In some cases, prejudice translates into violence against anyone known or suspected of being gay. As Rhonda Linde (1988) notes, AIDS becomes an excuse for society to heap more abuse onto groups that biased people would like to get rid of anyway (see also Blendon & Donelan, 1988). Thus, for people with AIDS or at high risk for AIDS, the origin of crisis is not as straightforward as in sudden infant death syndrome (SIDS), for example. Rather, as Daniel's and Sophia's cases illustrate, the origins are intertwined and produce personal crisis responses clearly related to the triple origins in the Crisis Paradigm, responses that sensitive crisis workers must be attuned to if the dangers of crisis are to be avoided. Certainly, individual behaviors are part of the picture, but attention to those outside of family and cultural context will have limited success (Bayer, 1994). And the more socially disadvantaged people targeted for prevention are, the less chance there is for individualistic approaches to be applied successfully (Mann, 1993).

Personal Crisis Manifestations

The person afflicted with AIDS will experience most of the common emotional responses to a traumatic life event. Anger springs not simply from being stricken by the ultimate misfortune of facing an untimely death but also from unfair or violent treatment by a society with limited tolerance for anyone who is different or is perceived as receiving deserved punishment for a deviant lifestyle. Besides feeling angry, persons who get AIDS through a blood transfusion may feel self-righteous as they compare their misfortune to those they perceive as afflicted because of their own behavior. Anxiety is felt not only for one's own health and welfare but also for one's lover or previous partners whom one may have infected. "Survivor guilt," as noted for Holocaust survivors in Chapter Ten, may also surface for those who have lost partners and loved ones to AIDS. Some may also feel guilt or shame over their gay lifestyle, having incorporated societal homophobia (Blumenfeld, 1992). Sophia says, for example, "I can't take pride in too many things I've done," but she does not wallow in guilt, nor is she ashamed of being lesbian even though her family condemns her for it.

Denial of the medical facts and the need for behavioral change, especially if accompanied by free-floating anger at being infected, may result in irresponsible sexual behavior and the risk of infecting others. On the other hand, when Sophia was told she had AIDS (after being tested without her consent), no one told her about cleaning her needles with bleach or practicing safer sex. She regrets that she may have infected others, but if she did, it was out of ignorance, not malice. In general, the most ethical approach is to inform a sex partner of one's infection status. Crisis counseling and support are clearly indicated for infected persons who act out their anger by placing others at risk. Sexual decision making is a complex process often not amenable to a simplistic, "just say no" approach (Gochros, 1988, p. 255).

Sadness over loss of health and impending death is compounded by fear of losing friends or lovers and the necessary support to face early death. These fears have not materialized in either Dan's or Sophia's cases, but occasionally Dan has an anxiety attack when people who promise to do things for him either forget or are late.

Anxiety's usual interference in cognitive functioning during crisis may be exacerbated with AIDS because of the fear of dementia. For example, normal forgetting may be interpreted as a first sign. AIDS Dementia Complex (ADC) may sometimes be the only sign of AIDS (Joyce, 1988). Sophia is clearly planning for this possibility by arranging for a friend to act with power of attorney on her behalf. In the case of Charlie, another person dying with AIDS, flashes of awareness and clarity pierced his general comatose state so that he could convey his wish not to be kept alive with heroic measures.

In general, the emotional and biophysical stress responses common during any life crisis are exaggerated here because of sociocultural facets of the crisis that are usually beyond the control of an individual to manage alone. Additionally, the physical toll that the disease exacts usually includes drastic energy reduction, which in turn increases stress because of inability to engage in physical stress reduction activities.

While these general crisis responses to the trauma of AIDS are illustrated in the lives of people like Daniel, Sophia, and their families, we must remember that AIDS is different for each person. This fact underscores the importance of careful individual assessment to ascertain effective and ineffective coping with the crisis and lays the groundwork for assistance tailored to the interrelated origins of this crisis. Table 14.1 summarizes effective and ineffective coping with AIDS and forms the foundation for planning crisis management strategies with the affected person and his or her family, lover, and other network members.

Aids to Positive Crisis Resolution

Soon after Daniel was diagnosed with AIDS, a psychiatrist walked into his hospital room. Dan asked, "Why are you here?" The psychiatrist responded, "Your doctor thought you . . ." Dan said, "Tell him to talk to me." In the traditional psychiatric model, this response would have been interpreted as resistance. In the crisis model, Daniel's response is considered normal. And engaging a psychiatric consultant without Dan's consent runs counter to the premise of the crisis model proposed here that planning must be done *with* the person in crisis.

But if Dan rejected the help of a psychiatrist and was on bad terms with the hospital social worker, what else was available to help him cope as effectively as he did with the crisis of AIDS? Daniel explained, "Sure, I was angry, sure I was scared . . . but they don't understand that throughout my life I've had to turn to myself. Once I can face it, I have to help my family and friends to understand." But does this mean that Dan needed no outside help? Not at all. Rather, it underscores the often repeated position of this book: people have been managing crises since

TABLE 14.1. EFFECTIVE AND INEFFECTIVE CRISIS COPING
BY PERSON WITH AIDS AND FAMILY MEMBER(S).

Person in Crisis	Personal Crisis Manifestations	Crisis Coping	
		Ineffective	Effective
Person with AIDS	Emotional	Denial of medical facts and probability of death Repression Depression Hatred of self	Grief work Communication of feelings with caring persons
	Biophysical	Additional stress symptoms of emotional origin	Physical symptoms limited to opportunistic infections Resistance to additional stress symptoms
	Cognitive	Conviction of being punished for lifestyle or sexual orientation Failure to accept reality of illness	Recognition and acceptance of the reality and horror of the disease and all it implies
	Behavioral	Irresponsible sexual behavior placing others at risk Violence Substance abuse	Safer sex practices Preventive health practices: diet, rest, exercise, relaxation Acceptance of love and necessary assistance Preparation for death
Family member of person with AIDS	Emotional	Denial of medical facts Inappropriate self-blame for child's sexual orientation	Grief work Unconditional acceptance regardless of sexual orientation or lifestyle
	Biophysical	Additional stress symptoms of emotional origin Burnout from failure to care for self	Resistance to additional stress symptoms and burnout through self-care and acceptance of support and respite
	Cognitive	Perception of AIDS as a "gay" disease Clinging to myths about contagion, etc.	Recognition and acceptance of medical facts about AIDS
	Behavioral	Judgment and blaming of person with AIDS Avoidance and withholding of support and love	Expression of caring through communication, hugging, etc. Material support and assistance with activities of daily living

the beginning of time (natural crisis management). Also, in spite of his spirit of independence Dan recognized his need for support and accepted it. He said that the hospital nurses were wonderful and that friends and his overall attitude helped the most. Also, Dan said that he was greatly strengthened by helping his friends face death. Many volunteers cite a similar growth process in their support work with people with AIDS (Stulberg & Smith, 1988). One "buddy" with Boston's AIDS Action Committee said, "Sometimes I feel guilty because it seems like I get more than I give." He also said of standing by a man dying of AIDS, "I've never been so compelled by anything in my whole life. . . . What a gift it was to be able to be with him. . . . Nothing I've done since has been as honest."

What about Sophia? Precisely what did she have or receive that assisted her along the path of constructive coping with AIDS? Sophia tells of being hospitalized for abscesses, violating hospital rules by shooting up drugs on the ward, and leaving the hospital only to collapse shortly afterward. She knew that without treatment she would probably die, but having a drug fix at the time seemed more important. Later she checked back into the hospital and was confronted by the head nurse who said: "You ruined my day. . . . I can help you, but here are the rules. . . . Are you willing to keep them?" Sophia said, "You know, that nurse did me a real favor. She was furious with me and I don't blame her, but instead of burying her anger she confronted me and I could tell that she did it because she cared." Sophia contrasted the nurse's response to that of a dentist who refused to treat her but also refused to wear gloves: "I sent the dentist an AIDS information packet and a note: 'I'm sad for you that your ignorance is putting you at risk.'"

These responses highlight the repeated point made by people with AIDS: they are not victims and do not want to be treated as victims; they are people in crisis. Dan's case reveals that those with poorer psychological health than his prior to a traumatic life event are more vulnerable to possible negative outcomes of crisis. Thus, Dan's healthy self-concept was a buffer against absorbing society's prejudice in the form of guilt and self-blame. Rather than blaming himself, Dan says that "AIDS made me aware of the strength and courage I have." When someone in the hospital suggested, "You're being punished," Dan said, "Excuse me, but I've received a blessing you'll never understand." For those of us less ready for death than Dan is, it is important to remember that emotional healing from life's traumatic events requires the individual in crisis to make sense out of the experience and to process it within his or her personal meaning system. In Dan's case, his relationship to God is a definite aid to his continuous coping with the disease and its old and new demands, as well as his success in finding meaning in life despite his suffering. For example, when Dan's immune system became weaker and weaker, he was advised to discontinue volunteer work at the men's shelter to protect himself from further infections. He then substituted his on-site volunteering with a monthly monetary donation out of his meager welfare funds (see Haney, 1988; van Servellen, et al., 1993).

Similarly, Sophia finds meaning in her suffering and a reason to keep going for the sake of her child as well as for the influence she can have on the drug problem and the help she can give health professionals as they learn about AIDS. Her lifelong proximity to suffering and pain has apparently heightened her sensitivity to the needs and pain of others. Assistance to Dan, Sophia, and many like them during crisis is available primarily through groups like the AIDS Action Committee in Boston. They provide housing and hospice care as well as neighborhood people who help as needed with tending the lawn, keeping the sidewalks clear, and tilling the garden. With this kind of assistance, Dan and others in his hospice house are able to live a normal life in the community and face their impending deaths with greater comfort than institutional care would provide. Dan has great fear of being put in an institution, saying he would rather be dead. His residence in a hospice house allows him to use his remaining strength to the greatest possible capacity. For him, this includes activism on behalf of other people with AIDS (especially speaking engagements and interviews) and liaison work at a hospital. The gradual return of his old friends has also helped, and Dan has made new friends as well. Relationships with some of his family members remain strained, but Dan is not consumed with guilt, anxiety, or pain about this. While he loves his family dearly and regrets his emotional distance from some of them, he does what he can to help them understand and simply hopes that for their own sake they will come to understand him better before he dies. Dan's family has rejected offers of support groups to help them through the crisis of Dan's illness. Sophia's family also rejects such support. While Sophia also mourns her family's emotional distance from her, she is grateful that they pay her rent and provide her with a car.

Positive Crisis Resolution

The crisis management strategies that have helped Daniel correspond to the interrelated origins of his crisis: situational, transitional, and social-cultural. Together, they have led to growth and development; for example, he says that getting AIDS has been the occasion for him to resolve with his ex-wife old issues around his bisexuality. He is no longer rushed and overworked. He feels needed and wanted by the homeless men and others with AIDS and has a healthy circle of friends, including a cadre of mental health professionals who enjoy rapping with him. His adjustment to a healthy interdependence allows him to maintain as much independence as he can, while he does not hesitate to ask for the help he needs. Dan says that AIDS has forced him to take a "closer, more intense look at life, so now I'm more ready to leave it." In fact, Dan is not unlike the top performing artists Goodman studied (1981) who had "won the race with death." Like them, Dan feels fulfilled, ready to die, and has no desire to return.

For Sophia, in addition to her educational work with health professionals and the importance of being there for her son as long as possible, she says: "There's a reason for this. . . . I went on the radio and made $53,000 for the AIDS Action

Committee. It makes it meaningful. I feel robbed by this disease, but it's an opportunity to plan my time and get closure, and that's good."

Avoiding Negative Crisis Outcomes

For Jesse, one of Dan's friends with AIDS, things did not go as well—at least temporarily. Jesse had Kaposi's sarcoma. His skin was dying; he was being eaten away. Jesse also had neurological involvement and some beginning symptoms of dementia. He found it humiliating to have people do things for him that he was used to doing for himself. Dan helped out by putting reminders up around the house to compensate for Jesse's growing mental impairment. One day Jesse declared to Dan that he just could not go on any more: "I want to kill myself." Dan's response was, "Jes, no matter how bad this hits us, let's face it together. . . . I'm in pain, too. You know where I'm at. . . . Let's share it. You're strong . . . Look at what you've done for others." Jesse did not commit suicide, but died in the hospital a few weeks later. Jesse's death is not unlike the one described earlier, which was such an inspiration to a buddy with the AIDS Action Committee. The fortitude and acceptance with which Charlie faced death was experienced as a gift by all those who stood by him to the end, even though it was a strain—an agony that even the buddy wanted to be over.

As we examine the interchange between Dan and Jesse, it is clear that Dan did not simply talk Jesse out of suicide. First of all, the issue of suicide for people dying of AIDS raises all the ethical issues discussed in Chapter Six. In the case of AIDS, it might be easier for people to favor "rational suicide" than in other crisis situations. Thus, many would argue for the right of people dying with AIDS to commit suicide rather than suffer the horrors of physical and mental deterioration. However, as tragic as AIDS is, Daniel, Sophia, and thousands like them tell us that life can be meaningful and worthwhile in spite of great suffering. Also, if those afflicted with AIDS experience insult added to injury through antigay scorn and violence and then decide to commit suicide, those of us left can well ask whether we have in some sense "manipulated" such suicides, even those considered to be rational (Battin, 1980), through our failure to respond to those in crisis with the necessary, nonjudgmental care. If a caretaker or friend of a person dying of AIDS requests assistance to commit suicide, the caretaker must not only be familiar with ethical and legal issues regarding suicide but should consider hidden messages as well. For example, a person in severe pain may not consider suicide the only option if provided with pain relief measures. Clear communication and understanding of the real message are crucial here. Dealing with such a request requires peer support and possibly consultation with a mental health professional experienced in work with suicidal people.

While the topic of suicide and AIDS is not yet thoroughly researched, it appears that people with AIDS, like most people dying of cancer, do not wish to kill themselves even though some individual and couple suicides have occurred. Perhaps the greatest challenge for supporters of people with AIDS is to help create a milieu that will make it unnecessary for them to choose suicide. It is altogether remarkable and inexcusable that some people in excruciating pain in modern medical facilities still do not receive adequate medication. An appropriate environment, either at home or in a hospice house, would underscore the love and caring that helps the dying put their material affairs in order; say goodbye to lovers and family after reconciliation and, it is hoped, healing; and be recognized and valued for their place on this earth, and thus be ready for life's final stage.

Women and Children with AIDS

Gena Corea's (1992) book, *The Invisible Epidemic,* is credited with doing for women what Randy Shilts (1987) did especially for the gay men's community (see also Dorn, 1992). As already noted, the fastest-growing risk group is women from fifteen to forty-four. In the United States, African-American women in this age group are fourteen times more likely to be infected than their white counterparts, while the risk for Hispanic women is nine times higher (McLaughlin, 1994, citing the U.S. Surgeon General). Estimates are that AIDS will be the third leading cause of death in this age and gender group by the year 2000 (Bianco, 1992).

Even though women constitute a smaller percentage of people with AIDS in Western countries, African women (primarily heterosexual) have always constituted at least 50 percent of the total number of people affected (Berer & Ray, 1993). The marked difference between African and Western rates of AIDS among heterosexuals has been attributed to infected blood transfusions; increased incidence of vaginal bleeding during intercourse among women with scar tissue from clitoridectomy and infibulation (Hosken, 1981); greater vulnerability to HIV infection due to poverty and generally poorer health status; lack of sterile technique in traditional circumcision rites and possibly in poor hospitals. Research has yet to confirm these possible explanations, though there is a growing consensus about these social factors and AIDS (see Mann, 1993; Root-Berstein, 1993).

The general neglect of women with AIDS worldwide is part of the larger picture of inadequate health care and research on *all* facets of women's health. There is, however, a growing recognition that progress in improving public and personal health indicators is intricately tied to attention to women in their central role as major caretakers in both domestic and public domains.

Sophia and Daniel illustrate commonalities among people with AIDS: shock, anger, loss, and mourning a shortened life. But women, whether sick with AIDS or as caretakers, face several special issues. For example, because of cultural messages regarding body image, women may experience greater stress around appearance as they deteriorate physically. Women have the additional stress of worrying about becoming pregnant and possibly transmitting the virus to offspring. Fortunately, having her child infected with the AIDS virus was not one of Sophia's many stressors. Women who are HIV-positive generally are advised not to become pregnant. However, while there is support for a sperm-washing procedure for men who wish to have children, there is no corollary support for women with the same desire.

While the efficiency of male-female versus female-male transmission of HIV is still unknown, researchers generally believe that the virus is less easily transmitted from woman to man than the other way around (Richardson, 1987). Thus, female prostitutes have more to fear from their clients than their clients do from them, despite the publicly expressed concern about prostitutes as a major source of spreading the virus. Similar risk factors operate for the female sex partners of intravenous drug users with AIDS. In Western countries, only about 5 percent of men with AIDS do not fall into known risk groups (gay, bisexual, intravenous drug users, hemophiliacs, or recipients of a blood transfusion). It is difficult to know whether the source of their infection is from visiting an infected prostitute or not, since many men would rather admit to visiting a prostitute than desiring a man for sex (Richardson 1987, p. 37). Because of the general inattention to women in research, this pattern of neglect influences AIDS prevention as well, in the limited research on chemical and barrier methods women might use to protect themselves (Stein, 1993). Research and prevention trends have also slighted the fact of women's unequal power at personal, family, and social levels worldwide (Bianco, 1992). Women's continued inequality has major implications for risk not only of contracting AIDS from their male partners demanding sex but also of violence if they urge the use of condoms.

Female prostitutes, perhaps more so than gay men, are scorned by most in society, as Sophia's case amply illustrates. Thus, it is easy to scapegoat them for spreading AIDS. In Africa, where AIDS is distributed equally between women and men in the heterosexual population, female prostitutes in particular have been blamed for its transmission, while male promiscuity is rarely mentioned. Prostitutes who have AIDS or are HIV-positive already receive discriminatory treatment. Blaming them for AIDS also reveals the double standard regarding prostitution—arresting the women, but rarely their patrons—and the economic disadvantages of women that drive many of them into prostitution in the first place. Similar dynamics operate in regard to the traffic in sex, for example, women who are kidnapped, raped, and sent to places like Japan or Europe and forced into prostitution to service tourists (Barry, 1979). Women like this who get AIDS are in crisis not only because of a fatal illness, but primarily because of the worldwide sexual and economic exploitation of women (Bianco, 1992; Seager & Olson, 1986). In other words, their crises around AIDS are primarily of social and cultural origin.

A problem faced by those prostitutes and many other women who attempt to have safer sex by using condoms is that many men refuse to cooperate. When that happens, a woman is at a disadvantage not only because of inadequate female barrier methods but she is also at risk of physical abuse if she asserts herself—a contemporary version of the traditional responsibility for contraception being borne primarily by women. This issue highlights the additional danger presented by AIDS if people ignore the imperative to change stereotypical sex roles and accept equal responsibility for safer sex.

An additional hazard for women with AIDS is linked to the pregnancy risk. That is, if they are also intravenous drug users (the largest group of women with AIDS) and fail to prevent pregnancy, their ability to take care of a child will be even more limited because the problems connected with drug use are added to the debilitating effects of AIDS. Sophia's foresight in this area moved her to place her child with a stable family when she was unable to overcome her addiction. Additionally, a woman whose child has AIDS will probably feel guilty and angry whether she does or does not have AIDS herself.

Lesbian women, while in the lowest-risk group for AIDS, are nevertheless at risk for the same reasons other women are, and the number of lesbians with AIDS is rising (Hollibaugh, 1994). Sophia, for example, traces her infection to dirty needles to support her drug habit, not her lesbian status. Lesbian women are affected by the crisis in other ways as well. As significant others for gay men, some lesbians will suffer the loss of friendships through the deaths of these men. They are similarly affected by greater antigay discrimination and violence, primarily because of inaccurate portrayals by the media and public ignorance about how AIDS is spread. Lesbians are also concerned if they are considering artificial or self-insemination. Finally, lesbians are among the majority of AIDS caretakers.

The tragedy of AIDS is even more poignant with respect to children. While an adult with AIDS can come to terms with the inevitability of death and work through the crisis, including its implications for his or her previous and future sexual behavior, children with AIDS obviously cannot. This implies an additional challenge for people with AIDS to prevent pregnancy and for caretakers to treat and care for children with AIDS with extraordinary compassion. Attention should also be paid to the disenfranchised parents who brought them into the world—blacks, Hispanics, intravenous drug users, and the poor in general (AIDS: Report of the Surgeon General, 1987).

Similarly poignant and tragic is the fear of HIV infection following rape. While this double crisis affects male victims of rape, the majority of rape victims are women. The emotional trauma for such victims is overwhelming, particularly in the face of continuing public attitudes of blaming the crime of rape on its victims and prosecuting very few assailants. If these attitudes prevail, rape victims may continue to blame themselves not only for the rape but for AIDS as well; in addition, they must face all that any other person with AIDS confronts in an untimely death.

The Worried Well, AIDS Anxiety Syndrome, and Testing

Anxiety about AIDS is not restricted to those in known high-risk groups. Men who have visited a prostitute once may fear HIV infection and consider suicide a more desirable option than revealing marital infidelity. Or a suburban housewife may feel guilt about an affair, which is expressed in unrealistic concern about AIDS infection. AIDS thus becomes the "coat rack" on which to hang all kinds of unresolved issues (Linde, 1988; Krieger, 1988, p. 264). Of the 301 undiagnosed gay men surveyed by Stulberg and Smith (1988), those in monogamous relationships experienced less psychological stress than those without a stable, intimate relationship. In this same group, older gays (between twenty-six and fifty) were twice as likely as younger gays to have thought about suicide because of AIDS. In another version of the stress-illness cycle, some of the "worried well" feel compulsively driven to perform preventive health practices like jogging in the hope of warding off either acquiring or activating the HIV infection.

The challenge in this area is to unbundle realistic concern about AIDS from anxiety about various other issues such as sexual practice, sexual identity, or traumatic events like the Vietnam War. Krieger (1988, pp. 263–264) suggests five steps in a counseling approach to persons with heightened anxiety about AIDS and fears about sexual transmission of AIDS: (1) obtain accurate information; (2) assess fear of prior exposure; (3) learn to protect oneself and others; (4) gather strong peer support; and (5) address related issues such as homophobia, addictive attachments to dangerous sex, or guilt over sexual or drug use behavior. Everyone working with the worried well and people in high-risk groups for AIDS should be thoroughly familiar with the clues to suicide, risk assessment techniques, and strategies of suicide prevention discussed in Chapters Six and Seven.

This leads to consideration of the controversial issue of testing for HIV infection. If testing were more definitive than it is, opinion might be less divided. Testing reveals infection with the virus but not whether a person has AIDS. Since it takes some time for antibodies to form, even if a person were exposed yesterday, tests might be negative today, thus potentially conveying false reassurance. In general, opinion is equally divided between the advantages and disadvantages of testing. Since a positive test can send psychologically unstable people into panic and possible suicide, testing should be carefully considered in each case. Also, people who may have absorbed society's homophobia and feel self-loathing may request testing to prove, in effect, that they are "sinful" or "immoral." Thus, counseling and ongoing support services for those who either are considering testing or have been tested are essential. Such services are available through groups like the AIDS Action Committee and health centers that are sensitive to the AIDS crisis. As public knowledge about AIDS increases and hysteria decreases, testing is a less heated issue. Also, self-testing kits are available now, although their use is controversial because of concern about access to emotional support when receiving results.

While the issue of testing will probably remain controversial as long as we lack a vaccine and adequate drugs to treat AIDS-related diseases, testing is definitely indicated when pregnancy is being considered for one who has symptoms and a differential diagnosis is needed (Linde, 1988). In all cases, however, individuals should have a choice about being tested (Galea, Lewis, & Baker, 1988). Those who are psychologically healthy enough to deal with the unknown and who have greater tolerance for ambiguity may choose not to be tested. On the other hand, some people embarking on a new relationship may decide jointly to be tested before engaging in sex. The situation is similar to that faced by people at risk for various genetically transmitted diseases.

Caring for People with AIDS

Former U.S. Surgeon General C. Everett Koop predicted in AIDS' first decade that there will be no cure for AIDS, and that a vaccine will not be discovered before the end of this century. While we may hope that this prediction will be proved false, we should also attend to what we know of how other major epidemics have been controlled, that is, through public health measures and the improvement in people's general health, economic, and social status. Presently, a twofold approach to the problem (macro and micro) is needed: (1) the worldwide implementation of poverty relief in concert with massive public health measures; and (2) caretakers' application of knowledge, skill, compassion, and caring on behalf of individuals and families affected by AIDS. We have seen from our opening case examples that Daniel and Sophia have come through the first crises of AIDS to the point of peace and acceptance of eventual death. They managed to do so with a combination of natural and formal crisis management strategies. We have also seen that their personal coping abilities compensated in part for the extra stress they endured because of less than ideal approaches by some health care providers, and that they understand and accept those around them who cannot understand.

Others with fewer resources, however, may not come through life's final passage to death with peace, fulfillment, and the comfort of family and friends without extraordinary assistance from various caretakers. Families and lovers in crisis over the impending loss of loved ones and the emotional cost of caring need similar help. In short, providing for others whose needs are very great also demands caring and understanding for the caretakers.

While women outside Africa are less at risk for AIDS, large numbers of women have joined the gay men's community in mobilizing care for people with AIDS. And in the family network, it is not uncommon for mothers of gay or bisexual men to know about their sons' sexual identity while fathers remain unaware. This results in a large emotional burden for these women that they have not been able to share with their husbands. Similarly, in the case of infants and children with AIDS, the major burden of care falls on mothers because of continued inequality in society over caretaking roles in the family. In hospitals as well, women provide most of the care for the acutely ill and dying; in addition, they face the stress of overwork because of fiscal constraints and health reform measures that leave nurses and low-wage workers vulnerable because of their historic disempowerment within the system (Rachlis & Kushner, 1994). As so often in the past, so now with AIDS, the cost of caring is born disproportionately by women (Sommers & Shields, 1987). Significantly, as the gay men's community mobilized to support their sick and dying members, they were joined chiefly by lesbian and heterosexual women. This fact reveals that much work lies ahead in assuming equal responsibility for meeting society's need for caretaking roles, regardless of gender or sexual orientation.

In caring for people with AIDS, extraordinary stressors must be dealt with: fear of contagion (though this is decreasing with increased education); stigmatization stemming from association with devalued members of society (Goffman, 1963); confrontation with issues of sexual identity, one's own risk of AIDS, and death; assuming power of attorney roles; dealing with suicide issues; and finally, simple overload from association with the depths of pain and tragedy surrounding people with AIDS, their families, and lovers. Meisenhelder's (1994) study of 114 randomly selected registered nurses revealed homophobia, fear of the unknown, and lack of emotional involvement as the strongest predictors of their fear of contagion; adequate knowledge and extended contact with a person with AIDS were suggested as the most effective interventions for decreasing nurses' fear of contagion. When nurses and other workers are accidentally exposed to possible infection through pin pricks or contact with body fluids, counseling should be readily available, as for any "worried well." The enthusiasm of thousands of volunteers and others who have mobilized around the AIDS crisis certainly acts as a buffer to some of the stress because, as many caretakers attest, new meaning has entered their lives through their work with people with AIDS. This is no small accomplishment in a death-denying society.

The principle of providing ongoing support for all AIDS crisis workers and family members must be applied in order to prevent burnout, compassion fatigue, and the eventual loss of needed staff (Hoff & Miller, 1987). Also, among families, the ability to care for a dying loved one varies, requiring that professionals provide what families may not be able to (McGaffic & Longman, 1993). A general lack of knowledge about caring for an AIDS patient implies the need for a comprehensive system of respite service for families offering care at home, in addition to skilled home nursing assistance. This is particularly important in view of the Centers for Disease Control and Prevention (CDC) and the World Health Organization (WHO) projections of future AIDS cases. The challenge of facing great numbers of new cases in the United States and worldwide will probably not be met if the general caretaking issue and national health insurance crisis are not addressed at a societal level. This includes providing appropriate work conditions and monetary incentives to attract people to caretaking professions such as nursing. The challenge is even more dramatic in rural and other communities where "difference" is less tolerated and resources often scarcer (Rounds, 1988). One response to this challenge is the increased employment of nurse practitioners as primary-care providers (Aiken, et al., 1993).

Groups in the forefront of the AIDS crisis (SHANTI in San Francisco, Gay Men's Health Crisis in NYC, AIDS Action Committee in Boston) have recognized the stressors on caretakers and have provided support groups and staffing arrangements that offer respite from the stress of caring for dying people. People working with persons with AIDS cite the following factors as most significant for self-care and the prevention of burnout from the constant giving and confrontation with loss and death:

- Support groups
- Being connected to a community of caring people
- Reading, taking time to smell the roses, watch the sunset
- Calling people "when I need them, when they need me"
- Unconditional acceptance of love on both sides
- Realizing there is more to life than material riches

These support and coping strategies apply to both formal and informal caretakers: volunteers, nurses, physicians, family members, friends, lovers, and anyone caring for people with AIDS. As one volunteer says, however, "Caretaking is very painful. . . . Don't go into it if you don't want to grow. By seeing other people's pain you grow yourself." Betty Clare Moffat (1986) writes poignantly about this growth process for herself, her family, and friends after learning about her son's diagnosis of AIDS and after standing by him to the end. The current QUILT and NAMES project stands as a national symbol of caring, grieving, and growth through AIDS (Ruskin, Herron, & Zemke, 1988).

Some families, however, are too afraid, lack information, or for other reasons seem unable to respond compassionately to people with AIDS. For example, the parents of one young man, Bob, dying of AIDS at home, planned a birthday party for him, expecting it would be his last. They invited 100 relatives, but not a single one came. When Bob died, however, everyone came to the funeral. The parents felt bitter for a time against their relatives and their church for not being there when Bob and they needed them most. They explained their relatives' behavior on the basis of Bob's gay identity. But they have finally worked through the worst part of their grief and are grateful for the opportunity to have had Bob with them, to care for him, to support him while dying. This experience has given new meaning to their life and now they give public talks about it, hoping to influence other parents not to reject a dying child and to set aside their fears and biases about sexual orientation. Fortunately, with public education the attitudes of church representatives and others are changing to greater compassion. For example, ecumenical healing services in various churches are becoming common. People who might otherwise despair under the weight of the AIDS crisis are finding new meaning and community support in these ritual gatherings—examples of contemporary rites of passage (see Figure 14.1, Box 3, lower circle).

While some have the choice of volunteering to work directly with people with AIDS, most families and those in the health and social service professions do not.

The global nature of the AIDS crisis and its embeddedness in social disadvantage means that practically everyone is affected, at least indirectly, and the enormity of caretaking needs demands that the burden be shared within the human community. This will probably not happen, however, without learning all we can about AIDS, without attention to caring for ourselves to prevent burnout, and without acceptance of the challenge to grow from humane involvement with the AIDS crisis. Concern about these needs of the caretakers of people with AIDS is expressed in the AIDS Action Committee requirement that volunteers attend support group meetings at least twice a month. Similar support sessions are available for family members and nurses routinely caring for AIDS patients in homes, hospitals, and hospice houses (Robinson, Skeen, & Walters, 1987). As the numbers of people with AIDS increase, necessary care must increasingly be absorbed by mainstream health and social services and not be left primarily to alternative agencies such as the AIDS Action Committee. Similarly, support services for caretakers should become a routine part of the total service program if we are to meet the challenge of providing all the care demanded by this ongoing crisis.

Opportunities and Dangers for Society

Clearly, judgmental attitudes and moralistic diatribes against a community's most vulnerable members compound the pain and crisis of individuals, their families, lovers, and others most closely affected by AIDS. Not only do such responses harm various suffering individuals but they damage the detractors as well, since one mark of a humane and civilized society is its ability to care for the sick, the "different," and the suffering and dying in a compassionate manner. As already noted, there is evidence of a beginning paradigm shift. Bianco (1992, p. 61), recapping her address to the international AIDS conference states:

> Despite repeated calls and protests by women all over the world, despite international conferences and the United Nations Convention on Elimination of All Forms of Discrimination Against Women, inequality is still ignored when political and social decisions are made. Will AIDS be the detonator needed to end this inequality?

And from activists (e.g., Murphy, 1994) to scientists (Root-Berstein, 1993) to mainstream public health, this theme is gaining visibility. Jonathan Mann (1993, p. 1379), discussing the 1993 international AIDS conference, said:

> We are all Berliners—because to the extent that societies can reduce discrimination, they will be able to uproot the HIV/AIDS pandemic, rather than addressing only its surface features. . . . The world needs—and is now ready for—a far-reaching transformation of our approach to the global epidemic of AIDS.

Rarely has the world community had such an opportunity through the paradigmatic crisis of AIDS to mobilize together, combine efforts, and reconsider policies and the distribution of national and international resources. Yes, there is danger of compassion fatigue and xenophobia (fear or hatred of foreigners) in the face of this crisis. But aside from the horrors of this crisis, AIDS can be viewed as a catalyst to address issues that we might otherwise continue to ignore, such as universal health care, widening inequality between rich and poor nations, the caretaking crisis, and advocating equal rights for all. As the AIDS crisis unfolds into the next millennium for the individuals and families affected around the world, our attempts to understand people with AIDS and communicate compassionately with them and their families can increase the opportunities for personal and community growth and forestall such dangers as suicide, violence, bigotry, and the creation of scapegoats for societal problems and global inequalities.

Summary

AIDS brings into perspective the intersection between personal, family, community, and global issues. It typifies life crises as a whole as it touches major themes of the crisis experience: loss, grief, suicide danger, violence, and the need for social support. AIDS reveals starkly the relationship between situational, transitional, and sociocultural origins of crisis as depicted in this book's Crisis Paradigm. No, crisis intervention for people with AIDS, their families, and caretakers is not a panacea any more than it is for others in crisis. But besides being a necessary element of comprehensive care, serving such individuals in need provides an extraordinary opportunity to address the *socioeconomic* and *cultural* roots of this crisis. By thus situating the pain of individuals in global perspective, we can work toward the communal goal of preventing a similar plight for millions of others.

References

AIDS: Report of the Surgeon General's workshop on children with HIV infection and their families. (1987). Washington, D.C.: U.S. Department of Health and Human Services in conjunction with The Children's Hospital of Philadelphia.

Aiken, L. H., Lake, E. T., Semaan, S., Lehman, H. P., Cole, C. S., Dunbar, D., & Frank, I. (1993). Nurse practitioner managed care for persons with HIV infection. *Image: Journal of Nursing Scholarship, 25*(3), 172–177.

Antonovsky, A. (1980). *Health, stress, and coping.* San Francisco: Jossey-Bass.

Barry, K. (1979). *Female sexual slavery.* New York: Avon Books.

Barth, R. B., Pietrzak, J., & Ramler, M. (Eds.). (1993). *Families living with drugs and HIV: Intervention and treatment strategies.* New York: Guilford.

Battin, M. P. (1980). Manipulated suicide. In M. P. Battin & D. J. Mayo (Eds.), *Suicide: The philosophical issues.* (pp. 169–182). New York: St. Martin's Press.

Bayer, R. (1994). AIDS prevention and cultural sensitivity: Are they compatible? *American Journal of Public Health, 84*(6), 895–898.

Berer, M., & Ray, S. (1993). *Women and HIV/AIDS: The international source book*. London: Pandora/HarperCollins.

Bianco, M. (1992). How HIV/AIDS changes development priorities. *Women's Health Journal/Isis International, 4,* 58–62.

Blendon, R. J., & Donelan, K. (1988). Discrimination against people with AIDS: The public's perspective. *New England Journal of Medicine, 319*(15), 1022–1026.

Blumenfeld, W. J. (1992). *Homophobia: How we all pay the price*. Boston: Beacon Press.

Centers for Disease Control. *AIDS weekly surveillance report*. Atlanta: Department of Health & Human Services.

Corea, G. (1992). *The invisible epidemic: The story of women and AIDS*. New York: HarperCollins.

Dorn, N. (Ed.). (1992). *AIDS: Women, drugs, and social care*. Bristol, Penn.: Taylor & Francis.

Durham, J. D., & Cohen, F. L. (1987). *The person with AIDS: Nursing perspectives*. New York: Springer.

Galea, R. P., Lewis, B. F., & Baker, L. A. (1988). Voluntary testing for HIV antibodies among clients in long-term substance-abuse treatment. *Social Work, 33*(3), 265–268.

Gochros, H. S. (1988). Risks of abstinence: Sexual decision making in the AIDS era. *Social Work, 33*(3), 254–265.

Goffman, E. (1963). *Stigma*. Englewood Cliffs, N.J.: Prentice-Hall.

Goodman, L. M. (1981). *Death and the creative life*. New York: Springer.

Haney, P. (1988). Providing empowerment to the person with AIDS. *Social Work, 33*(3), 251–253.

Hoff, L. A., & Miller, N. (1987). *Programs for people in crisis: A guide for educators, administrators, and clinical trainers*. Boston: Northeastern University Custom Book Program.

Hollibaugh, A. (1994, June). Transmission, transmission, where's the transmission? *Sojourner: The Women's Forum*, pp. 5P, 7P.

Hosken, F. (1981). Female genital mutilation and human rights. *Feminist Issues, 1*(3), 3–23.

Hughes, A., Martin, J. P., & Franks, P. (1987). *AIDS home care and hospice manual*. AIDS Home Care and Hospice Program, VNA of San Francisco.

Joyce, C. (1988). Assault on the brain. *Psychology Today, 22*(3), 38–44.

Krieger, I. (1988). An approach to coping with anxiety about AIDS. *Social Work, 33*(3), 263–264.

Linde, R. (1988). Keynote address at workshop: AIDS and mental health professionals. Boston.

Mann, J. M. (1993). We are all Berliners: Notes from the ninth international conference on AIDS. *American Journal of Public Health, 83*(10), 1378–1379.

McGaffic, C. M. (1993). Connecting and disconnecting: Bereavement experiences of six gay men. *Journal of the Association of Nurses in AIDS Care, 4*(1), 49–57.

McGaffic, C. M., & Longman, A. J. (1993). Connecting and disconnecting: Bereavement experiences of six gay men. *Journal of the Association of Nurses in AIDS Care, 4*(1), 49–57.

McLaughlin, L. (1994, April 14). The women with AIDS. *Boston Globe*, p. 15.

Meisenhelder, J. B. (1994). Contributing factors to fear of HIV contagion in registered nurses. *Image: Journal of Nursing Scholarship, 26*(1), 65–69.

Moffat, B. C. (1986). *When someone you love has AIDS: A book of hope for family and friends*. Santa Monica, Calif.: IBS Press.

Murphy, B. (1994). The politics of AIDS. Unpublished manuscript.

Rachlis, M., & Kushner, C. (1994). *Strong medicine: How to save Canada's health care system*. Toronto: HarperCollins.

Radin, C. A. (1994, August 10). AIDS fight portrayed as a failure. *Boston Globe*, pp. 1,10.

Richardson, D. (1987). *Women and the AIDS crisis*. London: Pandora Press.

Robinson, B., Skeen, P., & Walters, L. (1987). The AIDS epidemic hits home. *Psychology Today, 21*(4), 48–52.

Root-Berstein, R. S. (1993). *Rethinking AIDS: The tragic cost of premature consensus.* New York: Free Press-Maxwell Macmillan International.

Rounds, K. A. (1988). AIDS in rural areas: Challenges to providing care. *Social Work, 33*(3), 257–261.

Ruskin, C., Herron, M., & Zemke, D. (1988). *The quilt: Stories from the names projects.* New York: Pocket Books.

Seager, J., & Olson, A. (1986). *Women in the world: An international atlas.* New York: Simon & Schuster.

Shilts, R. (1987). *And the band played on.* New York: St. Martin's Press.

Sommers, T., & Shields, L. (1987). *Women take care: The consequences of caregiving in today's society.* Gainesville, Fla.: Triad.

Sontag, S. (1978). *Illness as metaphor.* New York: Farrar, Straus & Giroux.

Stein, Z. A. (1993). Editorial: The double bind in science policy and the protection of women from HIV infection. *American Journal of Public Health, 82*(11), 1471–1472.

Stulberg, I., & Smith, M. (1988). Psychosocial impact of the AIDS epidemic on the lives of gay men. *Social Work, 33*(3), 277–281.

van Servellen, G., Padilla, G., Brecht, M. L., & Knoll, L. (1993). The relationship of stressful life events, health status, and stress-resistance resources in persons with AIDS. *Journal of the Association of Nurses in AIDS Care, 4*(1), 11–22.

SELECTED BIBLIOGRAPHY

Anderson, C. M., & Stewart, S. (1994). *Flying solo: Single women at midlife.* New York: W.W. Norton.

Antonovsky, A. (1980). *Health, stress, and coping.* San Francisco: Jossey-Bass.

Antonovsky, A. (1987). *Unraveling the mystery of health.* San Francisco: Jossey-Bass.

Bagley, C., & King, K. (1990). *Child sexual abuse: The search for healing.* London: Routledge.

Bartholet, E. (1993). *Family bonds: Adoption and the politics of parenting.* Boston: Houghton Mifflin.

Battin, M., & Mayo, D. (Eds.). (1980). *Suicide: The philosophical issues.* New York: St. Martin's Press.

Becker, H. S. (1963). *Outsiders: Studies in the sociology of deviance.* New York: Free Press.

Bennis, W. G., Benne, K. D., & Chin, R. (Eds.). (1985). *The planning of change* (4th ed.). New York: Holt, Rinehart & Winston.

Berer, M., & Ray, S. (1993). *Women and HIV/AIDS: The international source book.* London: Pandora/HarperCollins.

Bertman, S. L. (1991). *Facing death: Images, insights, and interventions.* Washington: Hemisphere.

Blumenfeld, W. J., & Raymond, D. (1993). *Looking at gay and lesbian life* (2nd ed.). Boston: Beacon Press.

Boston Women's Health Book Collective. (1992). *The new our bodies, ourselves.* New York: Simon & Schuster.

Braswell, L. (1989). *Quest for respect: A healing guide for survivors of rape.* London: Pathfinder Press.

Breggin, P. (1992). *Beyond conflict: From self-help and psychotherapy to peacemaking.* New York: St. Martin's Press.

Breggin, P., & Breggin, G. R. (1994). *Talking back to Prozac: What doctors won't tell you about today's most controversial drug.* New York: St. Martin's Press.

Brendtro, L. K., Brokenleg, M., & Van Bockern, S. (1990). *Reclaiming youth at risk.* Bloomington, Ind.: National Educational Service.

Brown, G. W., & Harris, T. (1978). *The social origins of depression.* London: Tavistock.

Burgess, A. W., & Hartman, C. (Eds.). (1989). *Sexual exploitation of patients by health professionals.* New York: Praeger.

Burstow, B. (1992). *Radical feminist therapy: Working in the context of violence*. Newbury Park: Sage.

Burgess, A., & Holmstrom, L. L. (1979). *Rape: Crisis and recovery*. Bowie, Md.: Brady.

Cade, B., & O'Hanlon, W. H. (1993). *A brief guide to brief therapy*. New York & London: W.W. Norton.

Campbell, J. D., & Humphreys, J. H. (Eds.). (1993). *Nursing care of survivors of family violence*. St. Louis: Mosby.

Canter, L., & Canter, M. (1988). *A proven step-by-step approach to solving everyday behavior problems* (Rev. ed.). Santa Monica: Lee Canter & Associates.

Capponi, P. (1992). *Upstairs in the crazy house*. Toronto: Penguin.

Chernin, K. (1985). *The hungry self: Women, eating, and identity*. New York: Harper & Row.

Chesler, P. (1986). *Mothers on trial: The battle for children and custody*. Seattle: Seal Press.

Conrad, P., & Kern, R. (Eds.). (1990). *The sociology of health and illness: Critical perspectives*. New York: St. Martin's Press.

Corea, G. (1992). *The invisible epidemic: The story of women and AIDS*. New York: HarperCollins.

Corea, G. (1985). *The mother machine*. New York: Harper & Row.

Dobash, R. P., & Dobash, R. E. (1979). *Violence against wives: A case against the patriarchy*. New York: Free Press.

Dohrenwend, B. S., & Dohrenwend, B. P. (Eds.). (1984). *Stressful life events and their context*. New Brunswick, N.J.: Rutgers University Press.

Doress, P. B., & Siegal, D. L. (1987). *Ourselves, growing older*. New York: Simon & Schuster.

Dowrick, S. (1994). *Intimacy and solitude*. New York: W.W. Norton.

Dunne, E. J., McIntosh, J. L., & Dunne-Maxim, K. (Eds.). (1987). *Suicide and its aftermath*. New York: W.W. Norton.

Edleson, J. L., & Tolman, R. M. (1992). *Intervention for men who batter: An ecological approach*. Newbury Park, Calif.: Sage.

Eggert, L. (1994). *Anger management for youth: Stemming aggression and violence*. Bloomington, Ind.: National Education Service.

Ehrenreich, J. (Ed.). (1978). *The cultural crisis of modern medicine*. New York: Monthly Review Press.

Ericsson, S. (1993). *Companion through the darkness: Inner dialogues on grief*. New York: Harper Perennial.

Erikson, E. (1963). *Childhood and society* (2nd ed.). New York: W.W. Norton.

Erikson, K. (1994). *A new species of trouble*. New York: W.W. Norton.

Eyre, L., & Eyre, R. (1993). *Teaching your children values*. New York: Simon & Schuster.

Fagerhaugh, S. Y., & Strauss, A. (1977). *Politics of pain management*. Menlo Park, Calif.: Addison-Wesley.

Farberow, N. L. (Ed.). (1975). *Suicide in different cultures*. Baltimore: University Park Press.

Farberow, N. L., & Shneidman, E. S. (Eds.). (1961). *The cry for help*. New York: McGraw-Hill.

Feifel, H. (Ed.). (1977). *New meanings of death*. New York: McGraw-Hill.

Fried, N. N., & Fried, M. H. (1980). *Transitions: Four rituals in eight cultures*. New York: W.W. Norton.

Gans, H. (1962). *The urban villagers*. New York: Free Press.

Gelles, R. J., & Loseke, D. R. (1993). *Current controversies on family violence*. Newbury Park, Calif.: Sage.

Gil, D. (1970). *Violence against children*. Cambridge, Mass.: Harvard University Press.

Glaser, B. G., & Strauss, A. (1965). *Awareness of dying*. Chicago: Aldine.

Goffman, E. (1963). *Stigma*. Englewood Cliffs, N.J.: Prentice-Hall.

Golan, N. (1981). *Passing through transitions*. New York: Free Press.

Gondolf, E. W. (1987). *Man against woman: What every woman needs to know about violent men*. Bradenton, Fla.: Human Services Institute.

Goodman, L. M. (1981). *Death and the creative life*. New York: Springer.

Goodman, L. M., & Hoff, L. A. (1990). *Omnicide*. New York: Praeger.

Gove, W. (Ed.). (1975). *The labeling of deviance*. New York: John Wiley.

Greenspan, M. (1983). *A new approach to women in therapy*. New York: McGraw-Hill.

Grollman, E. (1977). *Living—when a loved one has died*. Boston: Beacon Press.

Haley, J. (1987). *Problem-solving therapy*. San Francisco: Jossey-Bass.

Halleck, S. (1987). *The mentally disordered offender*. Washington, D.C.: American Psychiatric Press.

Hansell, N. (1976). *The person in distress*. New York: Human Sciences Press.

Hatton, C., Valente, S., & Rink, A. (1984). *Suicide: Assessment and intervention* (2nd ed.). New York: Appleton-Century-Crofts.

Herman, J. (1982). *Father-daughter incest*. Cambridge: Harvard University Press.

Herman, J. (1992). *Trauma and recovery: The aftermath of violence*. New York: Basic Books.

Hoff, L. A. (1990). *Battered women as survivors*. London: Routledge.

Hoff, L. A. (1995). *Violence issues: An interdisciplinary curriculum guide for health professionals*. Ottawa: Health Canada, Health Services Directorate. Available from National Clearinghouse on Family Violence. Health Canada, Ottawa, Ontario K1A 1B5 Canada.

Hoff, L. A., & Miller, N. (1987). *Programs for people in crisis: A guide for educators, administrators, and clinical trainers*. Boston: Northeastern University Custom Book Program.

Hoff, L. A., & Wells, J. O. (Eds.). (1989). *Certification standards manual* (4th ed.). Denver: American Association of Suicidology.

Hoff, M. D., & McNutt, J. G. (Eds.). (1994). *The global environmental crisis*. Aldershot, England: Avebury.

Holinger, P. C., Offer, D., Barter, J. T., & Bell, C. C. (1994). *Suicide and homicide among adolescents*. New York: Guilford.

Holland, H. (1994). *Born in Soweto*. London: Penguin.

Holmstrom, L. L., & Burgess, A. W. (1978). *The victim of rape: Institutional reactions*. New York: Wiley.

Illich, I. (1976). *Limits to medicine*. Middlesex, England: Penguin.

Jacobs, D. J., & Brown, H. N. (Eds.). (1989). *Suicide: Understanding and responding*. Madison, Conn.: International Universities Press.

Jaffe, P., Wolfe, D., & Wilson, S. (1990). *Children of battered women*. Newbury Park, Calif.: Sage.

Jencks, C. (1994). *The homeless*. Cambridge, Mass.: Harvard University Press.

Joan, P. (1986). *Preventing teenage suicide: The living alternative handbook*. New York: Human Sciences Press.

Johnson, A. B. (1990). *Out of bedlam: The truth about deinstitutionalization*. New York: Basic Books.

Kastenbaum, R., & Aisenberg, R. (1976). *The psychology of death*. New York: Springer.

Kottler, J. (1994). *Beyond blame: A new way of resolving conflicts in relationships*. San Francisco: Jossey-Bass.

Kozel, J. (1988). *Rachel and her children: Homeless families in America*. New York: Crown.

Kübler-Ross, E. (1975). *Death, the final stage of growth*. Englewood Cliffs, N.J.: Prentice-Hall.

Landy, D. (1977). *Culture, disease, and healing*. New York: Macmillan.

Leach, P. (1994). *Children first: What our society must do—and is not doing—for our children today*. New York: Knopf.

Leenaars, A. A., & Wenckstern, S. (1991). *Suicide prevention in schools*. New York & Washington: Hemisphere.

Levine, S., & Scotch, N. (1970). *Social stress*. Chicago: Aldine.

Levinson, D. J., Darrow, C. N., Klein, E. B., Levinson, M. H., & McKee, B. (1978). *The seasons of a man's life*. New York: Knopf.

Lifton, R. J. (1993). *The protean self: Human resilience in an age of fragmentation*. New York: Basic Books.

MacLean, M. (Ed.). (1995). *Abuse and neglect of older Canadians*. Toronto: Thompson Educational Publishing.

Maltsberger, J. T. (1986). *Suicide risk: The formulation of clinical judgment.* New York: New York University Press.

Maris, R. (1981). *Pathways to suicide.* Baltimore: Johns Hopkins University Press.

Maris, R. W., Berman, L. L., Maltsberger, J. T., & Yufit, R. I. (Eds.). (1991). *Assessment and prediction of suicide.* New York: Guilford.

Marks, I., & Scott, R. (Eds.). (1990). *Mental health care delivery: Innovations, impediments, and implementation.* Cambridge: Cambridge University Press.

Marris, P.: (1974). *Loss and change.* London: Routledge & Kegan Paul.

Marris, P. (1987). *Meaning and action: Community action and conceptions of change* (2nd ed.). London: Routledge & Kegan Paul.

Maslow, A. (1970). *Motivation and personality* (2nd ed.). New York: Harper & Row, 1970.

Mawby, R. I., & Walklate, S. (1994). *Critical victimology.* London: Sage.

McCamant, K., & Durrett, C. (1988). *Cohousing: A contemporary approach to housing ourselves.* Berkeley: Ten Speed Press.

McElroy, A., & Townsend, P. K. (1985). *Medical anthropology in ecological perspective.* Boulder & London: Westview Press.

McKenry, P. C., & Price, S. J. (Eds.). (1994) *Families and change: Coping with stressful events.* Thousand Oaks, Calif.: Sage.

McNamee, S., & Gergen, K. J. (Eds.). (1992). *Therapy as social construction.* London: Sage.

Medoff, P., & Sklar, H. (1994). *Streets of hope: The fall and rise of an urban neighborhood.* Boston: South End Press.

Meloy, R. (1992). *Violent attachments.* Northvale, N.J.: Jason Aronson.

Mendel, M. P. (1994). *The male survivor.* Newbury Park, Calif.: Sage.

Miller, J. B. (1986). *Toward a new psychology of women* (Rev. ed.). Boston: Beacon Press.

Mills, C. W. (1959). *The sociological imagination.* Oxford: Oxford University Press.

Minuchin, S. (1993). *Family healing: Strategies for hope and understanding.* New York: Simon & Schuster.

Mitford, J. (1993). *The American way of birth.* New York: Dutton.

Monahan, J. (1981). *Predicting violent behavior: An assessment of clinical techniques.* Beverly Hills: Sage.

Mosher, L. R., & Burti, L. (1989). *Community mental health: Principles and practice.* New York: W.W. Norton.

Ngugi, W. (1965). *The river between.* London: Heinemann.

NiCarthy, G. (1989). *You can be free: An easy-to-read handbook for abused women.* Seattle: Seal Press.

Parad, H. J. (Ed.). (1965). *Crisis intervention: Selected readings.* New York: Family Service Association of America.

Parkes, C. M. (1975). *Bereavement: Studies of grief in adult life.* Middlesex, England: Penguin.

Perlin, S. (1975). *A handbook for the study of suicide.* Oxford: Oxford University Press.

Pfeffer, C. R. (1986). *The suicidal child.* New York: Guilford.

Pillemer, K. A., & Wolf, R. S. (Eds.). *Elder abuse: Conflict in the family.* Dover, Mass.: Auburn House.

Rachlis, M., & Kushner, C. (1994). *Strong medicine: How to save Canada's health care system.* Toronto: HarperCollins.

Remafedi, G. (Ed.). (1994). *Death by denial: Studies of gay and lesbian teenagers.* Boston: Alyson.

Renzetti, C. M. (1992). *Violent betrayal: Partner abuse in lesbian relationships.* Newbury Park, Calif.: Sage.

Richman, J. (1986). *Family therapy of suicidal individuals.* New York: Springer.

Root-Berstein, R. S. (1993). *Rethinking AIDS: The tragic cost of premature consensus.* New York: Free Press-Maxwell Macmillan International.

Rosenthal, T. (1973). *How could I not be among you?* New York: Braziller.

Ruddick, S. (1989). *Maternal thinking: Toward a politics of peace.* Boston: Beacon Press.

Russell, D. (1986). *Secret trauma: Incest in the lives of girls and women.* New York: Basic Books.

Ryan, W. (1971). *Blaming the victim.* New York: Vintage Books.

Sadker, M., & Sadker, D. (1994). *Failing at fairness.* New York: Charles Scribner's Sons.

Schor, J. B. (1993). *The overworked American: The unexpected decline of leisure.* New York: Basic Books.

Shilts, R. (1987). *And the band played on.* New York: St. Martin's Press.

Shneidman, E. S. (1976). *Suicidology: Contemporary developments.* New York: Grune & Stratton.

Shneidman, E. S. (1985). *Definition of suicide.* New York: Wiley.

Shneidman, E. S., & Farberow, N. L. (Eds.). (1957). *Clues to suicide.* New York: McGraw-Hill.

Sidel, R. (1986). *Women and children last: The plight of poor women in affluent America.* New York: Penguin.

Sommers, T., & Shields, L. (1987). *Women take care: The consequences of caregiving in today's society.* Gainesville, Fla.: Triad.

Sontag. S. (1978). *Illness as metaphor.* New York: Farrar, Straus & Giroux.

Thurer, S. L. (1994). *The myths of motherhood: How culture reinvents the good mother.* Boston: Houghton Mifflin.

Tolstoy, L. (1960). *The death of Ivan Illyich.* New York: New American Library.

Vaillant, G. E. (1993). *The wisdom of the ego: Sources of resilience in adult life.* Cambridge, Mass.: Harvard University Press.

VandeCreek, L., & Knapp, S. (1993). *Tarasoff and beyond: Legal and clinical considerations in the treatment of life-endangering patients* (Rev. ed.). Sarasota, Fla.: Professional Resource Press.

van der Kolk, B. A. (1987). *Psychological trauma.* Washington, D.C.: American Psychiatric Association.

van Gennep, A., (1960). *Rites of passage.* Chicago: University of Chicago Press (French edition 1909).

Van Ornum, W., & Mordock, J. B. (1987). *Crisis counseling with children and adolescents.* New York: Continuum.

Walsh, F., & McGoldrick, M. (Eds.). (1991). *Living beyond loss: Death in the family.* New York: W.W. Norton.

Waring, M. (1990). *If women counted: A new feminist economics.* New York: HarperSanFrancisco.

Warshaw, R. (1988). *I never called it rape.* New York: Harper & Row.

Watson, R. S., Poda, J. H., Miller, C. T., Rice, E. S., & West, G. (1990). *Containing crisis: A guide to managing school emergencies.* Bloomington, Ind.: National Educational Service.

West, C. (1993). *Race matters.* New York: Vintage Books.

Wolin, S. (1993). *The resilient self: How survivors of troubled families rise above adversity.* New York: Random House.

Worden, J. W. (1991). *Grief counseling and grief therapy: A handbook for the mental health practitioner* (2nd ed.). New York: Springer.

NAME INDEX

A

Adamowski, K., 339, 360
Adams, D., 295
Aguilera, D. C., 10, 11
Ahmed, F. E., 310–311
Ahrons, D., 137
Aiken, L. H., 451
Aisenberg, R., 423
Allen, K. R., 140
Allgeyer, L., 152
Alvarez, A., 190
Anders, R. L., 283, 297, 350
Anderson, B. G., 47, 48, 345
Anderson, C. M., 417
Antonovsky, A., 3, 19, 37, 46, 49, 133, 327
Apfel, R. J., 329, 332
Arditti, R., 404
Aries, P., 423
Armer, J. M., 377
Atkinson, J. M., 30, 169
Attala, J., 259
Attneave, C., 133
Aubry, J., 378
Avison, W. R., 10, 39, 45

B

Baber, K. M., 140
Baechler, J., 184
Bagley, C., 242
Baker, L. A., 450
Bane, M. J., 138
Baracos, H. A., 286
Bard, M., 112, 283
Barnes, R. A., 183, 187, 215
Barney, K., 23, 77, 126, 128
Barry, K., 447
Barth, R. B., 436
Bartholet, E., 403
Bates, J. D., 403
Bateson, G., 110
Battin, M. P., 175, 177, 229, 445
Baum, A., 43, 308, 325, 326
Baum, M., 43, 83, 236, 249
Bayer, R., 438, 440
Bebbington, P., 46
Beck, A. T., 196
Becker, H., 72, 173
Becktell, P. J., 342
Bell, C. C., 63, 239, 292, 293
Bellah, R., 381
Bellak, L., 27
Benne, K. D., 63, 64
Bennet, G., 317
Benson, H., 338
Berer, M., 446
Berger, P. L., 73
Berk, R. A., 294
Berkman, L. F., 133
Berlin, I. N., 168

Berman, A. L., 193, 204, 223
Bernstein, R. J., 37
Bertalanffy, L. von, 12
Bertman, S. L., 360, 423, 424, 425
Besharov, D., 237
Bianco, M., 446, 447, 453
Birnbaum, F., 321
Birnbaum, H. J., 297
Bishop, E. E., 137
Bittner, E., 73
Blanford, H., 320
Blendon, R. J., 440
Bloch, M., 423
Blumenfeld, W., 223, 407, 440
Boell, J. L., 250
Bograd, M., 13, 235, 256, 295
Bohn, C. R., 238
Bohnet, N., 178, 219, 347
Boissevain, J., 133
Bongar, B., 214, 215, 216, 217, 218, 224, 226
Boon, C., 44
Borg, S., 400
Borst, S. R., 167
Borysenko, J., 338
Bowles, R. T., 241
Brandt, R. B., 175, 179
Braswell, L., 249
Bredenberg, P., 342
Breed, W., 193
Breggin, G. R., 126

463

SUBJECT INDEX

A

Abortion, 400

Abuse: child, 241–247; elder, 267–272. *See also* Battering; Violence; Woman battering

Accountability, of batterers, 295

Action for Mental Health, 13–14, 15

Adolescents, 405–406; crisis intervention with, 407–413; developmental tasks of, 406; as parents, 402; rites of passage for, 394; sexual identity crisis in, 406–407, 408; and suicide, 167–168, 169, 178, 195, 221–222; violence by, 272–273, 290–292

Adoption, 403

Aggression, 281–282. *See also* Violence

Aid to Incarcerated Mothers (AIM), 298

AIDS, 160, 340, 414, 424, 425, 433–434, 454; anxiety about, 448–450; caretaking with, 450–453; coping with, 441, 442; loss with, 53; negative crisis outcomes with, 445–446; origins of crisis with, 438–440; paradigmatic shift with, 434–438; as personal crisis, 440–441; positive crisis resolution with, 441,

443–445; prevention of, 25; and rape, 254; and society, 453–454; suicide with, 195, 445–446; women and children with, 446–448

AIDS: Report of the Surgeon General, 448

Alcoholism, 354; attitudes toward, 356–357; crisis intervention with, 354–356. *See also* Drinking

Alienation, of youth, 291–292

Alliance for the Mentally Ill (AMI), 114

Alma Ata Declaration, 14

Ambivalence: of self-destructive people, 188. *See also* Lethality assessment

American Association of Suicidology (AAS), 6, 79, 230, 288; certification by, 30, 32–33; school prevention programs of, 221, 222

Anger management, 292

Antidepressants, 126, 201, 216–218. *See also* Drugs

Anxiety, 84, 85–86; about AIDS, 441, 448–450; with ambiguity, 388–389; in crisis development, 56–59; and perceptions, 86, 87; and suicide, 172, 213–214; tranquilizers for, 127. *See also* Feelings

Assault: assessing risk of, 282, 284–288; medicalization of,

288–290. *See also* Violence

Assessment: of assault and homicide risk, 282, 284–288; lethality, 188–189, 200, 288; victimization, 239–241. *See also* Crisis assessment; Suicide risk assessment

Attorney General's Task Force on Family Violence, 274

B

Batterers, 294; programs for, 294–296

Battering, 90; of homosexual and bisexual partners, 266–267; of husbands, 266; of parents and teachers, 272–273. *See also* Woman battering

Befrienders International, 15

Behavior: anti-social, 290–292, 299–301; chronic self-destructive, 170, 181–183, 354–357; with health status change, 345; of people in crisis, 88; suicidal, 196, 197–203, 204, 219–220

Birth: of handicapped child, 350–352; medicalization of, 401; rites of passage with, 394; of stillborn child, 399–401. *See also* Parents

Boston Women's Health Book

precipitated, 193

Homophobia, 205, 407

Hospice movement, 427–428

Hospitalization: of children, 343–344, 401; as crisis, 340–344; psychiatric, 28, 72, 76, 349–350; for suicide prevention, 176, 179, 196, 206, 223–224. *See also* Institutionalization

Hostage situations, 284

Housing crisis, 139, 142, 376–383. *See also* Homelessness

Human growth and development. *See* Growth and development

Human services, 9

Husband beating, 266

I

Iatrogenesis, 13

Illness, 47–48; of child, 343–344, 401; and stress and crisis, 49–52; and suicide risk, 195, 198. *See also* Health status change; Mental illness

Immigrants, 380

Institutionalization: of elderly, 421–423; with inadequate assessment, 72. *See also* Hospitalization

International Institute, 380

Intervention. *See* Crisis intervention; Prevention

Interviews: crisis assessment, 91–94; crisis intervention, 129–130; with suicide survivors, 229–230

Intimate relationships, 143–144, 394, 413–417

Isolation, 153, 176, 295; and suicide, 195–196, 198, 213

J

Job loss. *See* Retirement; Unemployment

L

Labeling theory, 73–76

Language, 108–109

Laws: and elder abuse, 268; and medicalization of crime, 289–290; on violence, 300. *See also* Public policies

Lesbians, and AIDS, 448, 451. *See also* Gays/lesbians/bisexuals

Lethality assessment: and assault and

homicide risk, 288; and suicide risk, 188–189, 200. *See also* Suicide risk assessment

Life crises, 387–388. *See also* Transition states

Life passages, 393, 428–429; in adolescence and young adulthood, 54–55, 405–413; birth and parenthood as, 396–405; death as, 423–428; in intimate relationships, 413–417; in middle age, 417–419; in old age, 419–423; rituals for, 389–398. *See also* Transition states

Lifeline, 224

Listening, 122. *See also* Communication

Loss, 11; with AIDS, 53; with disasters, 309; feelings of, 84; and grief work, 120–122; as "minideath," 424; with moves, 377; by people in crisis, 53; and suicide risk, 195, 198

M

Marriage, 391–392; and suicide risk, 194–195. *See also* Divorce; Families; Intimate relationships

Matrix program, 381–382

Medical approach: to crisis management, 31; to self-destructive people, 172–173

Medical emergency: crisis management in, 357–362; with suicidal people, 211–212

Medicalization, 7; of birth, 401; of crime, 288–290; of crisis intervention, 339; of middle age, 417, 418–419; and stress, 48; of violence, 236

Medicine wheel, 293

Menopause, 418–419

Mental health. *See* Community mental health

Mental health professionals, 6; and police, 286–287; violence against, 282–283. *See also* Crisis workers

Mental illness, 367; among battered women, 49–52; and crises, 4, 5, 6; and labeling, 75–76; and suicide risk, 171, 199; versus distorted perceptions, 86–87

Middle age, 395, 417–419

Migrants, 41, 378–380

Minnesota Multiphasic Personality Inventory (MMPI), 189

Minority groups, 292; suicide rates for, 167–168, 194. *See also* Culture; Ethnic groups; Native peoples

Miscarriage, 398

Motherhood. *See* Parents; Women

Moves, 376; anticipated, 377; unanticipated, 377–378

Myths: about people in crisis, 6–7; about rape, 248–249; about suicide, 171

N

National Center for Health Statistics, 168

National Committee on Youth Suicide, 220–221

National Institute on Drug Abuse (NIDA), 126

National Institute of Mental Health (NIMH), 320; Task Force on Youth Suicide, 220

National Organization for Victim Assistance (NOVA), 141, 274, 321

Native peoples: communities of, 142; self-destructive behaviors among, 183; suicide risk among, 167–168; youth violence prevention by, 293

Natural disasters. *See* Disasters

Needs: of abusive parents, 246; of AIDS caretakers, 451–452; basic human, 53, 366; intimacy as, 413–414; regarding self and social network, 143–144

No-suicide contract, 213

Nurses, 340, 359, 360, 421; crisis assessment interview by, 91–94; self-destructive behavior by, 170. *See also* Crisis workers

Nursing homes. *See* Institutionalization

O

Occupational changes, as crises, 367–370, 372–376

Old age. *See* Elderly people; Retirement

Ontario Psychiatric Survivors Association (OPSA), 114

P

Pan American Health Organization (PAHO), 18, 282